G. Alexander Rübel · Ewald Isenbügel · Pim Wolvekamp
Editors

Atlas of

Diagnostic Radiology of Exotic Pets

Small Mammals, Birds, Reptiles and Amphibians

Authors:
Karl Gabrisch · Fritz Grimm · Ewald Isenbügel · Phil Koblik
Joanne Paul-Murphy · Christian Peter Oschwald
Georg Alexander Rübel · Bernd-Joachim Schildger · Pim Wolvekamp

W. B. Saunders Company

Authors

Karl Gabrisch, DVM
Kleintierklinik am Ring
U 6/11
D-6800 *Mannheim 1*

Fritz Grimm, DVM
Institut für Geflügelkrankheiten
der Ludwig-Maximilians-
Universität München
Mittenheimer Straße 54
D-8042 *Oberschleißheim*

Ewald Isenbügel, DVM, Professor
Departement für Fortpflanzung
der Universität Zürich
Klinik für Zoo- und Heimtiere
Winterthurer Straße 260
CH-8057 *Zürich*

Phil Koblik, DVM
Radiology Department
School of Veterinary Medicine
University of California
USA-*Davis,* CA 95616

Joanne Paul-Murphy, DVM
Department of Medicine
School of Veterinary Medicine
University of California
USA-*Davis,* CA 95616

Christian Peter Oschwald
Kleintierklinik beim Stadtcasino
Haselstraße 7
CH-5400 *Baden*

Georg Alexander Rübel, DVM
Departement für Fortpflanzung
der Universität Zürich
Klinik für Zoo- und Heimtiere
Winterthurer Straße 260
CH-8057 *Zürich*

Bernd-Joachim Schildger, DVM
Zoologischer Garten Frankfurt
Alfred-Brehm-Platz 16
D-6000 *Frankfurt am Main*

Pim Wolvekamp, DVM, Ph D.
Department of Radiology
Veterinary Faculty
University of Utrecht
Yalelaan 10
NL-3584 *CM Utrecht-de Uithof*

Distributed in the United States and Canada by
W. B. Saunders Company
The Curtis Center
Independence Square West
Philadelphia, Pa. 19106-3399

ISBN 0-7216-3493-1

This is an international edition issued by Schlütersche, Hannover, Wolfe Publishing Limited, London and W. B. Saunders Company, Philadelphia.

Printed in Germany

Reprinted 1992

G. Alexander Rübel · Ewald Isenbügel · Pim Wolvekamp

Atlas of Diagnostic Radiology of Exotic Pets

Small Mammals, Birds, Reptiles and Amphibians

Contents

Preface 7
M. E. Fowler

Introduction 8
G. A. Rübel/E. Isenbügel/P. Wolvekamp

Radiographic Technique in Exotic Pets 9
G. A. Rübel/P. Wolvekamp

Small Mammals

P. Wolvekamp/Ch. Oschwald
Radiographic Technique 12

Guinea Pig: Radiographic Anatomy 14
Radiographic Abnormalities
Musculoskeletal System
Skull 18
Spine 19
Appendicular Skeleton 19
Thorax
Lungs 20
Abdomen
Gastrointestinal Tract 21
Urogenital Tract 23

Rabbit: Radiographic Anatomy 26
Radiographic Abnormalities
Musculoskeletal System
Skull 32
Spine 34
Appendicular Skeleton 36
Thorax
Lungs 38
Miscellaneous 40
Abdomen
Gastrointestinal Tract 43
Liver 45
Urogenital Tract 46
Miscellaneous 50

E. Isenbügel
Hamster: Radiographic Anatomy 52
Radiographic Abnormalities 54

Chinchilla: Radiographic Anatomy 56
Radiographic Abnormalities 58

Chipmunk: Radiographic Anatomy 62
Radiographic Abnormalities 63

Mouse: Radiographic Anatomy 64

Rat: Radiographic Anatomy 65

Gerbil: Radiographic Anatomy 66

Ferret: Radiographic Anatomy 68
Radiographic Abnormalities 70

Hedgehog: Radiographic Anatomy 72

Birds

G. A. Rübel
Radiographic Technique 76

Psittacines: Radiographic Anatomy
Internal Organs 80
Contrast Radiography of the Alimentary Tract 82
Appendicular Skeleton 83

J. Paul-Murphy/Ph. Koblik
Skull 84
Radiographic Abnormalities
Skull 86

G. A. Rübel
Appendicular Skeleton 90
Lungs 94
Air Sacs 98
Heart and Vessels 102
Esophagus and Proventriculus 104
Ventriculus 106
Intestine 108
Cloaca 110
Liver 112
Spleen 114
Kidneys 116
Genital Organs 120
Miscellaneous 124

F. Grimm
Contrast Radiography of the Alimentary Tract 126

G. A. Rübel
Raptors: Radiographic Anatomy
Internal Organs 138

F. Grimm
Contrast Radiography of the Alimentary Tract 140

G. A. Rübel
Axial Skeleton 142
Appendicular Skeleton 144

Contents

Raptors:

J. Paul-Murphy/Ph. Koblik

Skull 146

Radiographic Abnormalities

Skull 147

F. Grimm/G. A. Rübel

Appendicular Skeleton 148

Miscellaneous 150

Woodcock/ Raptors:

Radiographic Abnormalities

Miscellaneous 153

Hill-Mynah:

G. A. Rübel

Radiographic Anatomy 154

Radiographic Abnormalities 156

Pigeon:

F. Grimm

Radiographic Anatomy

Internal Organs 158

Contrast Radiography of the Alimentary Tract 159

Radiographic Abnormalities 160

Fowl:

Radiographic Anatomy 164

Radiographic Abnormalities 165

Waterfowl:

Radiographic Anatomy 166

Radiographic Abnormalities 168

Long-legged Birds:

Radiographic Anatomy 170

Radiographic Abnormalities 172

Reptiles and Amphibians

B.-J. Schildger/K. Gabrisch

Radiographic Technique:

Tortoises and Turtles 176

Lizards 178

Snakes 178

Amphibians 179

Tortoises and Turtles:

Radiographic Anatomy

Internal Organs and Skeleton 180

Contrast Radiography of the Alimentary Tract 184

Radiographic Abnormalities

Skeleton 188

Lungs 190

Gastrointestinal Tract 191

Urogenital Tract 194

Lizards:

Radiographic Anatomy

Internal Organs and Skeleton 196

Contrast Radiography of the Alimentary Tract 199

Radiographic Abnormalities

Skeleton 200

Gastrointestinal Tract 204

Urogenital Tract 206

Miscellaneous 208

Snakes:

Radiographic Anatomy

Internal Organs and Skeleton 210

Contrast Radiography of the Alimentary Tract 213

Radiographic Abnormalities

Skeleton 216

Gastrointestinal Tract 218

Urogenital Tract 220

Amphibians:

G. A. Rübel/B.-J. Schildger

Radiographic Anatomy 222

Radiographic Abnormalities 224

References of Radiographs

P. Wolvekamp, Utrecht: small mammals 1-7, 9-13, 15-17, 20-26, 28-36, 38-66, 68-71; birds 149, 150; reptiles 19, 39, 40, 57, 72.
Ch. Oschwald, Zurich: small mammals 8, 14, 18, 19, 27, 37, 67.
E. Isenbügel, Zurich: small mammals 72-110.
G. A. Rübel, Zurich: birds 1-5, 19-62, 64-85, 111, 112, 123-126, 131-133, 141, 143-147; reptiles 17, 28, 67; amphibians 79, 81.
Joanne R. Paul-Murphy/Ph. D. Koblik, Davis: birds 6-18 (Original paper: "Psittacine Skull Radiography: Anatomy, Radiographic Technic, and Patient Application", published in Veterinary Radiology 1990; 31 [4]: 218-224), 127-130.
G. Barandun, Chur: birds 63.
F. Grimm, Munich: birds 86-110, 113-122, 134-140, 142, 148, 151-178.
B.-J. Schildger, Frankfurt: reptiles 1-16, 18, 21-25, 27, 29-35, 38, 41-56, 58-63, 65, 66, 68, 69, 71, 74, 75; amphibians 76, 77, 80.
K. Gabrisch, Mannheim: reptiles 20, 26, 36, 37, 64, 70, 73.
G. Guex, Zurich: amphibians 78. — **Drawings** Jeanne Peter, Zurich.

Preface

There are numerous books published on nondomestic animals in both English and German language. None of these books do adequate justice to radiographic interpretation. Thus it is exciting to see this volume published.

Readers will find excellent radiographs of selected clinical cases in mammals, birds and reptiles along with the narration of pertinent clinical findings and radiographic film evaluations. The editors have selected clinicians and radiologists with considerable experience with their class of animals. The authors have categorized the cases according to species and organ systems. Obviously not every clinical condition nor species can be illustrated, but there is sufficient diversity to provide the reader with valuable information to deal with clinical problems.

Line drawings are used effectively to augment the radiographs by outlining important landmarks and lesions.

The broad species range covered has heightened the task of the editors to select those species and conditions that are most important for clinicians. Their objectives have been met.

MURRAY E. FOWLER, DVM

Introduction

Keeping small mammals, birds, reptiles and amphibians as exotic pets has become very popular over the last few years. A number of factors has caused this development: the great variety of equipment for pet animals provided by the pet industry for housing, feeding and caretaking, successful breeding in many species, a great deal of information on the variety of species, on their behavior and on recent advances of animal management. Marketed products and information do not always correspond with the specific needs for the comfort of the individual animal. Only too often dietary deficiencies or diseases result from inadequate management or feeding. The veterinarian is requested to provide prophylaxis and therapy to solve these problems. In the last few years, expert information about exotic pet medicine has been provided in veterinary schools, at congresses and in professional journals.

Radiographic examination has proven to be a revealing and essential diagnostic method in these species. Still, there is too little information concerning radiography in exotic pet medicine textbooks. Practitioners have expressed the wish to have at their disposal comparative radiographs. This Atlas of Diagnostic Radiology of Exotic Pets is meant to meet this need.

Introductory remarks on the radiographic technique of the different animal groups should allow the practitioner to more frequently use radiography as a diagnostic tool. The variety of species and diseases makes it impossible to be complete. The text to the radiographs is limited to information that allows their evaluation and interpretation. This should always be used in combination with a related medical textbook. The atlas was produced on the basis of the two textbooks edited by K. Gabrisch and P. Zwart "Krankheiten der Heimtiere" and "Krankheiten der Wildtiere". For clinical information and treatment, the reader should refer to one of these or another related textbook.

The radiographs come from the files of the various authors who have been practicing radiography in exotic pets for many years. The atlas focuses on normal radiographic appearance, and on the most frequent and typical physiologic and pathologic radiographic abnormalities in some of the more common species. With good radiographs, insufficient positioning of the animal has been tolerated. For better comprehension and interpretation of normal radiographic anatomy, explanatory drawings have been included. Incidentally, radiographic abnormalities are also illustrated this way.

In order to preserve radiographic detail in the illustrations, the radiographs were electronically processed using a LogEtronic® device prior to printing.

Following general rules, positional printing of the radiographs within each chapter is uniform and independent of the animal's position during the radiographic examination. Only with the pictures of normal radiographic anatomy the original projections are presented. In all chapters, lateral films are reproduced in *right lateral recumbent view,* with the head pointing to the left. In the small mammal and bird chapters, all dorsoventral and ventrodorsal films are printed in *ventrodorsal view,* with the left side of the animal on the right side of the page. In the chapters on reptiles and amphibians, the *dorsoventral view* is printed for reasons of convenience with interpretation. The cranial (rostral) part of the animal always points *upwards.*

We want to express sincere thanks to the co-authors, and their co-workers, for their contributions. We are very much indepted to Prof. Dr. P. F. Suter, Rolf Sandmeier, MD, Dr. M. Flückiger, Veterinary Faculty, University of Zurich, Switzerland; Prof. M. E. Fowler, DVM, Joanne Paul-Murphy, DVM and Victoria R. Davis, Veterinary School, University of Davis, California, and J. E. Cooper, FRCVS, and Lyn Thomson, The Royal College of Surgeons of England, London, for their kind advice and critical reading of the manuscript. Our special thanks go to Prof. Dr. G. Ueltschi, Ms. Christa Schulte and Ms. Anita Hug for their kind assistance in reproducing the films and Ms. Jeanne Peter for the drawings. We appreciate the excellent cooperation of the publisher Schlütersche Verlagsanstalt und Druckerei for the layout of this atlas. Last but not least, we like to thank Ms. Yvonne Vogt for her untiring efforts in typing the manuscript.

The Editors

Radiographic Technique in Exotic Pets

General Remarks

Radiography is one of the methods of investigation by which veterinarians examine small animals. In contrast to other diagnostic procedures, radiography is a noninvasive technique, providing excellent diagnostic information.

Technical Requirements

It is not necessary to have a very strong X-ray machine to produce good radiographs since most animals are small. However, it is helpful to have an equipment with high mA-capability and a short exposure time of 1/60 of a second or faster. The high mA-capacity allows the use of high resolution film-screen combinations that are recommended for identification of small detail. The short exposure time minimizes degradation of radiographic detail caused by motion of the animal. For the examination the patient should be fixed directly upon the cassette.

Exposure Factors

It is essential to keep the exposure time as low as possible (below 0.02 s) to avoid motion blurring. Exposure factors are mainly affected by the focal-film distance, the speed of the intensifying screens used and the choice of kVp- and mAs-setting. A grid is not needed. Focal-film distance must be at least 90 cm. Exposures are made at approximately 50 kVp, with mAs-settings adjusted to the film-screen combination. Detail recognition can be enhanced by use of high resolution, slow-speed intensifying screens.

Radiation Safety

The general rules of radiation safety, e.g. maximum distance from the primary beam, use of protective clothing such as lead aprons and gloves with 0.5 mm lead equivalent, and beam collimation using a collimator with illuminated exposure field also apply to radiography of small mammals (FIG. **A**).

Especially with these small animals where low kVp-settings are used, collimation of the X-ray beam according to the size of the animal and not to the size of the cassette is essential. Therefore, every diagnostic X-ray machine for veterinary use should have a beam limiting device with adjustable lead shutters and with field size illumination (FIG. **B**).

Persons holding animals can only stand at a safe distance from the primary beam if adequate restraint by using sedation, anaesthesia and/or positioning devices are used.

Interpretation of the Radiographs

When reviewing radiographs, it is essential to be systematic in order to avoid an incorrect diagnosis. The specific characteristics of the different species under examination should be taken into consideration.

The criteria for radiographic interpretation and evaluation of exotic pets are similar to those in domestic mammals and are as follows:

organ position
organ shape and delineation
organ density and homogeneity
comparative size of the organs
patient nutrition and overall body condition
gastrointestinal contents

A

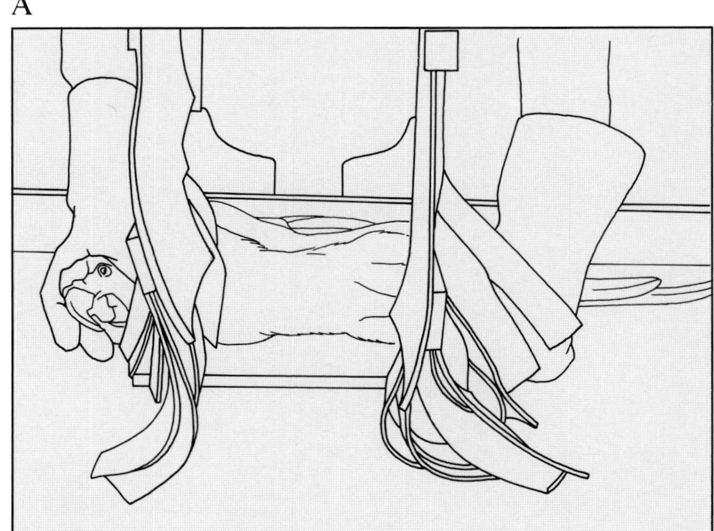

B

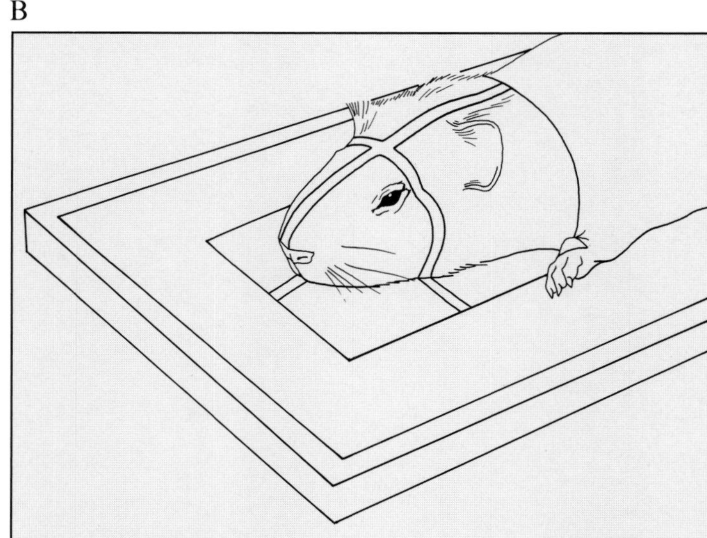

Contents

Small Mammals

Radiographic Technique 12

Guinea Pig:
Radiographic Anatomy 14
Radiographic Abnormalities
- Musculoskeletal System
  - Skull 18
  - Spine 19
  - Appendicular Skeleton 19
- Thorax
  - Lungs 20
- Abdomen
  - Gastrointestinal Tract 21
  - Urogenital Tract 23

Rabbit:
Radiographic Anatomy 26
Radiographic Abnormalities
- Musculoskeletal System
  - Skull 32
  - Spine 34
  - Appendicular Skeleton 36
- Thorax
  - Lungs 38
  - Miscellaneous 40
- Abdomen
  - Gastrointestinal Tract 43
  - Liver 45
  - Urogenital Tract 46
  - Miscellaneous 50

Hamster:
Radiographic Anatomy 52
Radiographic Abnormalities 54

Chinchilla:
Radiographic Anatomy 56
Radiographic Abnormalities 58

Chipmunk:
Radiographic Anatomy 62
Radiographic Abnormalities 63

Mouse:
Radiographic Anatomy 64

Rat:
Radiographic Anatomy 65

Gerbil:
Radiographic Anatomy 66

Ferret:
Radiographic Anatomy 68
Radiographic Abnormalities 70

Hedgehog:
Radiographic Anatomy 72

Preparation

Even tame small mammals are very shy in unknown surroundings and are afraid of all unknown objects and persons. They have a tendency to panic easily. For this reason, it is hardly ever possible to make radiographs without physical or chemical restraint of the animal. If the animals condition allows, chemical restraint is preferred.

For chemical restraint of small mammals, ketamine alone or in combination with xylazine is safe. The drugs are given intramuscularly in the dorsal part of the upper thigh. Caution must be taken not to damage the Nervus ischiadicus. Inhalation anesthesia with methoxyflurane may also be used for sedation.

For chemical restraint of small mammals during radiographic investigation, the following dosages are recommended:

Guinea pig:	ketamine 20 mg/kg bw + xylazine 4 mg/kg bw
Rabbit:	ketamine 20 mg/kg bw + xylazine 4 mg/kg bw + 0,5 ml atropine (1‰)
Hamster:	ketamine 20 mg/kg bw
Chinchilla:	ketamine 60 mg/kg bw
Chipmunk:	ketamine 80 mg/kg bw
Mouse:	methoxyflurane per inhalationem
Rat:	ketamine 40 mg/kg bw
Gerbil:	ketamine 20 mg/kg bw
Ferret:	ketamine 10 mg/kg bw
Hedgehog:	ketamine 20 mg/kg bw or methoxyflurane per inhalationem

A

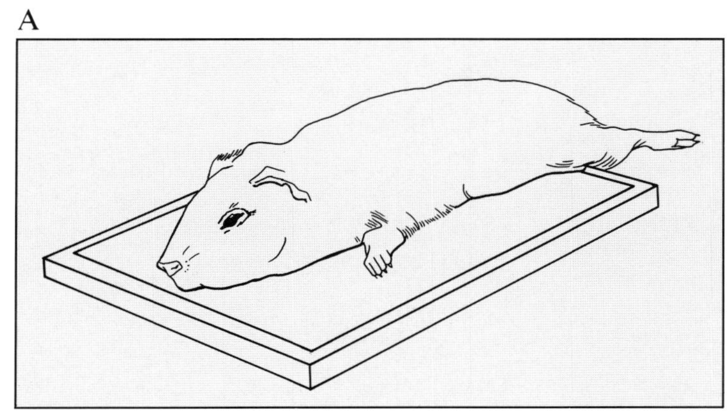

B

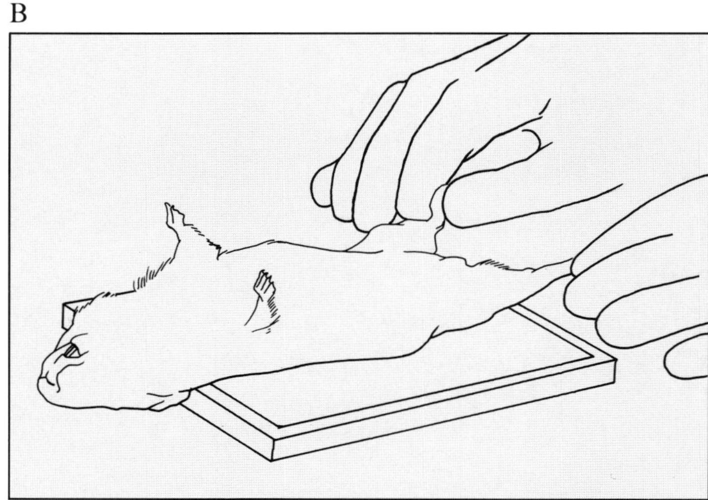

C

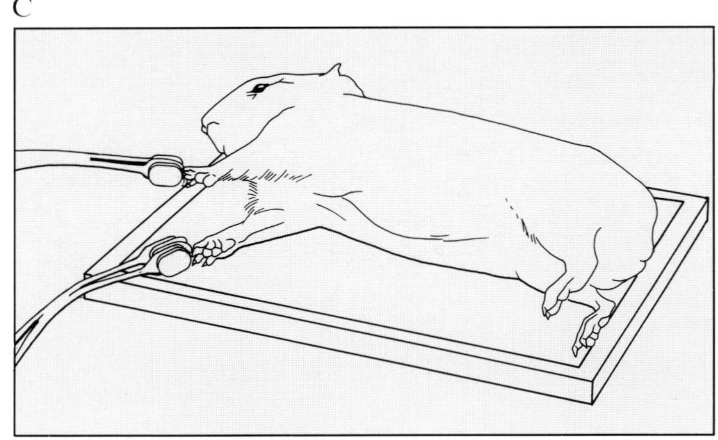

Positioning

For the radiographic examination of small mammals, tabletop technique is used. The well-sedated animal is positioned directly on the cassette (FIG. **A**). Additional manual assistance is only needed when exact or unusual positioning is required (FIG. **B**).

To prevent unwanted superposition of appendicular structures on the abdominal and thoracic images, the frontlimbs and hindlegs are pulled away from the body using small soft forceps or strings (FIG. **C**).

For laterolateral radiographs, the right lateral recumbent position should be selected (FIG. **D**). Additional radiographs include the dorsoventral (sternal recumbent) projection of the thorax and skull (FIG. **E**), the ventrodorsal (supine) projection of the abdomen, pelvic region and spinal column (FIG. **F**), and dorsopalmar (ap) or plantodorsal (pa) projections of the appendicular structures.

D

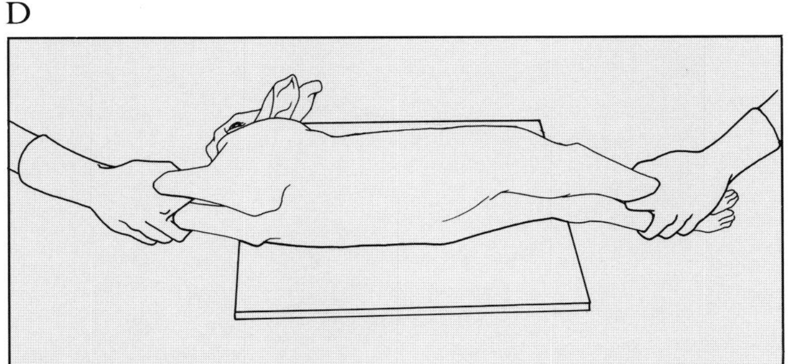

E

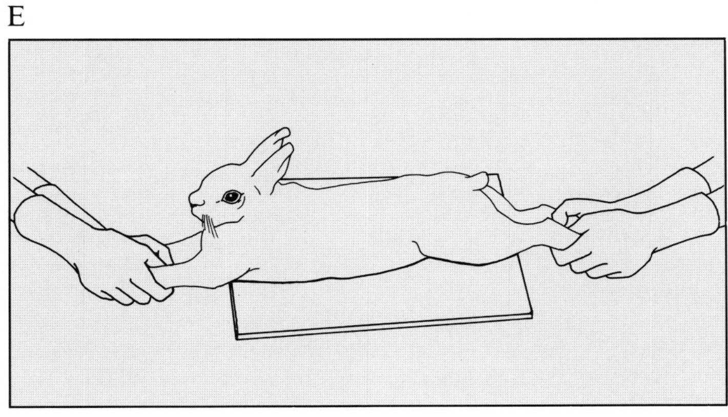

F

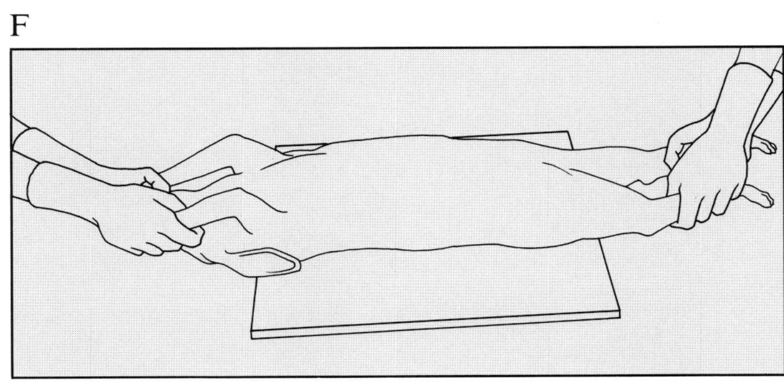

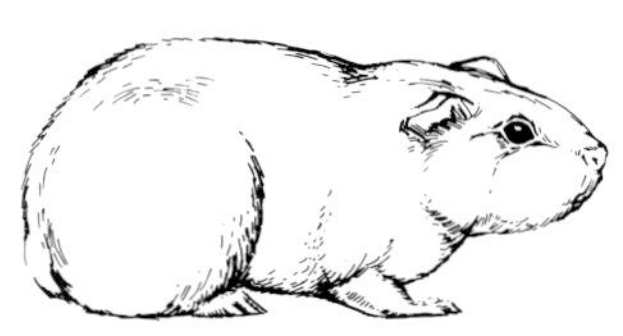

Small Mammals: Guinea Pig

Radiographic Anatomy

1

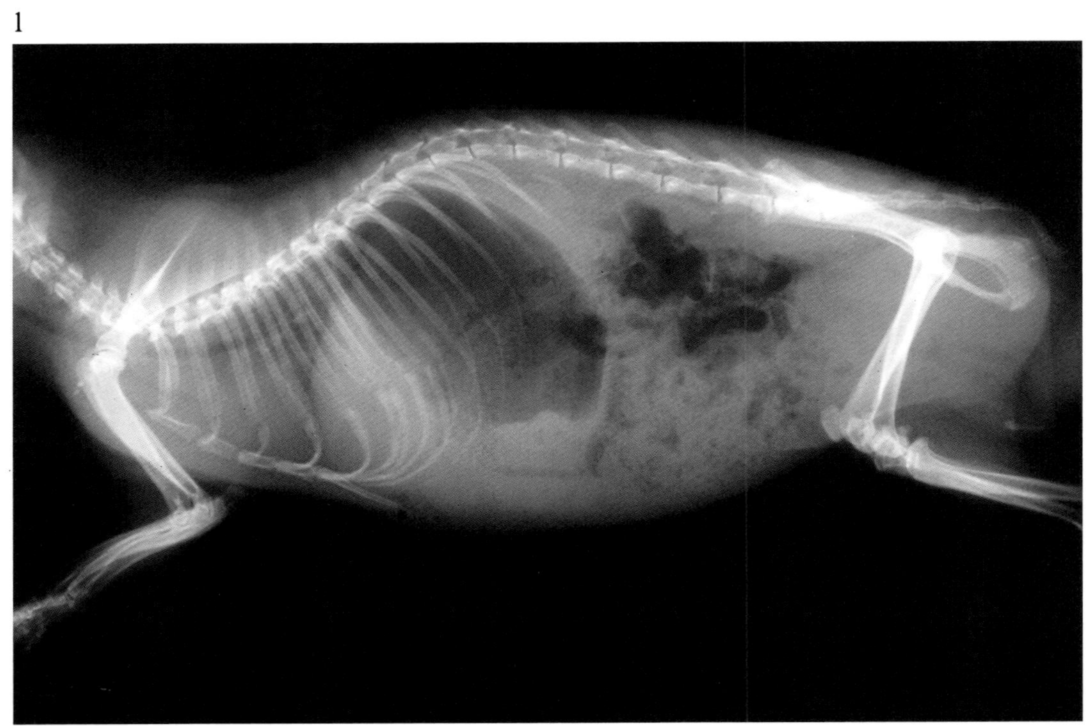

1 A

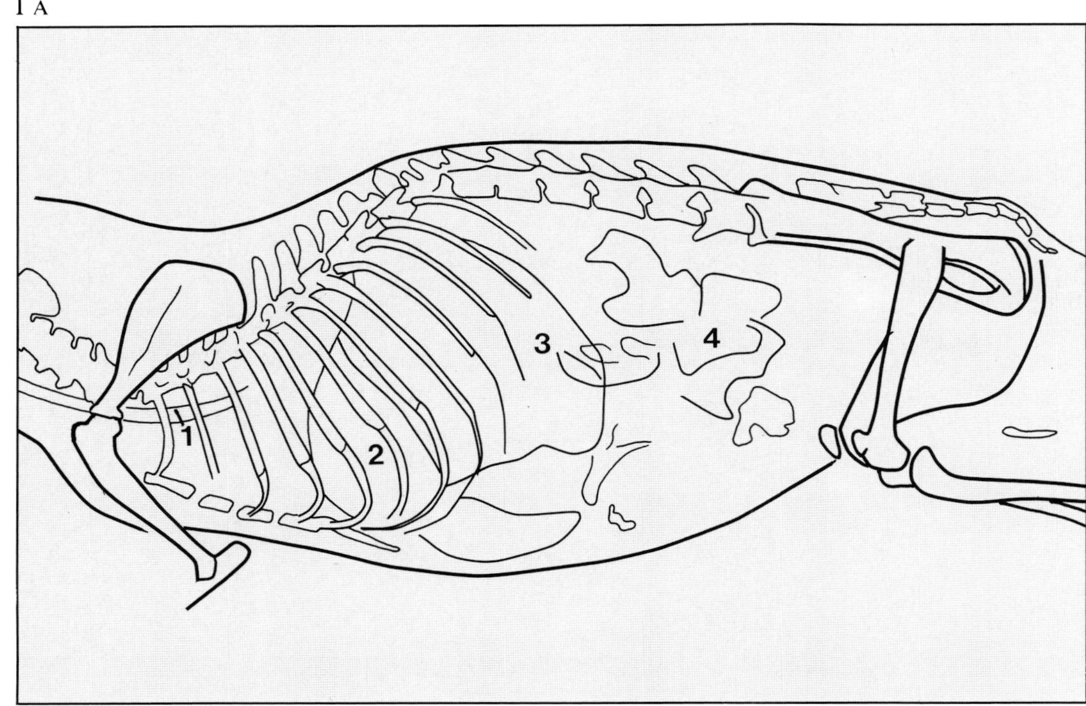

Small Mammals: Guinea Pig

Radiographic Anatomy

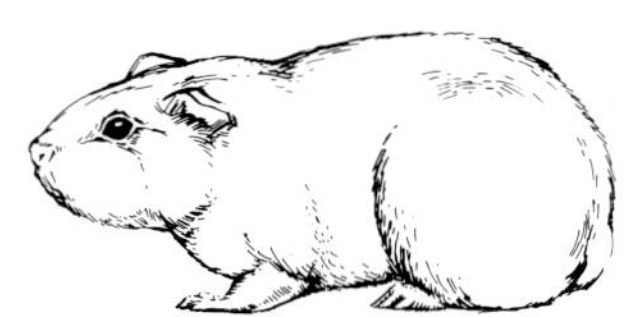

2

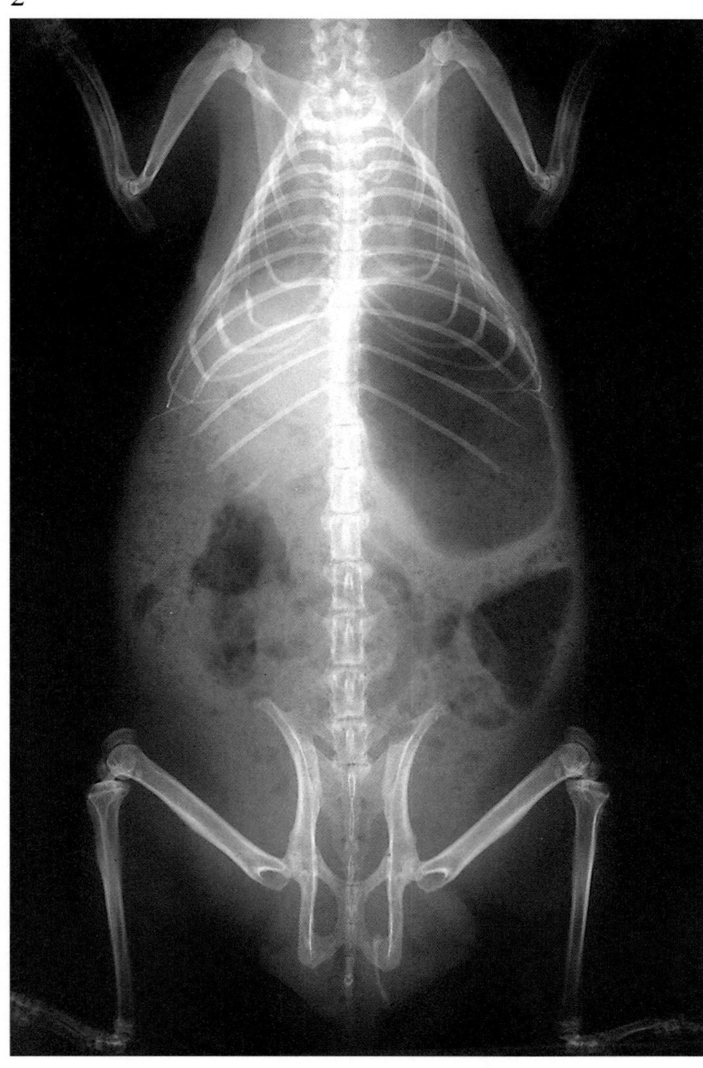

2 A

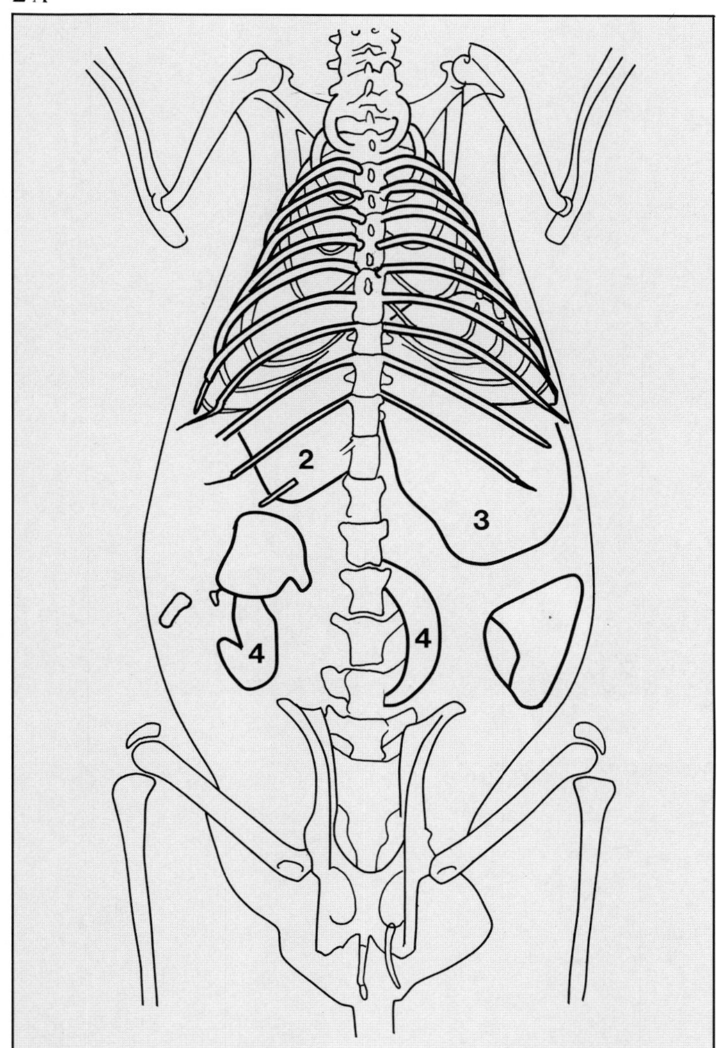

1/1A/2/2A Thorax and Abdomen: Normal Radiographic Appearance,
lateral and dorsoventral.

Guinea Pig *(Cavia aperea f. porcellus)*, male, adult.

The thoracic cavity is relatively small and reveals only a few details. The trachea (**1**) can be seen. Ventral to it, the cardiac shadow is only faintly delineated. Lungparenchyma and vasculature are difficult to evaluate because the lungs are small and not well-aerated.

Clearly visible are the extrathoracic structures such as ribs, sternum, spine and diaphragmatic outline.

In the abdominal cavity, the liver (**2**) is visible between the diaphragmatic outline and the gas-filled stomach (**3**). The small bowel and cecum are filled with food and gas (**4**).

Kidneys and urinary bladder cannot be distinguished individually due to absence of sufficient abdominal detail (lack of fat!).

3

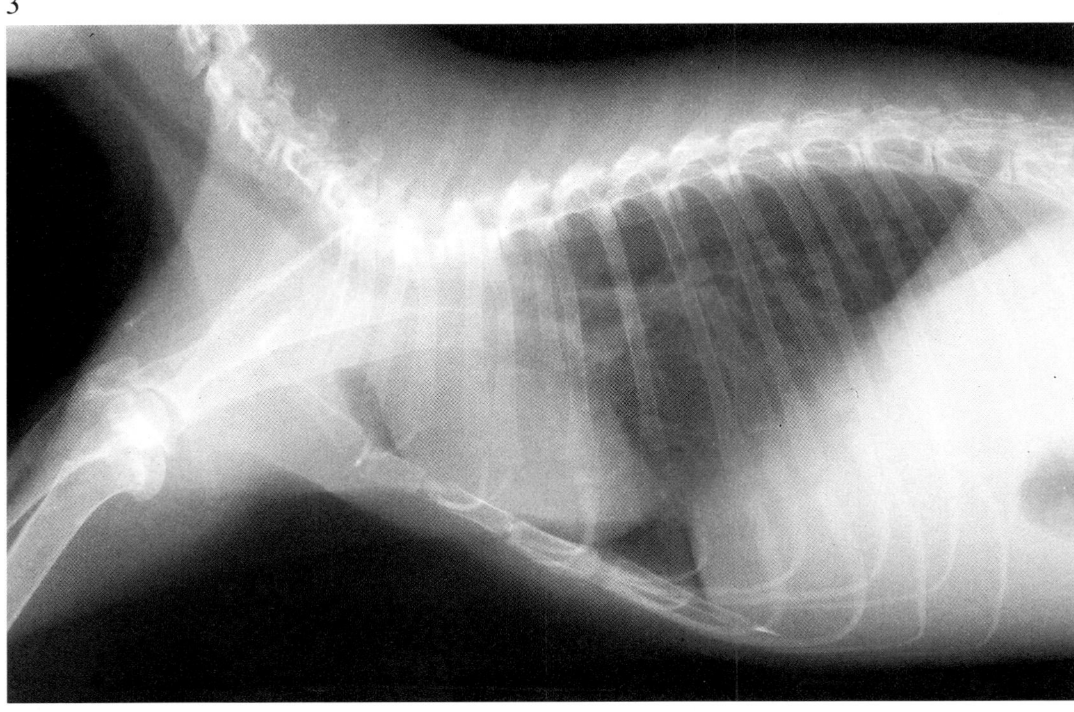

4

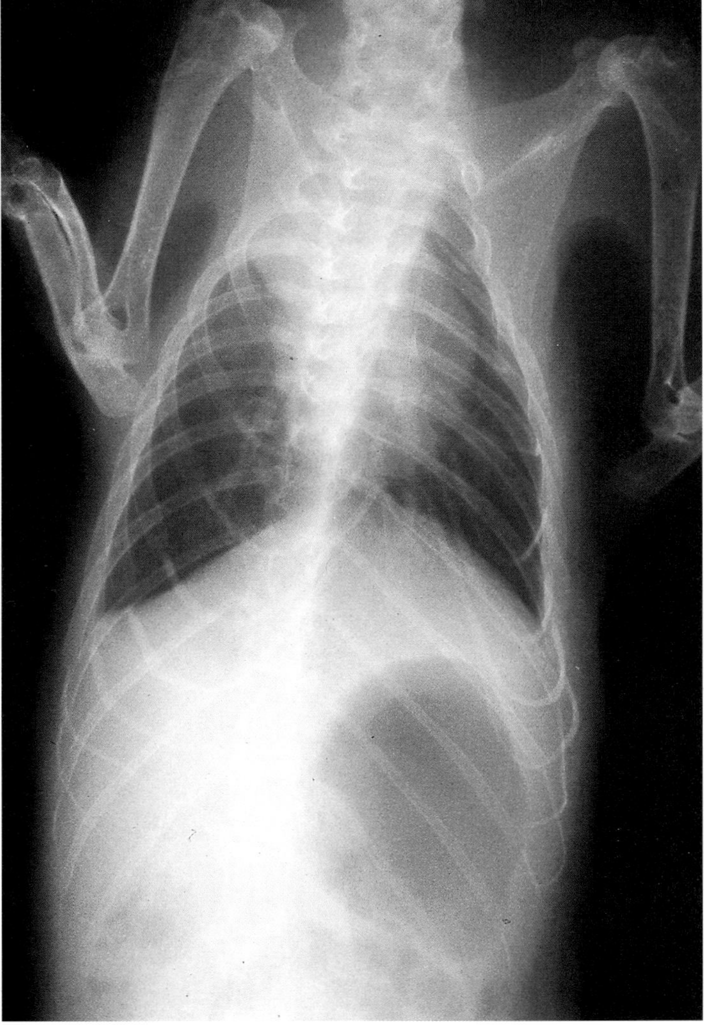

3/4 Thorax: Normal Radiographic Appearance, lateral and dorsoventral.

Guinea pig *(Cavia aperea f. porcellus)*, adult.

In this larger guinea pig, more intrathoracic detail is present. Size, shape and position of the heart can be evaluated. Notice the cranial position and ventrocranial inclination of the heart. The trachea and larger pulmonary arteries are visible. The dorsoventral projection shows symmetrical insufflation of both lungs and a wide cranial mediastinum.

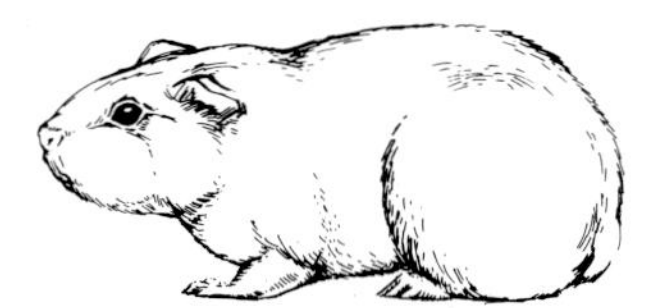

5

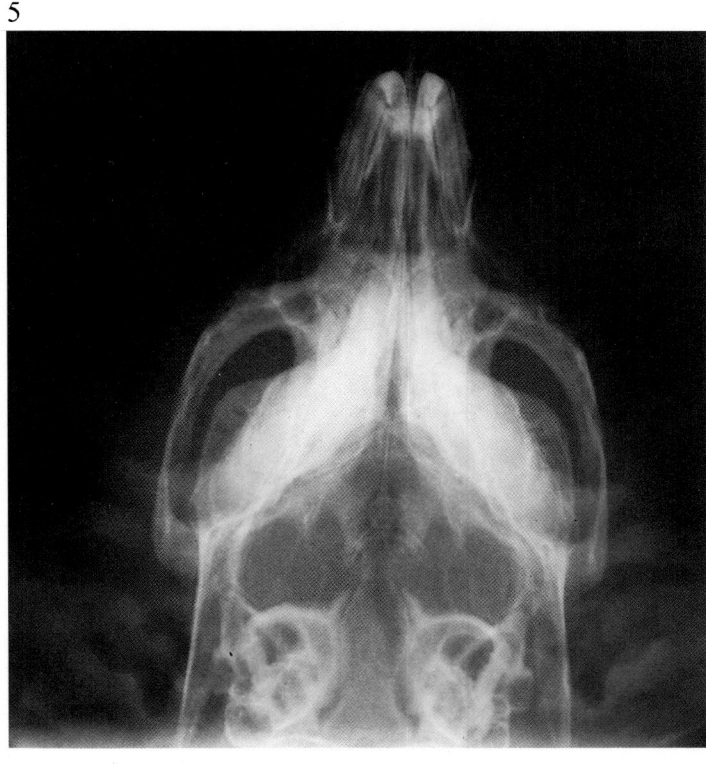

6

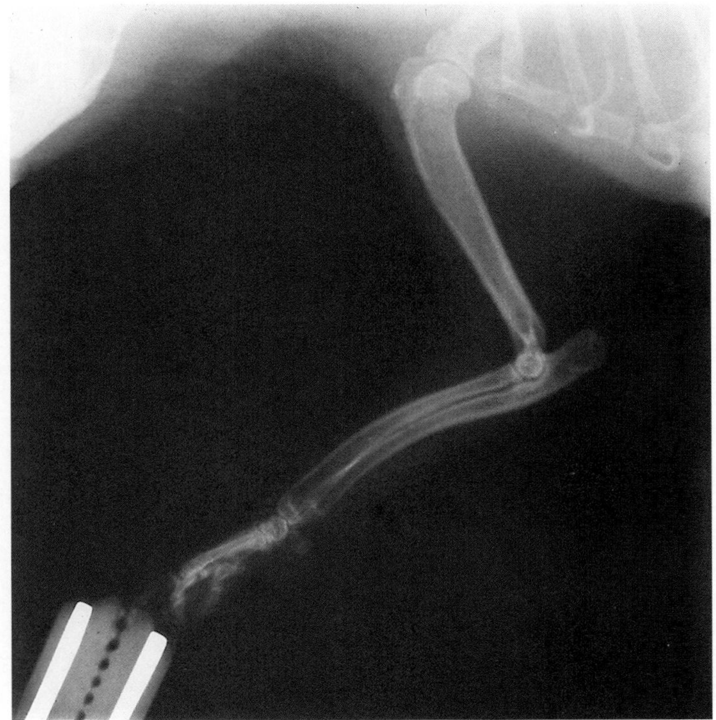

5 Skull: Normal Radiographic Appearance, dorsoventral.

Guinea Pig *(Cavia aperea f. porcellus)*, adult.

The tympanic bullae and zygomatic arches are clearly visible. However, superimposition of the mandibular arches prevents visualization of the structures of the maxilla and nasal cavity. For visualization of these structures, lateral and ventrodorsal open-mouth projections are required.

6 Foreleg: Normal Radiographic Appearance, mediolateral.

Guinea pig *(Cavia aperea f. porcellus)*, male, adult.

For radiographic examination of the forelimb, the leg has to be extended using a small, soft forceps or a string.

Anatomical detail of the bony structures is excellent.

7

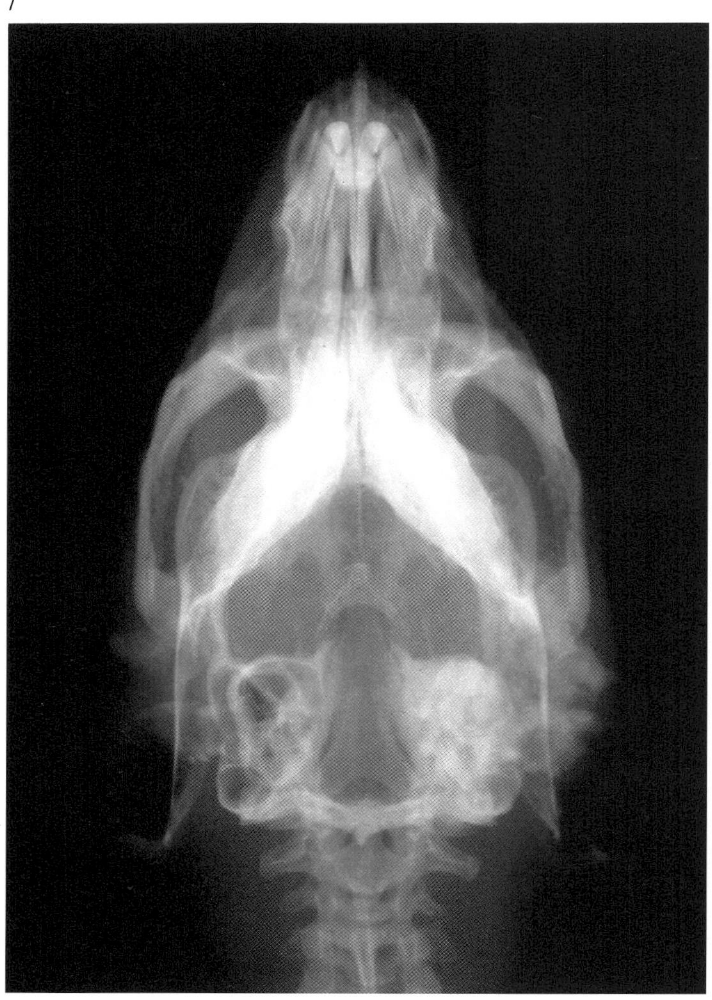

8

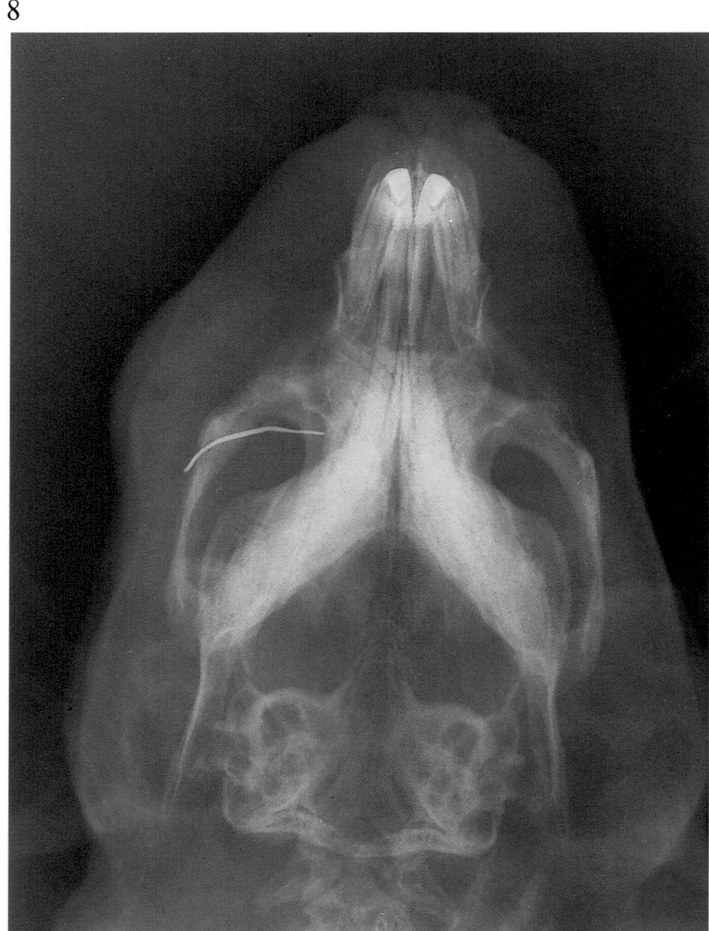

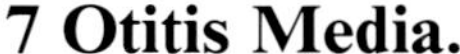

7 Otitis Media.

Guinea pig *(Cavia aperea f. porcellus)*, male, adult.

The left tympanic bulla has an increased radiopacity with loss of the finer internal structures. Compare this image with the normal right tympanic bulla that is air-filled and uniformly thin-walled.

The walls of the left external ear canal are also thickened and calcified indicating concomitant chronic otitis externa.

8 Foreign Body in the Skull.

Guinea Pig *(Cavia aperea f. porcellus)*, adult.

A linear metallic foreign body can be seen inside the boundaries of the right orbit, pointing at a right angle to the maxillary bone. Notice the soft tissue swelling.

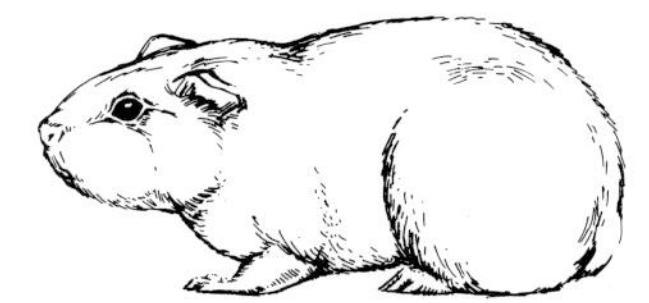

9

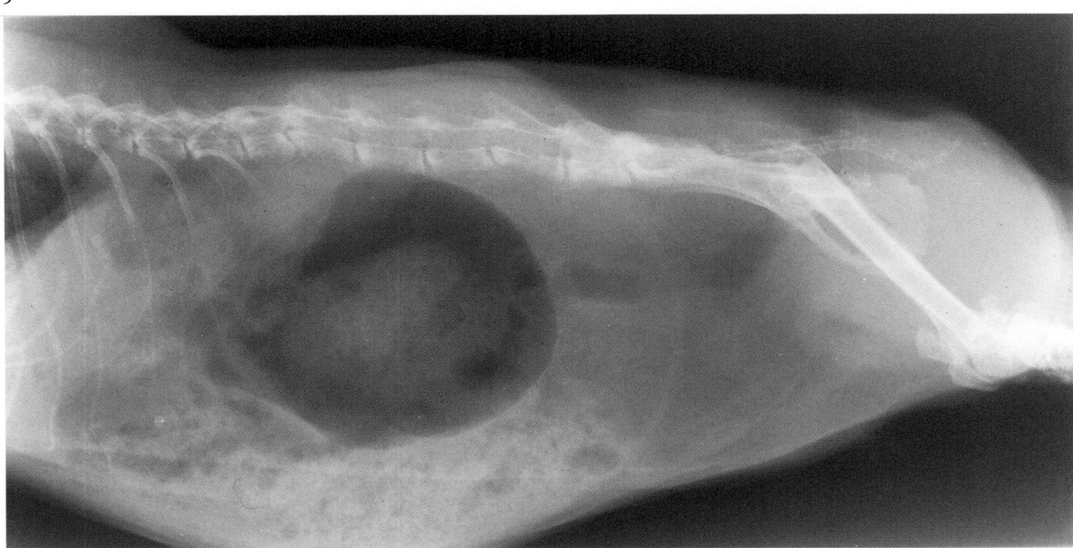

10

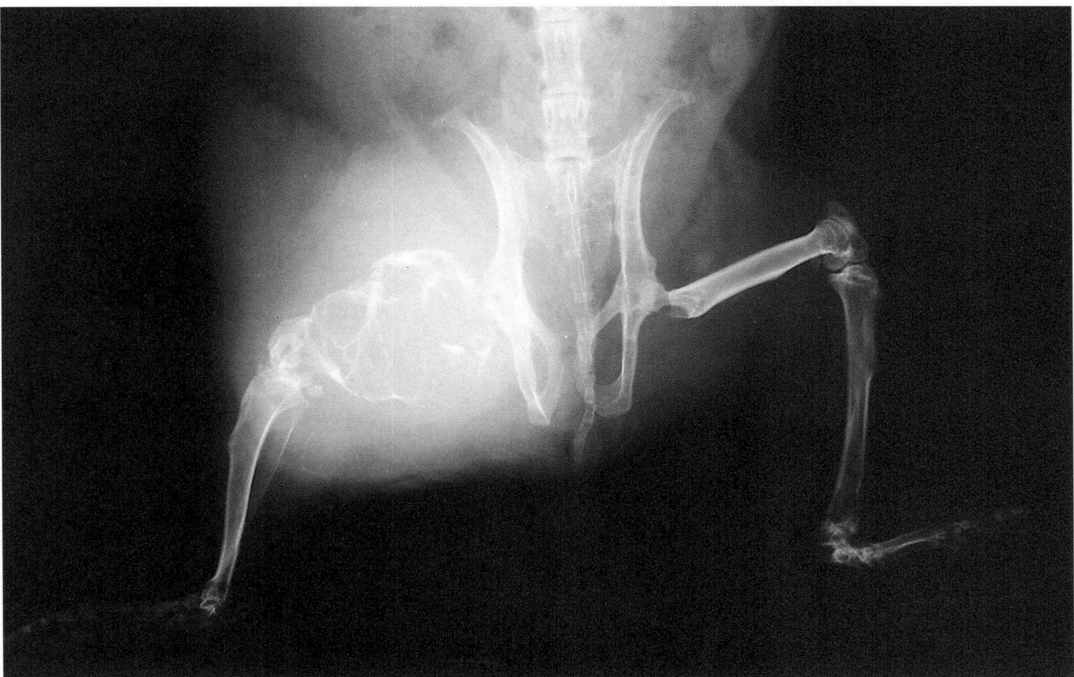

9 Spinal Malformation.

Guinea Pig *(Cavia aperea f. porcellus)*, female, 3 years.

The lumbar vertebral column shows a malformation due to the abnormal shape of several segments.

10 Osteosarcoma.

Guinea Pig *(Cavia aperea f. porcellus)*, female, adult.

Around the proximal part of the right hindleg an enormous soft tissue swelling is present. Inside this mass, the bony structures of the femur can barely be recognized due to extensive bone destruction combined with expansile deformation.

These radiographic signs are compatible with a primary bone tumor, usually an osteosarcoma.

11

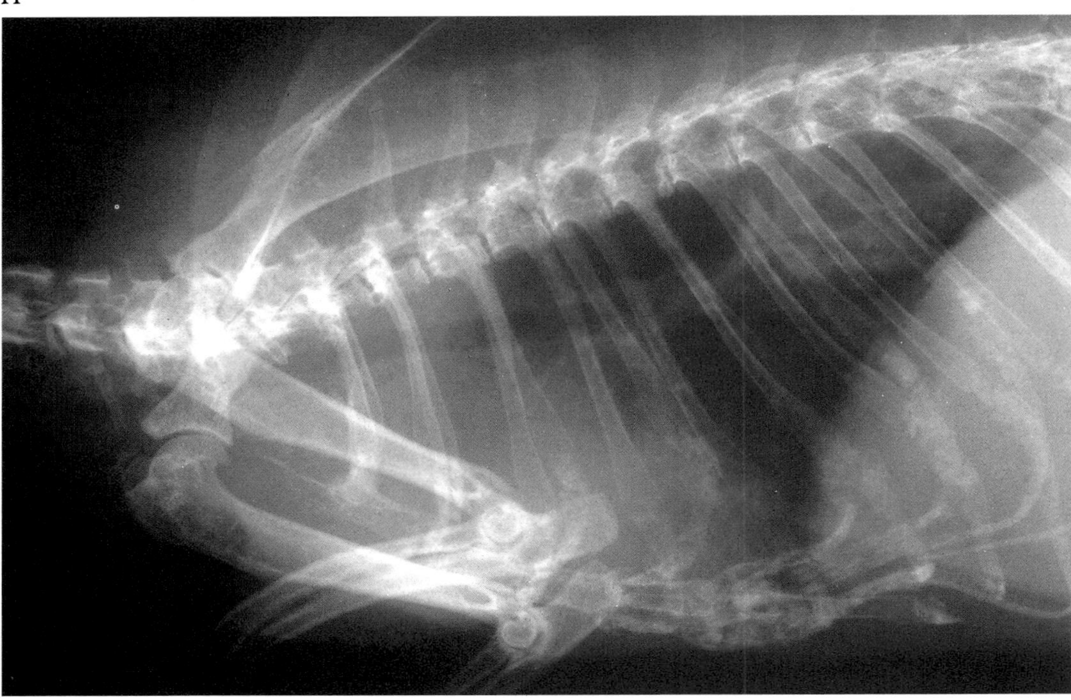

12

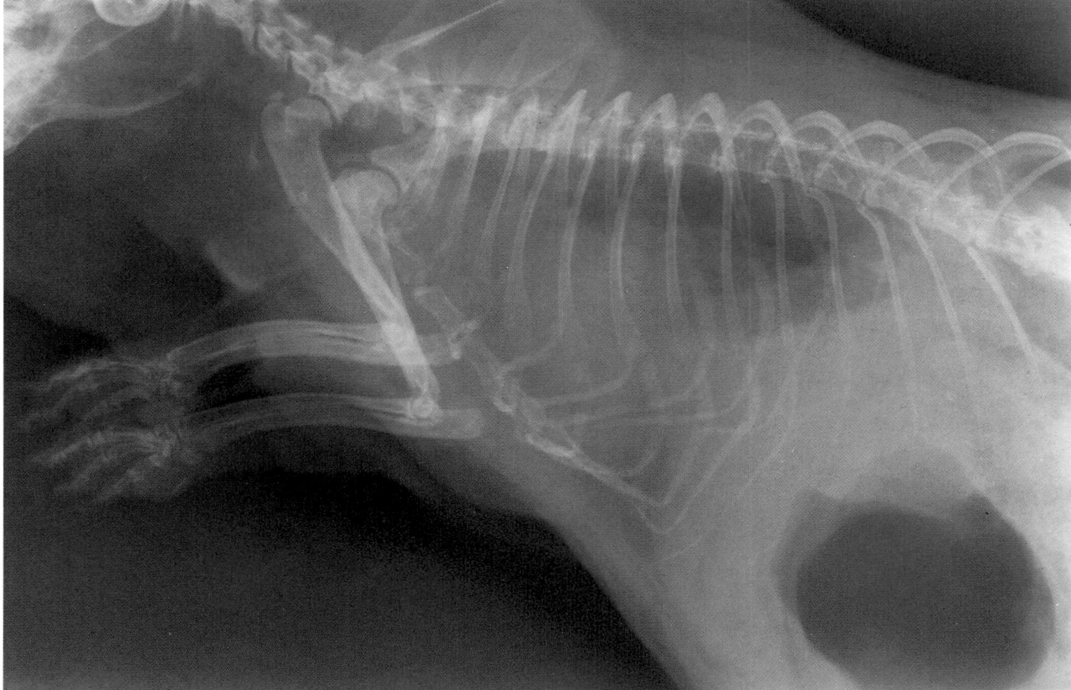

11 Pneumonia and Lungabscess.

Guinea Pig *(Cavia aperea f. porcellus)*, male, 3 years.

In the caudodorsal region of the thorax, an ill-defined radiodense mass is visible. This proved to be an abscess in the right caudal lobe of the lung.

Note: The haziness of the cranial lung lobes is caused by superposition of the soft tissues of the forelimbs.

12 Pulmonary Edema.

Guinea Pig *(Cavia aperea f. porcellus)*, male, 18 months.

Generalized increased pulmonary density and blurring of the cardiac and diaphragmatic outlines are present. This is due to cardiogenic edema. Notice the elevation of the trachea indicating cardiac enlargement.

Note: Due to severe dyspnea it was impossible to obtain a perfect radiograph.

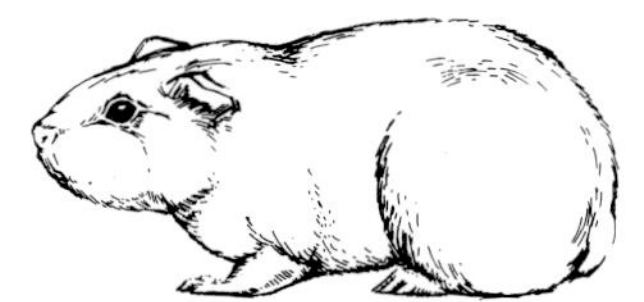

13

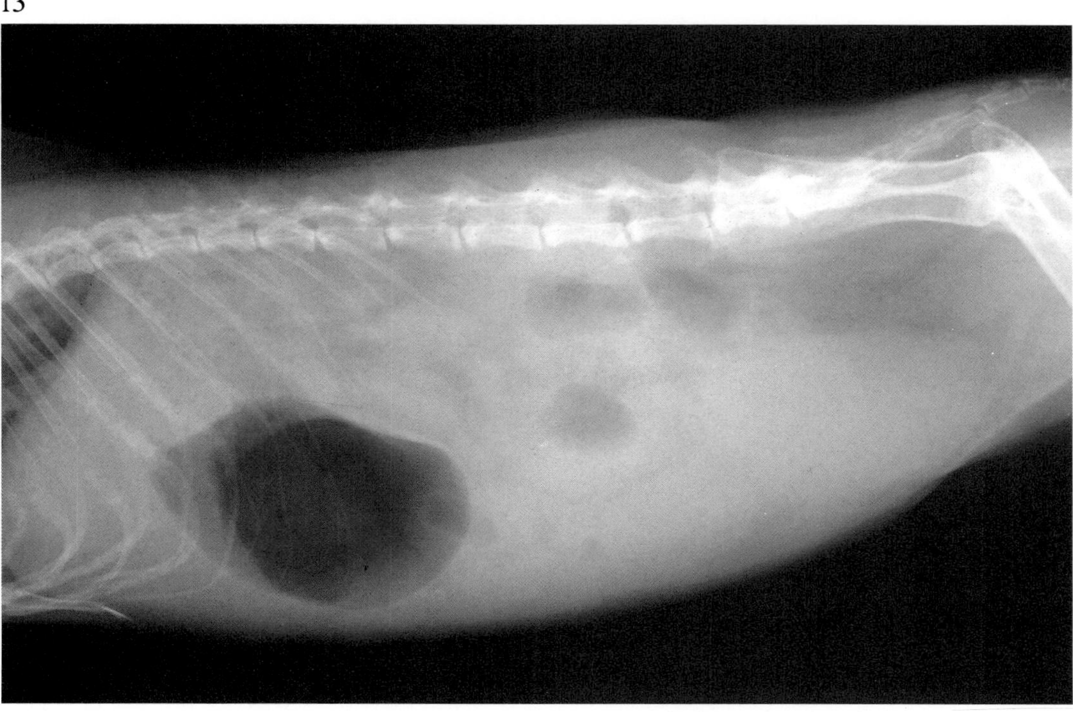

14

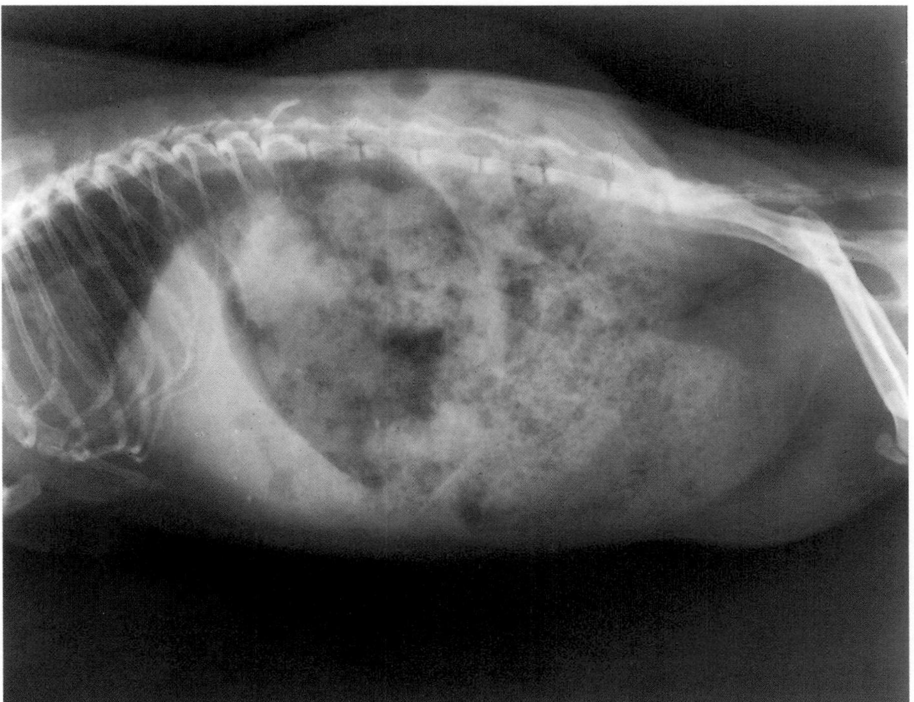

13 Enteritis.

Guinea Pig *(Cavia aperea f. porcellus)*, female, 2 years.

The haziness of the abdominal image results from large amounts of fluid in the intestines. This is a normal finding with chronic diarrhea. The stomach is empty and gas-filled.

14 Colonic Impaction.

Guinea Pig *(Cavia aperea f. porcellus)*, adult.

The intestinal tract is greatly distended and overfilled with granular food and stool.

Note: The liver is enlarged extending far caudally into the ventral abdominal cavity.

15

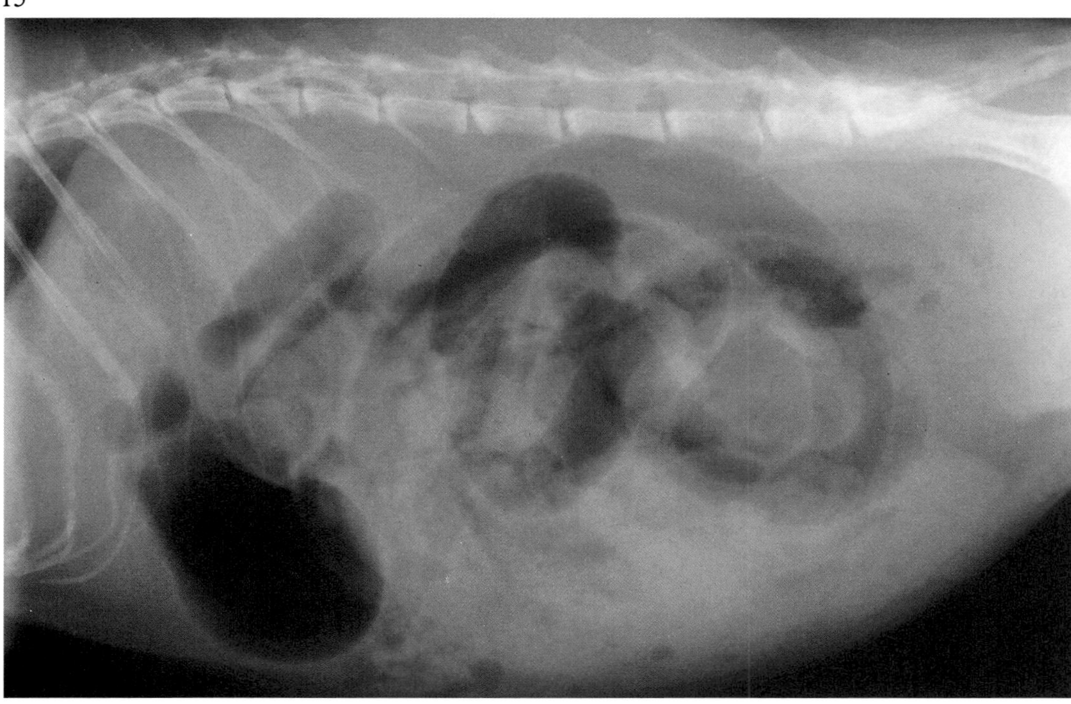

16

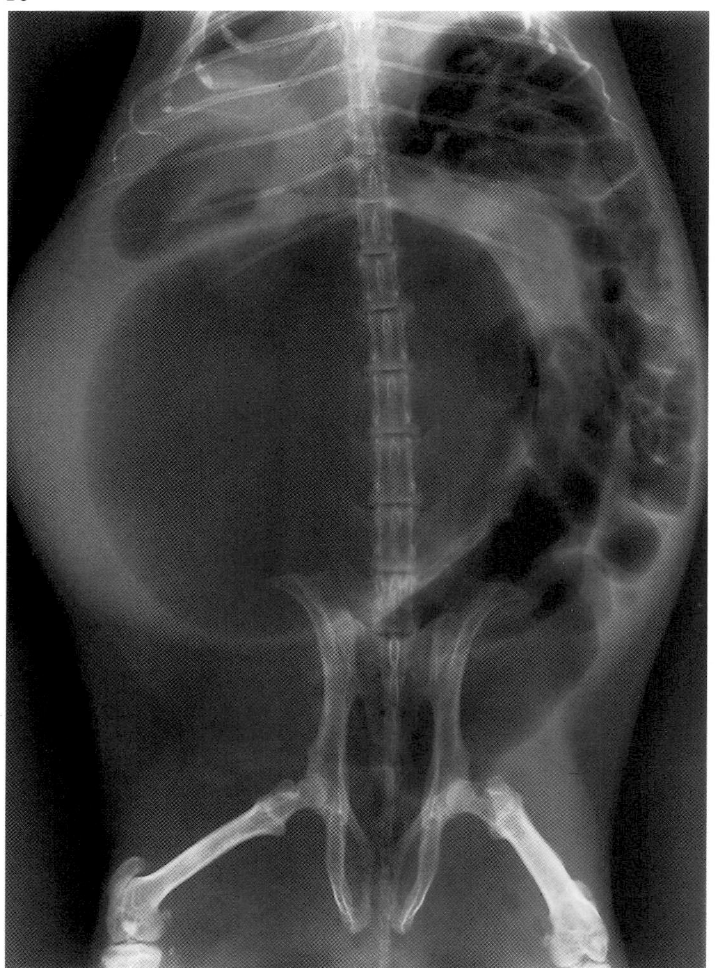

15 Ileus.

Guinea Pig *(Cavia aperea f. porcellus)*, female, 3 years.

Several dilated, gas-filled small intestinal loops are visible. The stomach contains gas. The soft tissue-dense mass in the ventral abdomen is caused by the accumulation of food remnants in distended small bowel loops, mimicking a well-filled cecum. The large bowel cannot be recognized. The origin of this obstructive ileus cannot be determined from this radiograph.

16 Gastric Dilatation and Volvulus.

Guinea Pig *(Cavia aperea f. porcellus)*, female, adult.

The stomach is greatly distended and gas- and fluid-filled. It is positioned abnormally occupying the right half of the abdominal cavity. The gas-filled small bowel loops are dislocated cranially and to the left side of the peritoneal cavity.

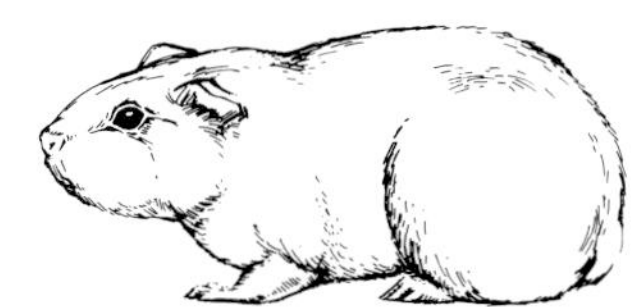

17

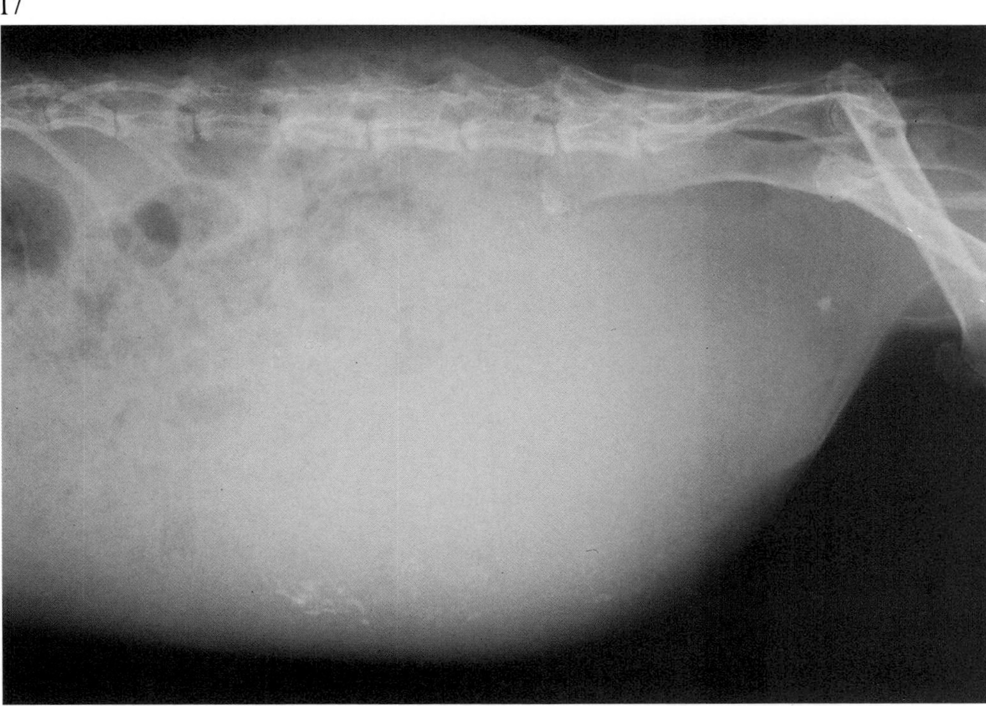

18

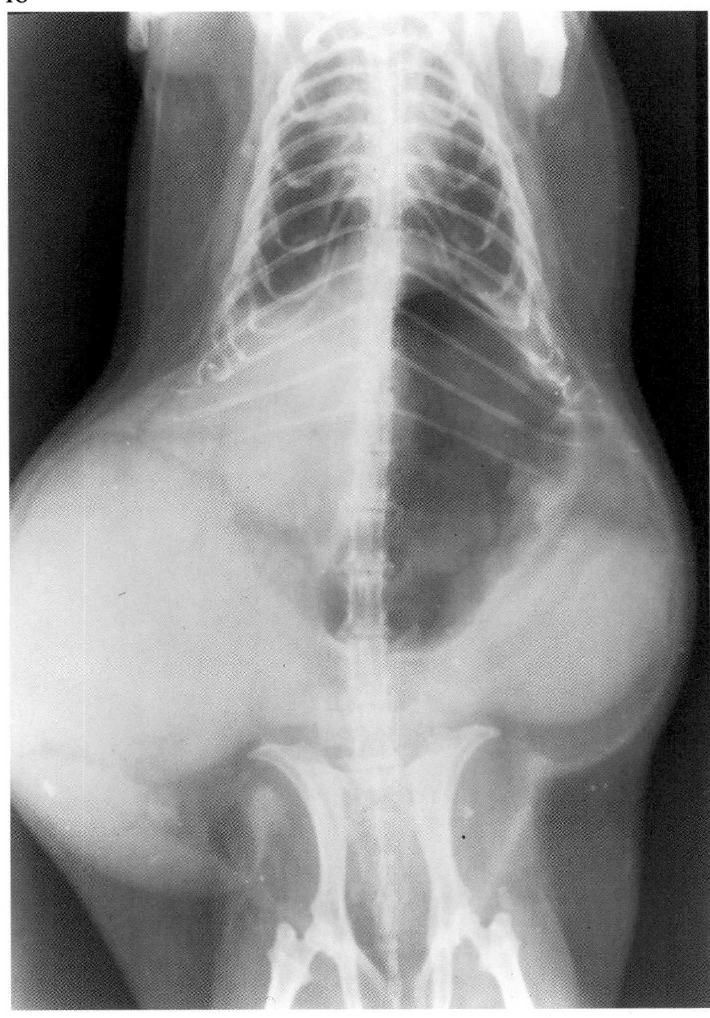

17 Urethral Obstruction.

Guinea Pig *(Cavia aperea f. porcellus)*, 4 years.

The caudal part of the abdominal cavity is occupied by a large fluid-dense structure that represents a severely distended urinary bladder. The bladder distension is due to an urethral obstruction by a small urinary calculus that is visible as a tiny radiopacity, just ventral to the hip joints.

More calcified material (urinary calculi) is visible at the cranioventral border of the distended bladder.

18 Ovarian Cysts.

Guinea Pig *(Cavia aperea f. porcellus)*, female, adult.

Two well-defined soft tissue masses are present on both sides of the abdominal cavity. These masses are located just caudal to the kidneys and represent large ovarian cysts.

19

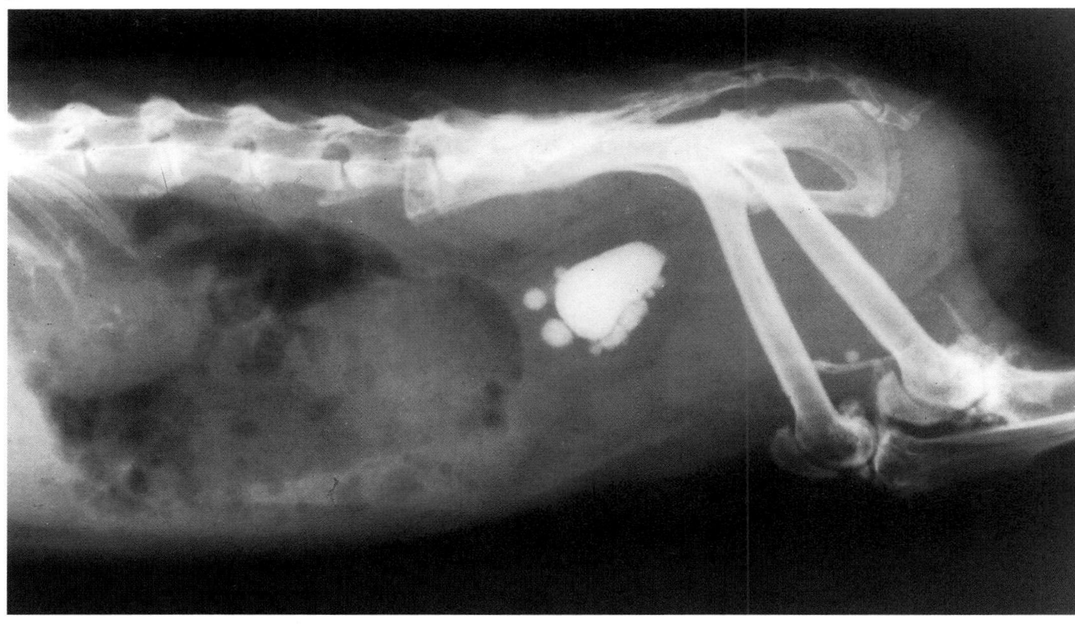

19 A

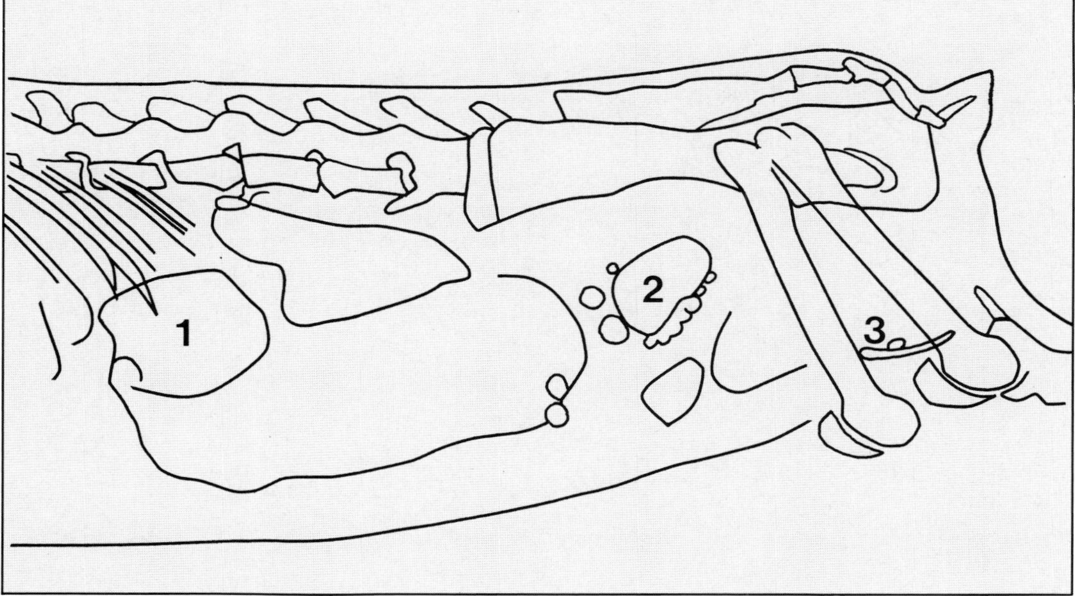

19/19A Urolithiasis (Cystic calculi).

Guinea Pig *(Cavia aperea f. porcellus)*, male, adult.

Multiple calcifications and several calculi are visible in different parts of the urinary tract:

(**1**) Calcific densities in the pelvic region of the kidneys,

(**2**) Multiple cystic calculi,

(**3**) A small calculus lodged in the urethra, visible as a small radiopacity just dorsal to the bony outline of the os penis.

Additional findings include collapse of the L_{2-3} disc space with endplate sclerosis and ventral vertebral spondylosis, and chronic osteoarthrosis of the right stifle joint.

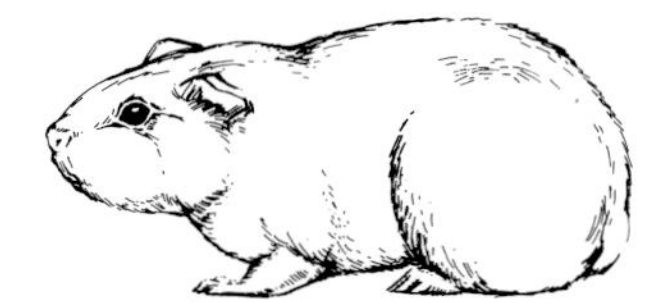

20

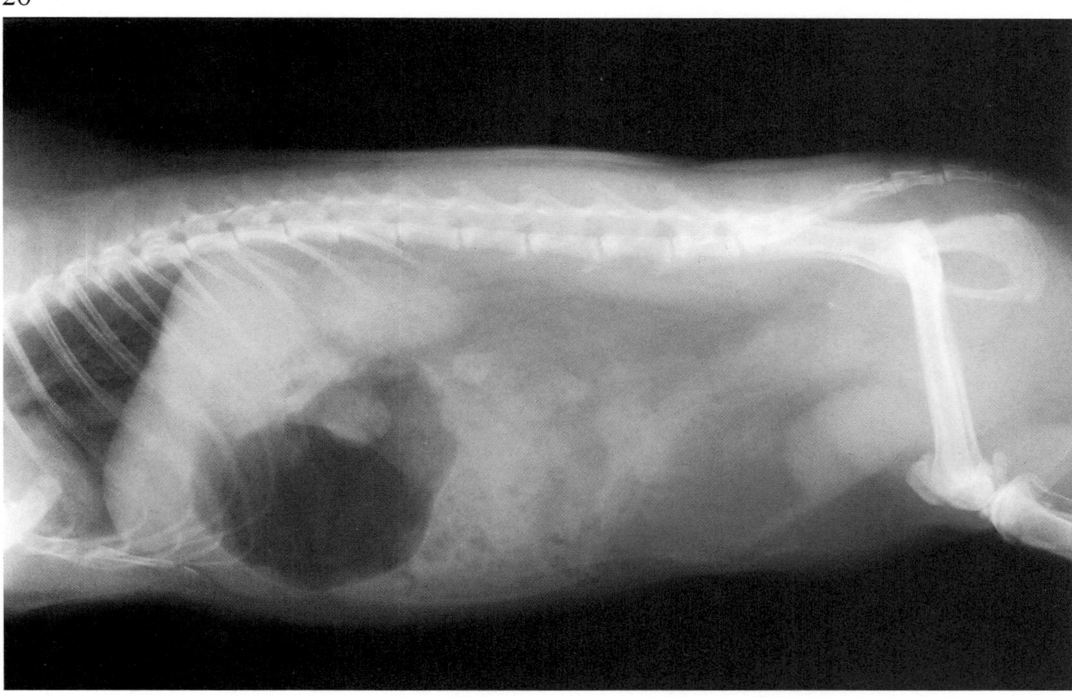

21

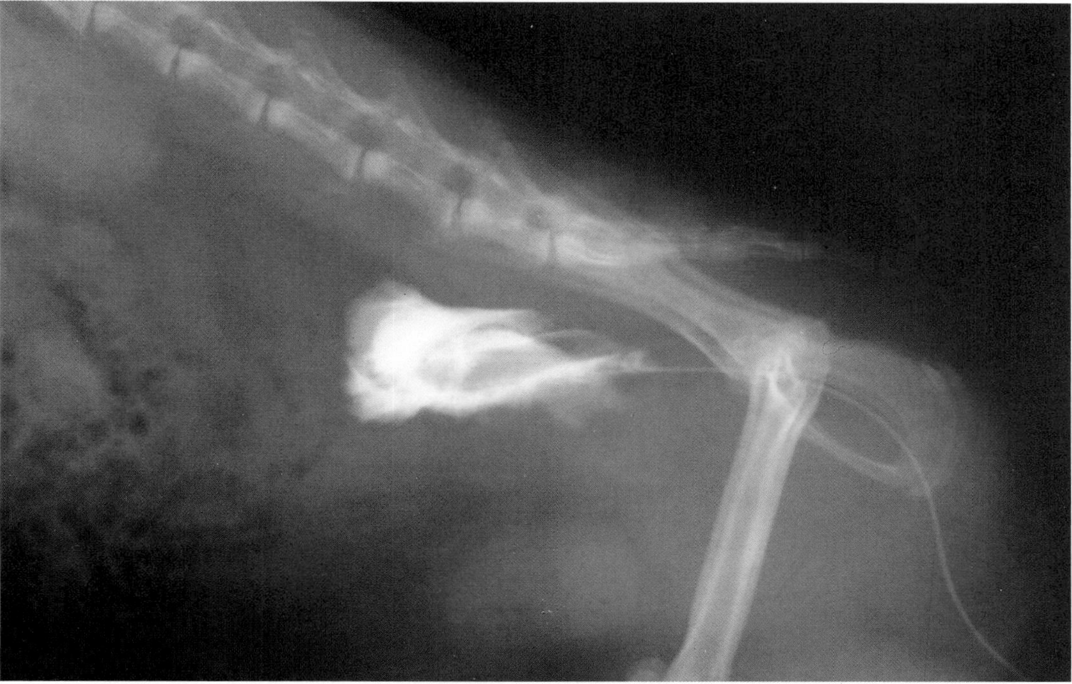

20/21 Bladder Perforation.

Guinea Pig *(Cavia aperea f. porcellus)*, male, 7 months.

The noncontrast film shows an ill-defined, empty urinary bladder. This is a strange finding because the abundant amounts of intra-abdominal fat should provide good anatomical detail.

A positive-contrast cystogram following catheterization of the urinary bladder and introduction of 5 ml of an iodinated contrast medium reveals an abnormally-shaped urinary bladder and leakage of contrast medium into the peritoneal cavity. The contrast-filled catheter marks the position of the urethra.

Note: The well-defined soft tissue density that is present on the ventral abdominal wall of the hypogastrium strongly resembles the urinary bladder, but is caused by the intra-abdominal presence of the testicles.

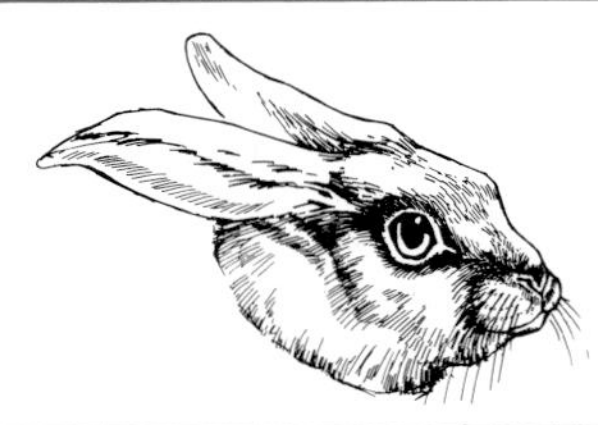

Small Mammals: Rabbit

22

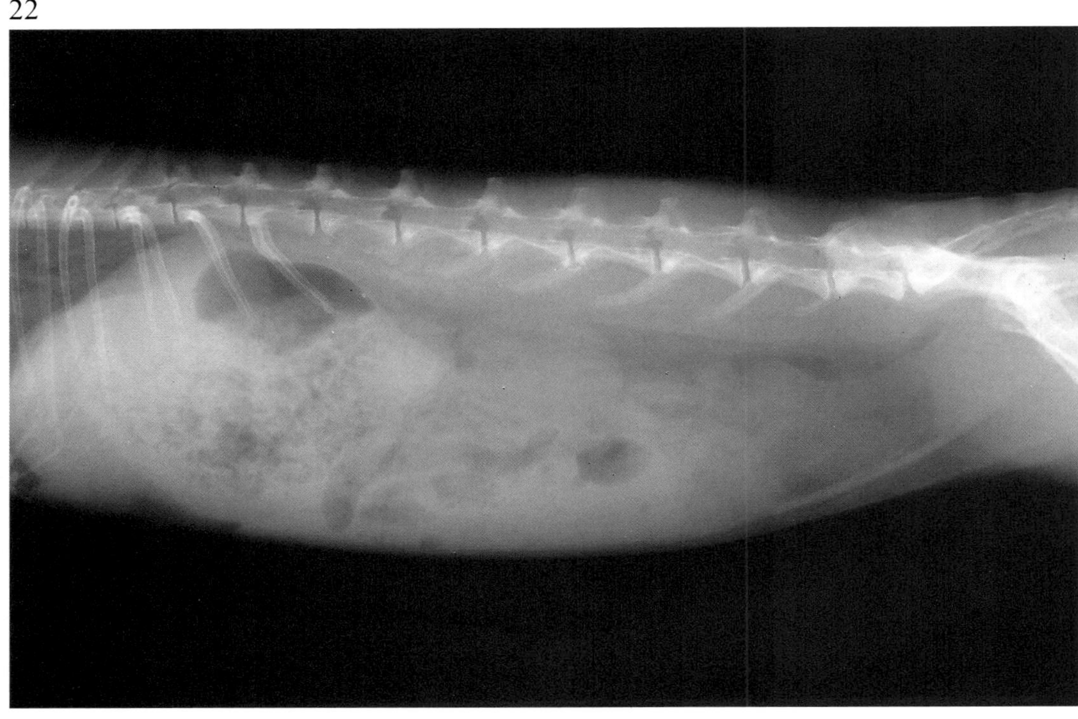

22 A

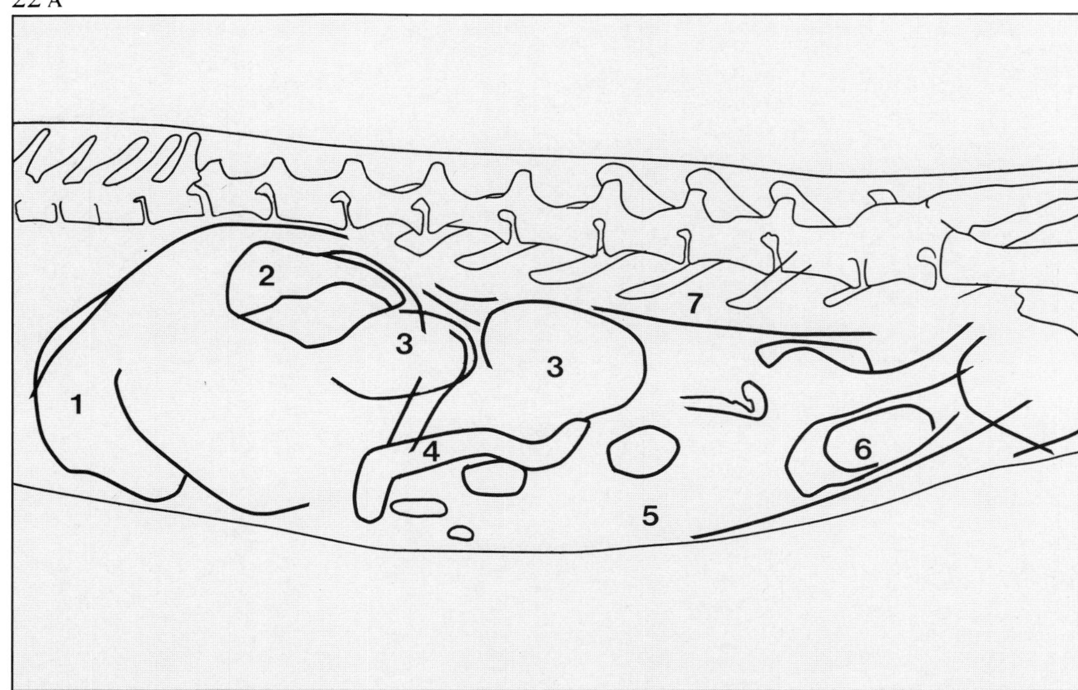

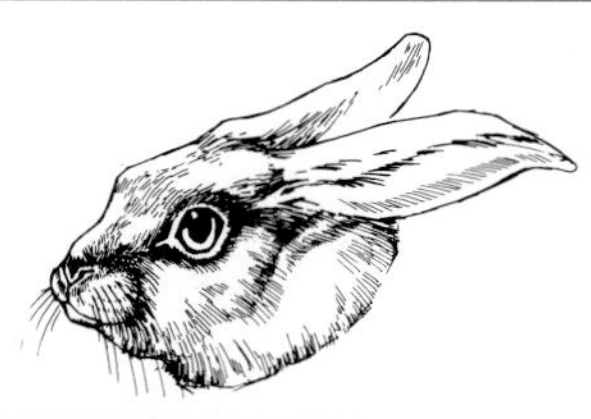

23

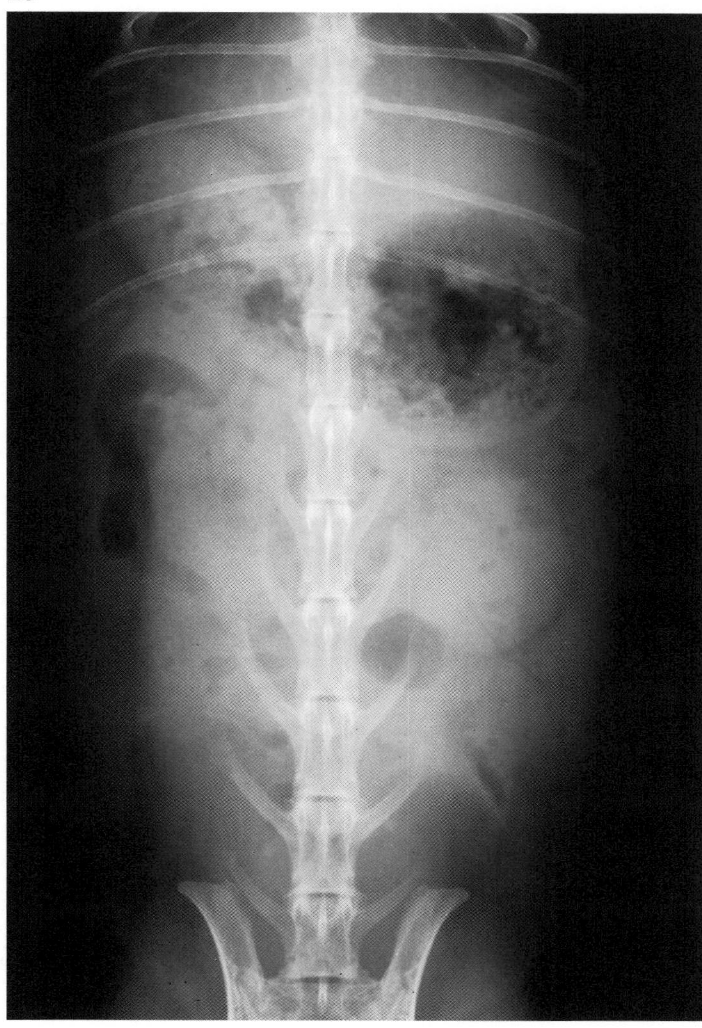

23 A

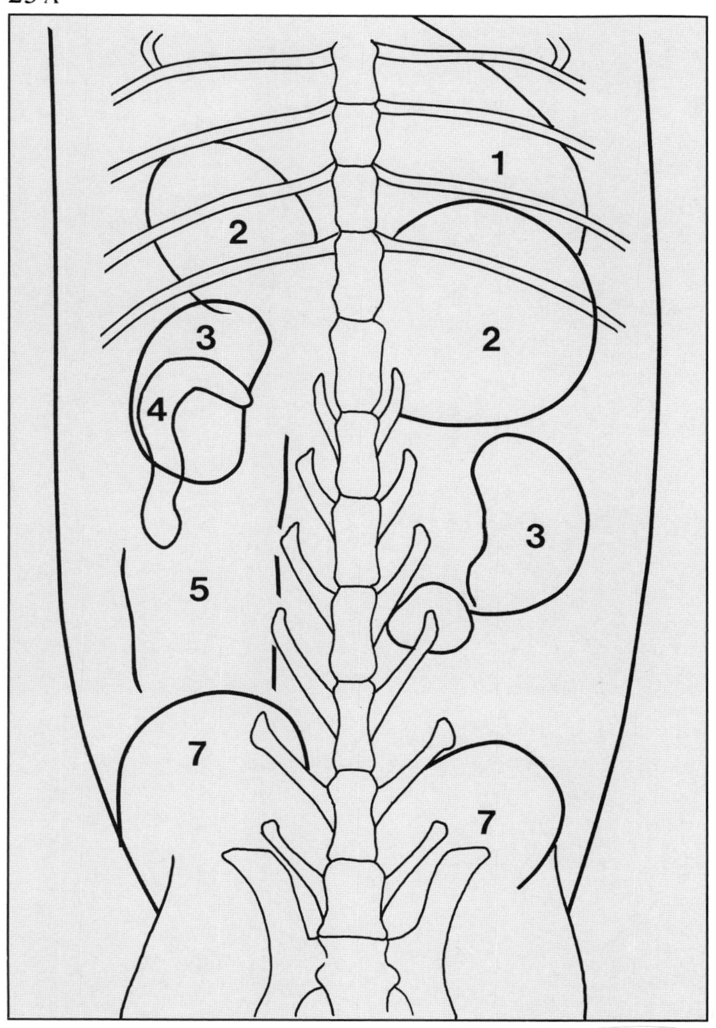

22/22A/23/23A
Abdomen: Normal Radiographic Appearance, lateral and ventrodorsal.

Rabbit *(Oryctolagus cuniculus)*, male, 8 years.

Several abdominal structures can be recognized:

liver (**1**), stomach filled with food and gas (**2**), kidneys (**3**), small bowel loops (**4**), cecum (**5**), urinary bladder (**6**) and intra-abdominal fat deposits (**7**).

24

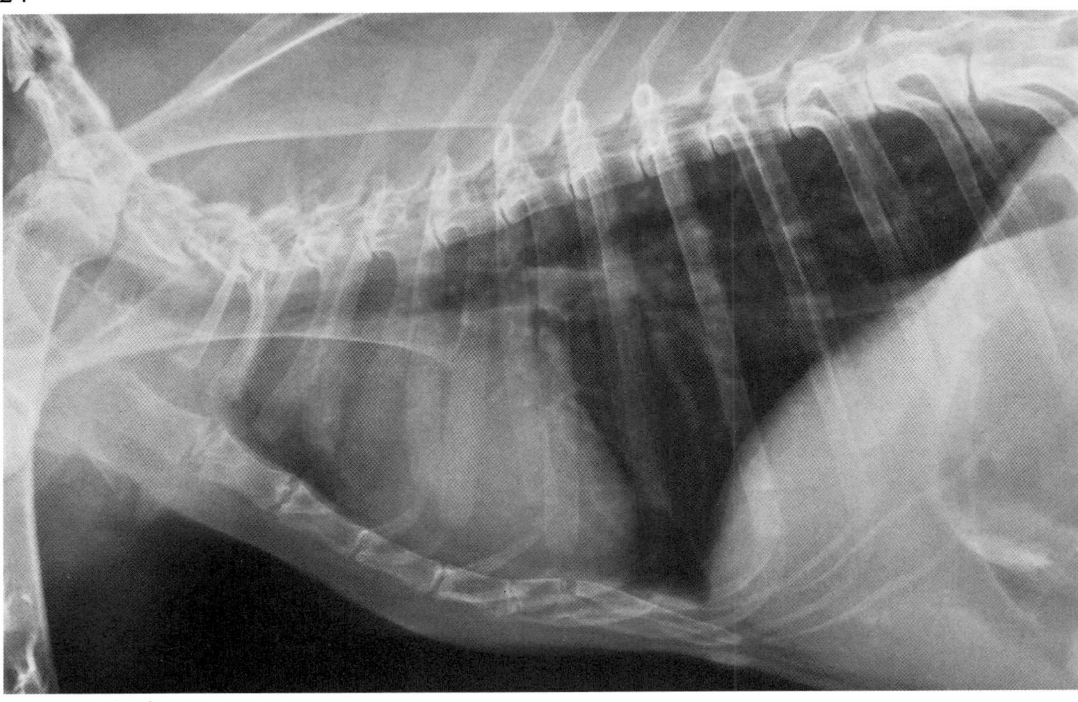

25

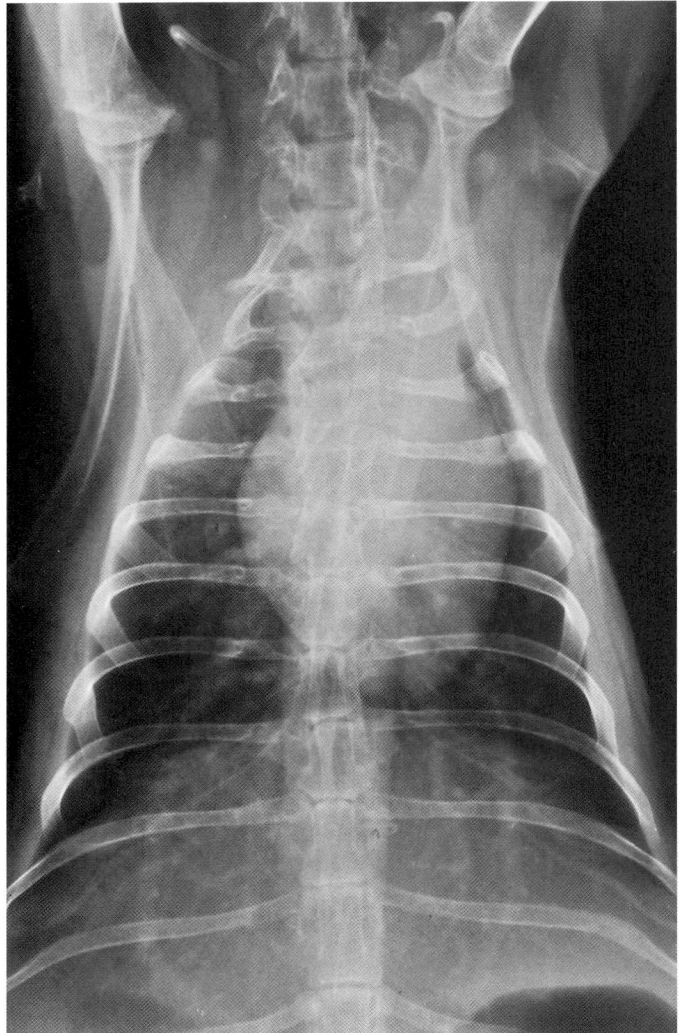

24/25 Thorax: Normal Radiographic Appearance, lateral and dorsoventral.

Rabbit *(Oryctolagus cuniculus)*, male, 8 years.

The heart is located between the fourth and sixth pairs of ribs. The cranial lung lobes are relatively small surrounding a wide cranial mediastinum. The caudal lung lobes are well aerated, with a detailed pulmonary vasculature. The aorta and caudal vena cava are clearly visible.

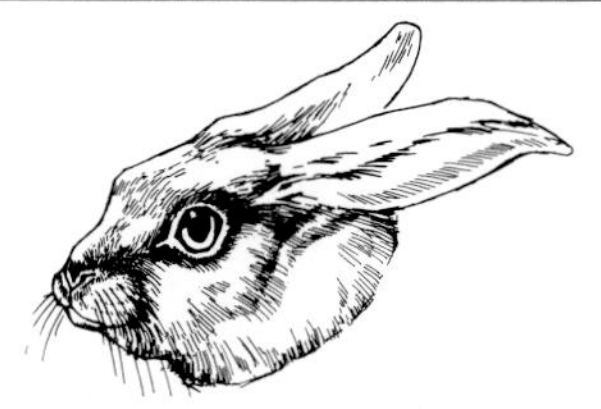

26

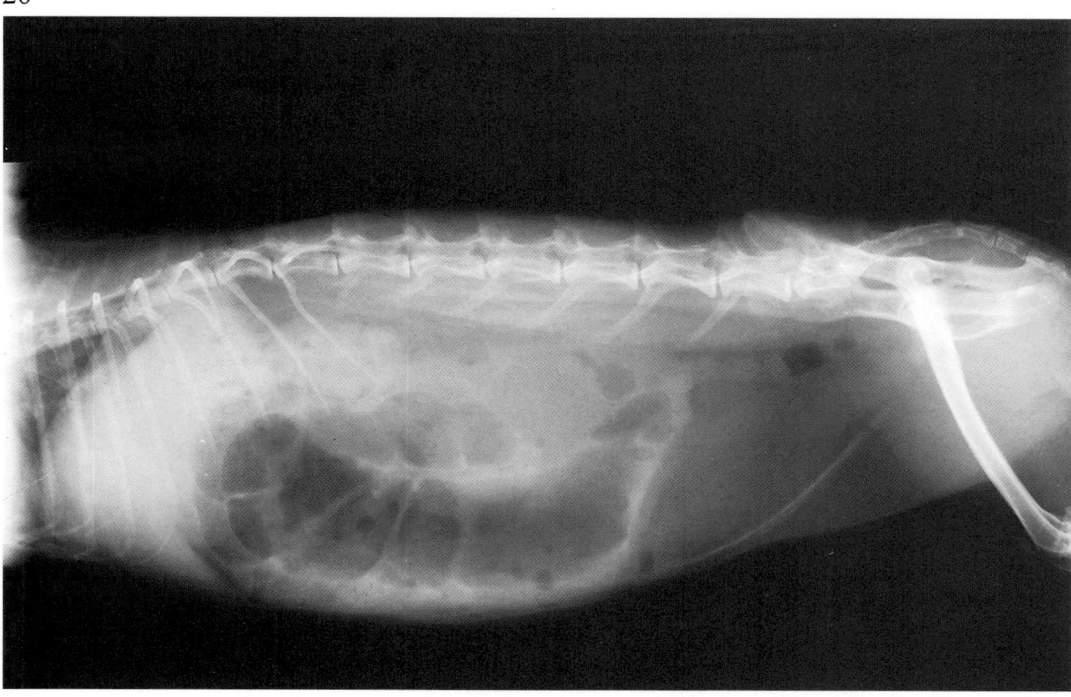

27

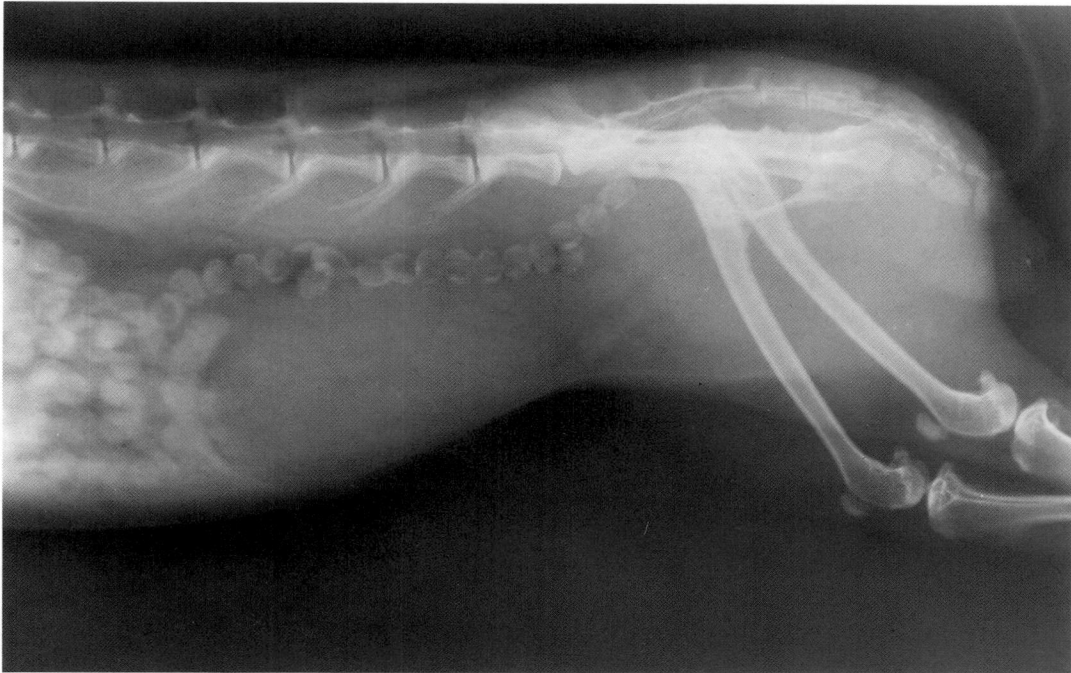

26 Abdomen: Normal Radiographic Appearance, lateral.

Rabbit *(Oryctolagus cuniculus)*, adult.

The ventral part of the abdominal cavity is mainly filled by the greatly distended, gas-filled cecum. Also visible are the liver, kidneys and urinary bladder.

27 Abdomen: Normal Radiographic Appearance, lateral.

Rabbit *(Oryctolagus cuniculus)*.

The large intestines, and especially the descending colon, are filled with characteristic small fecal balls. The urinary bladder is fully distended.

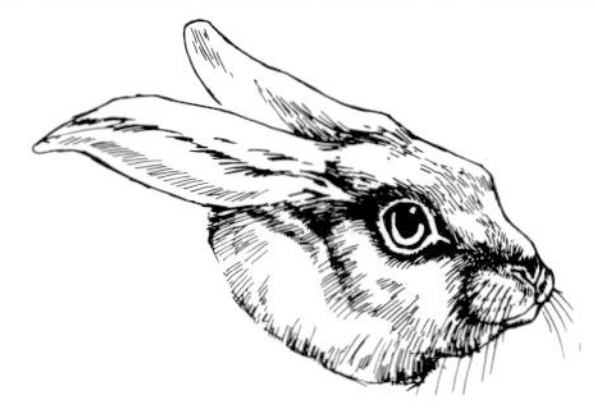

Small Mammals: Rabbit

Radiographic Anatomy

28

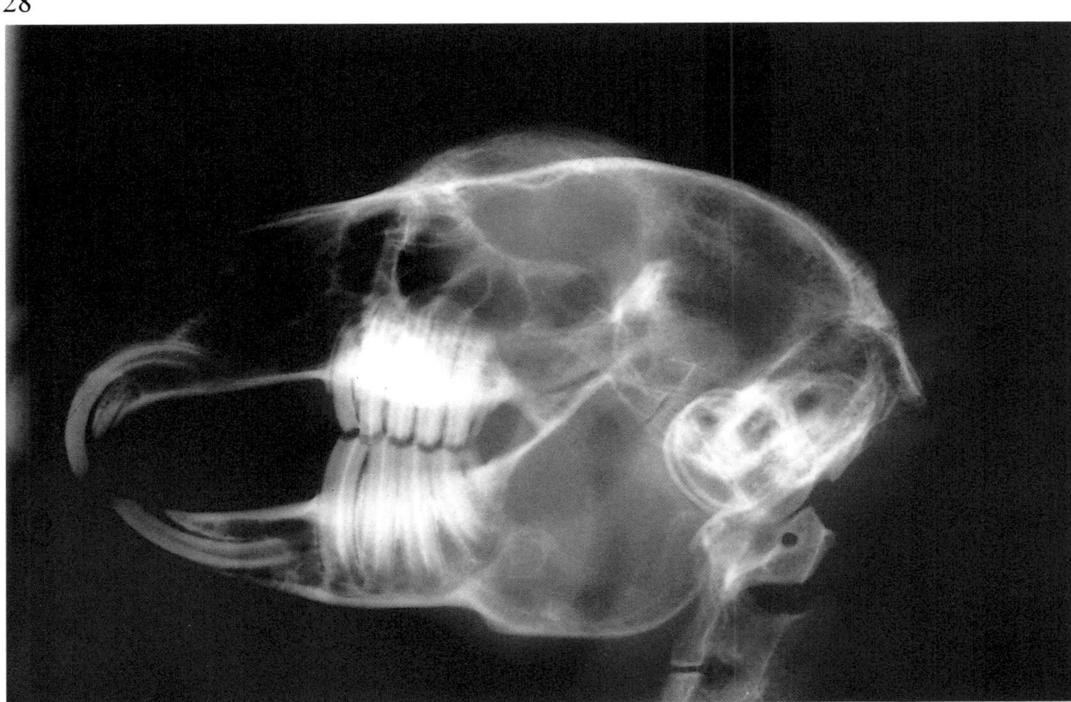

29

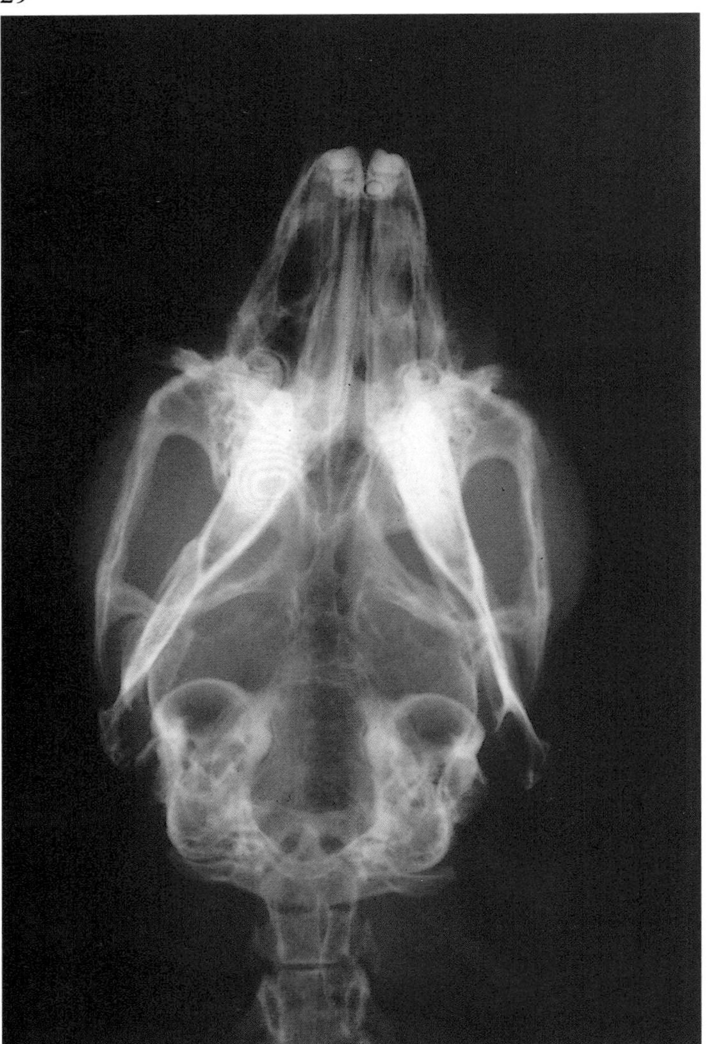

28 Skull: Normal Radiographic Appearance, lateral.

Rabbit *(Oryctolagus cuniculus)*, male, adult.

The normal dental formula of a rabbit is $\frac{2\,0\,3\,3}{1\,0\,2\,3}$.

The third upper molar is very small and hardly visible. The first two incisors of the upper jaw grow in a half circle towards the hard palate of the oral cavity. The lower incisors prevent this by rubbing constantly on the upper pair. Therefore, incisors of upper and lower jaw must be in good alignment with each other. All upper premolars and molars grow parallel to each other. In the lower jaw, the last two molars grow at a slight angle towards the other teeth.

The angular processes of the mandibles are large, but paper-thin and appear almost radiolucent. The nasal cavity is well-aerated, with very delicate structures.

29 Skull: Normal Radiographic Appearance, dorsoventral.

Rabbit *(Oryctolagus cuniculus)*, male, adult.

Superimposition of the mandibular rami hinders the interpretation of the nasal cavity and other maxillar structures. For this purpose, a ventrodorsal open-mouth projection is required. The bony structures of the middle ears and the tympanic bullae are well visualized. For comparison of the two sides, exact symmetrical positioning is essential.

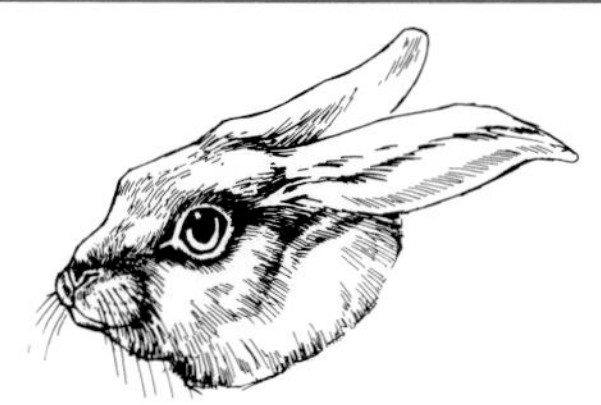

30

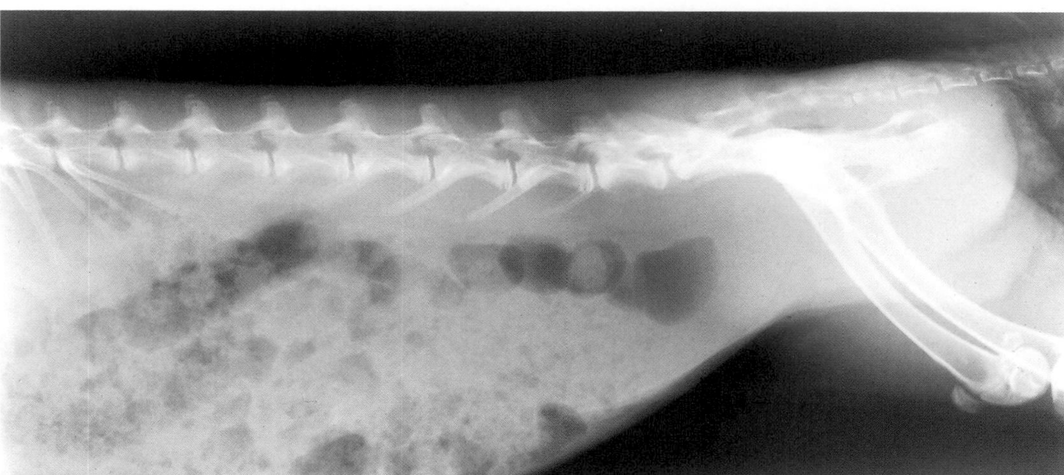

31

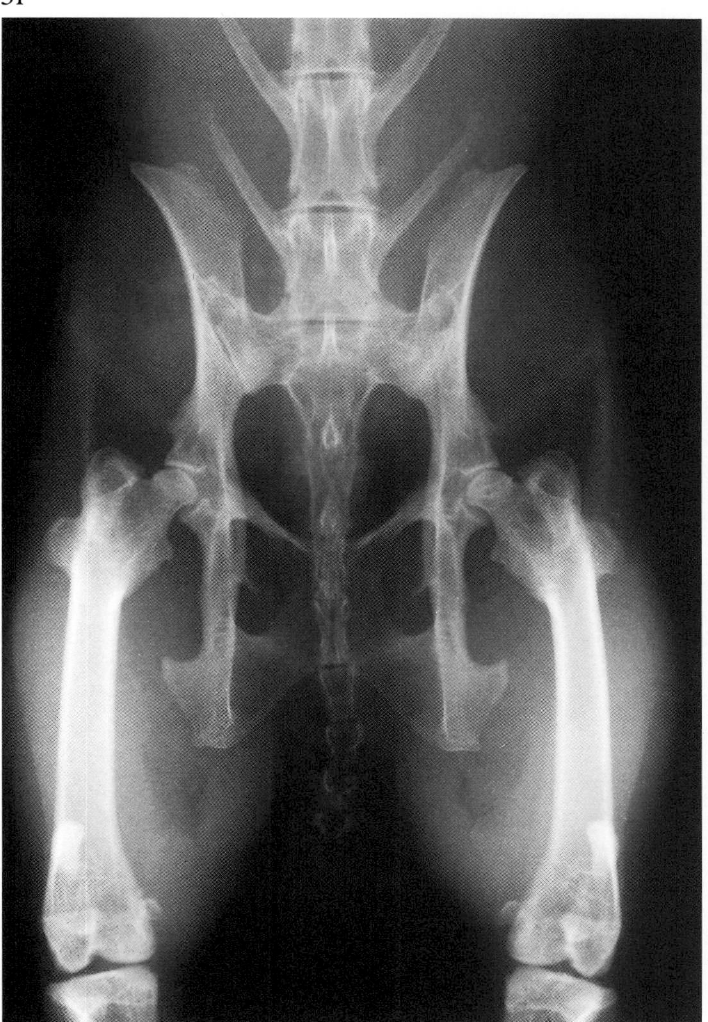

30 Lumbar Spine: Normal Radiographic Appearance, lateral.

Rabbit *(Oryctolagus cuniculus)*, male, 4 months.

The rabbit has 7 cervical, 12 or 13 thoracic and 7 lumbar vertebrae. The first 7 pairs of ribs are fused with the sternum, the 8th and 9th pairs are attached to the 7th pair. The last ribs end free in the muscles of the abdominal wall. In young animals, the cranial and caudal growth plates of the vertebral bodies can be seen.

31 Pelvis and Femora: Normal Radiographic Appearance, ventrodorsal.

Rabbit *(Oryctolagus cuniculus)*, female, 4 years.

For this radiograph, the animal is positioned in dorsal recumbency, without too much tilting of the pelvis. Special attention is given to a symmetrical projection by pulling both legs backwards in parallel position.

The hip joints are relatively small and the foramina obturatoria are very large. Notice the prominent muscles of the thighs.

32

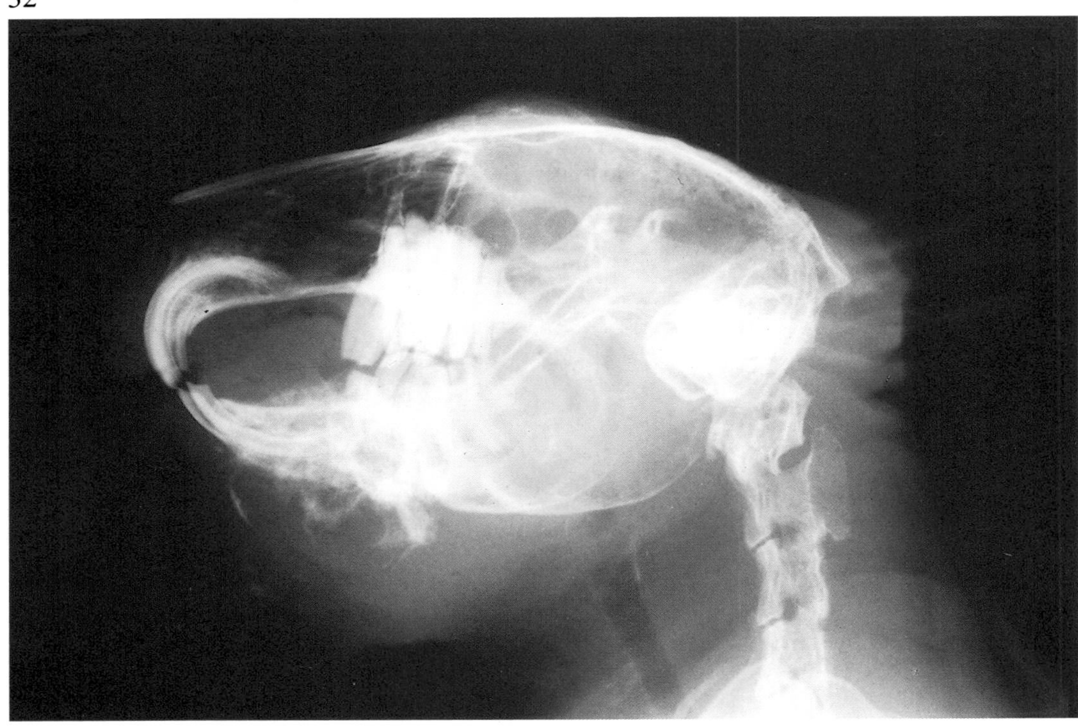

33

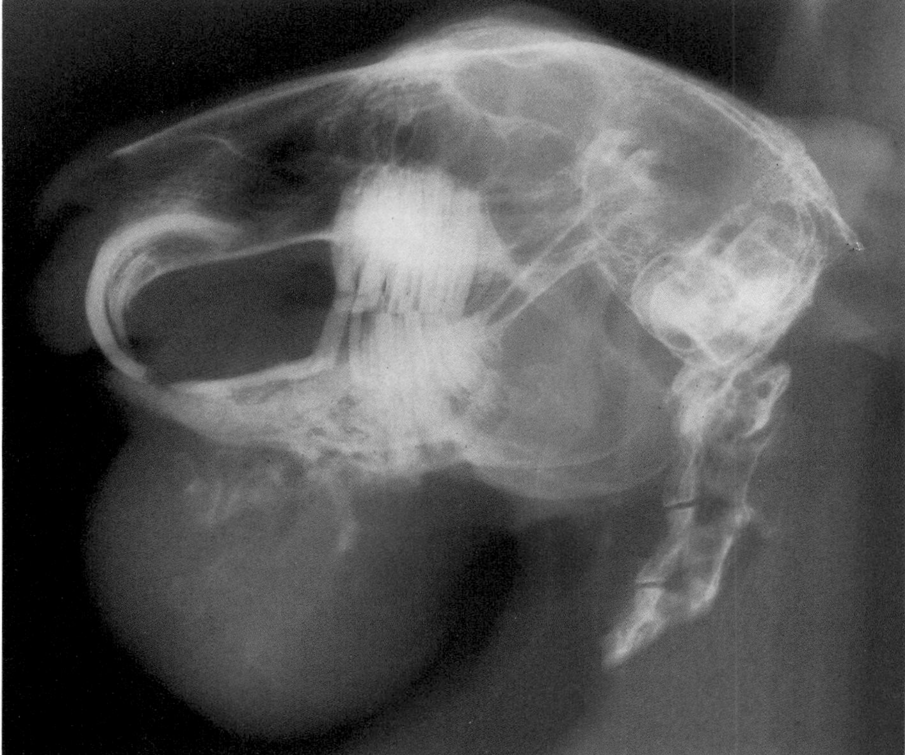

32/33 Mandibular Abscesses.

Rabbit *(Oryctolagus cuniculus)*, male, adult.

Mandibular abscesses are characterized by extensive soft tissue swelling under the mandibular rami, often containing extensive calcifications. Depending upon the duration of the lesion, the ventral borders of the rami mandibulares appear abnormal due to a combination of bony lysis and new bone formation that extends into the surrounding soft tissue. The roots of the mandibular molars are irregularly outlined due to chronic (peri)alveolitis. Sometimes gas pockets are visible in large abscesses.

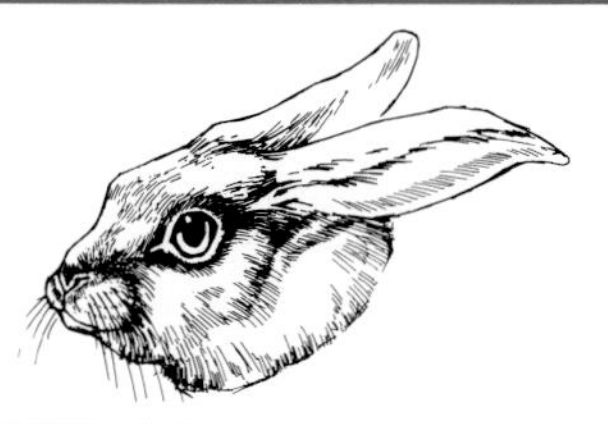

34

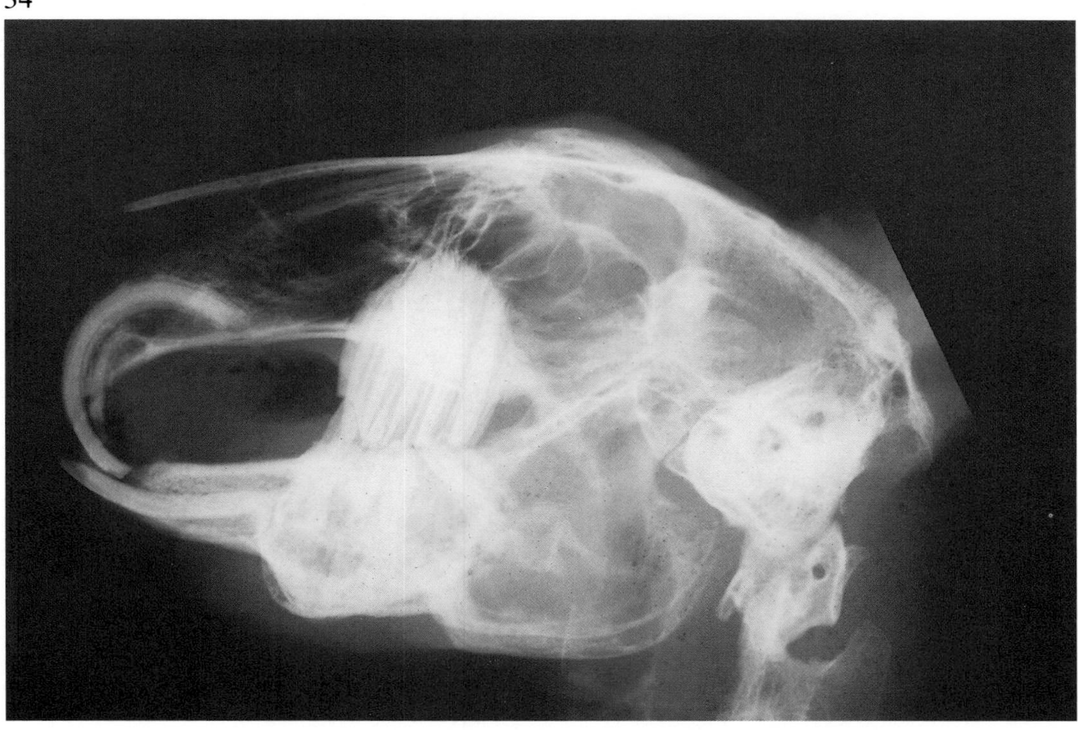

35

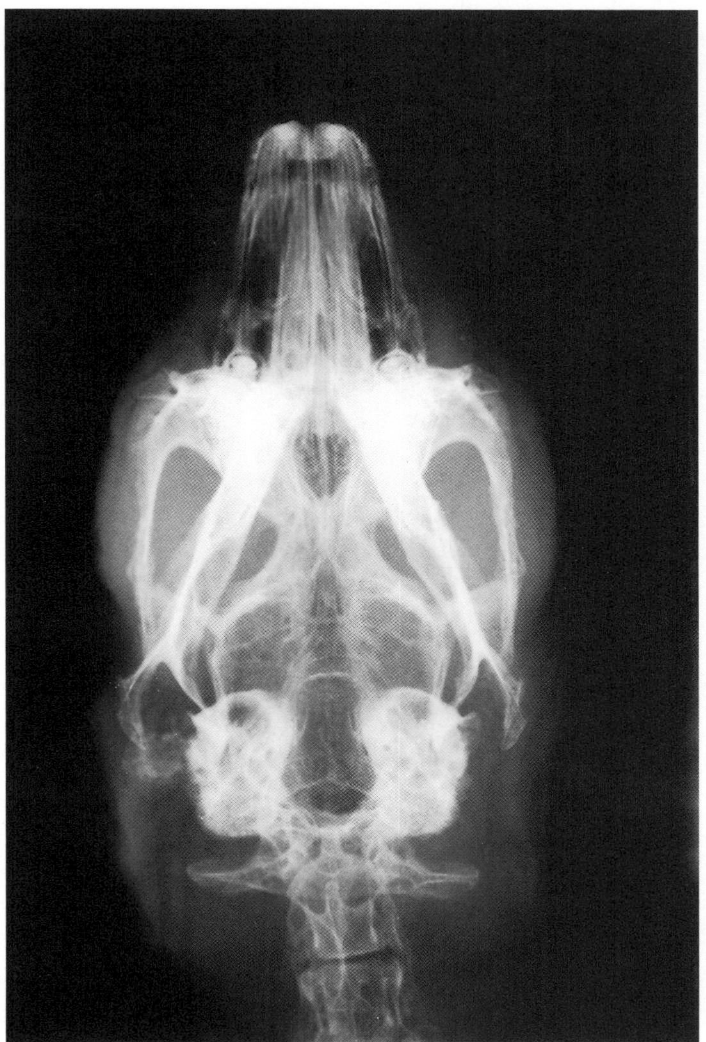

34 Malocclusion of Incisors.

Rabbit *(Oryctolagus cuniculus)*, 6 months.

There is abnormal alignment of the incisors, with an overgrowth in length of the incisors of the upper jaw. This is prognathia superior.

Note: There are also abnormalities of the roots of the mandibular molars visible.

35 Otitis Media.

Rabbit *(Oryctolagus cuniculus)*, male, 2 years.

The density of both tympanic bullae, especially the left one, is increased. The right external ear canal is calcified.

These radiographic findings are indicative of chronic bilateral otitis media.

36

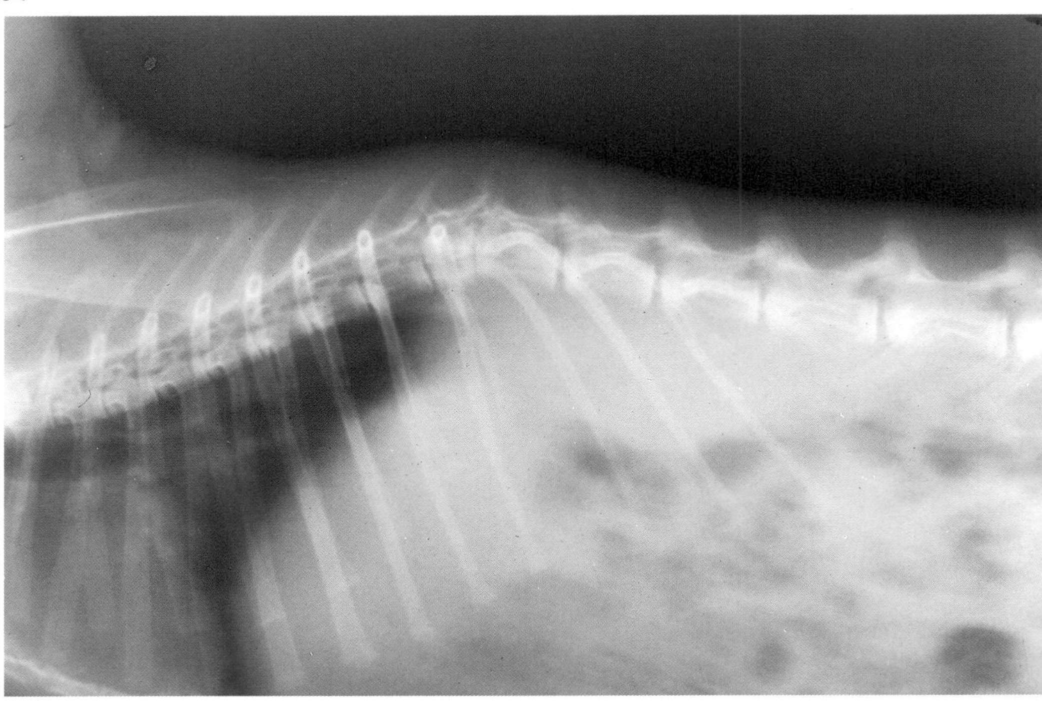

37

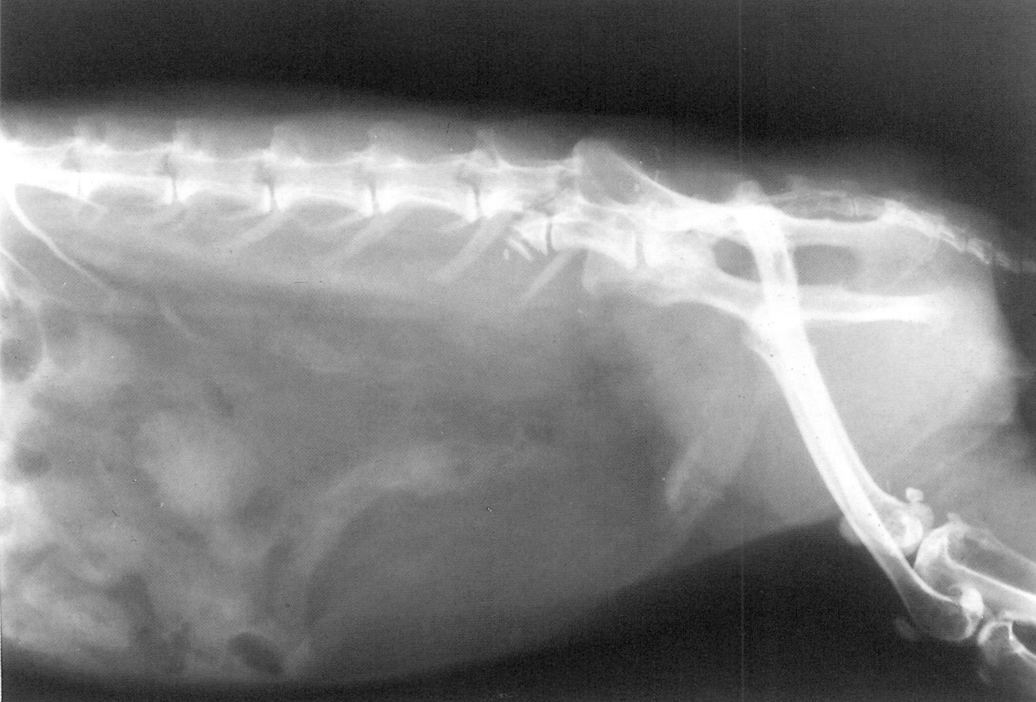

36 Spinal Infraction Fracture.

Rabbit *(Oryctolagus cuniculus)*, 4 months.

Size and shape of the 10th thoracic vertebra are abnormal due to an infraction (compression) fracture. There is also a marked spinal kyphosis, however, the alignment has been maintained.

37 Comminuted Vertebral Fracture.

Rabbit *(Oryctolagus cuniculus)*, adult.

Due to a comminuted fracture of the vertebral body of L_6 there is complete loss of normal alignment of the vertebral column at the fracture site and ventral dislocation of the caudal segment. As an accidental finding, calcified material in the urinary bladder is noted.

Note: Evaluation for pelvic trauma requires a ventrodorsal radiograph.

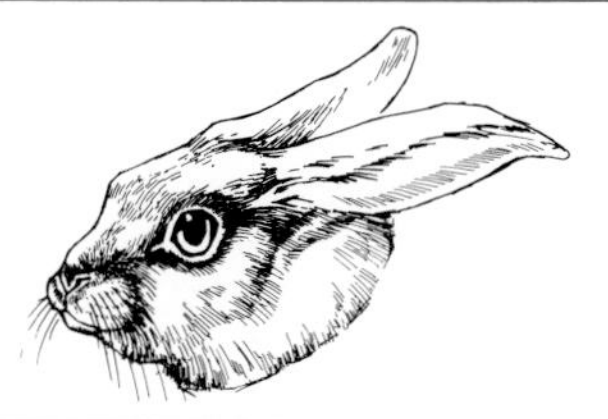

38

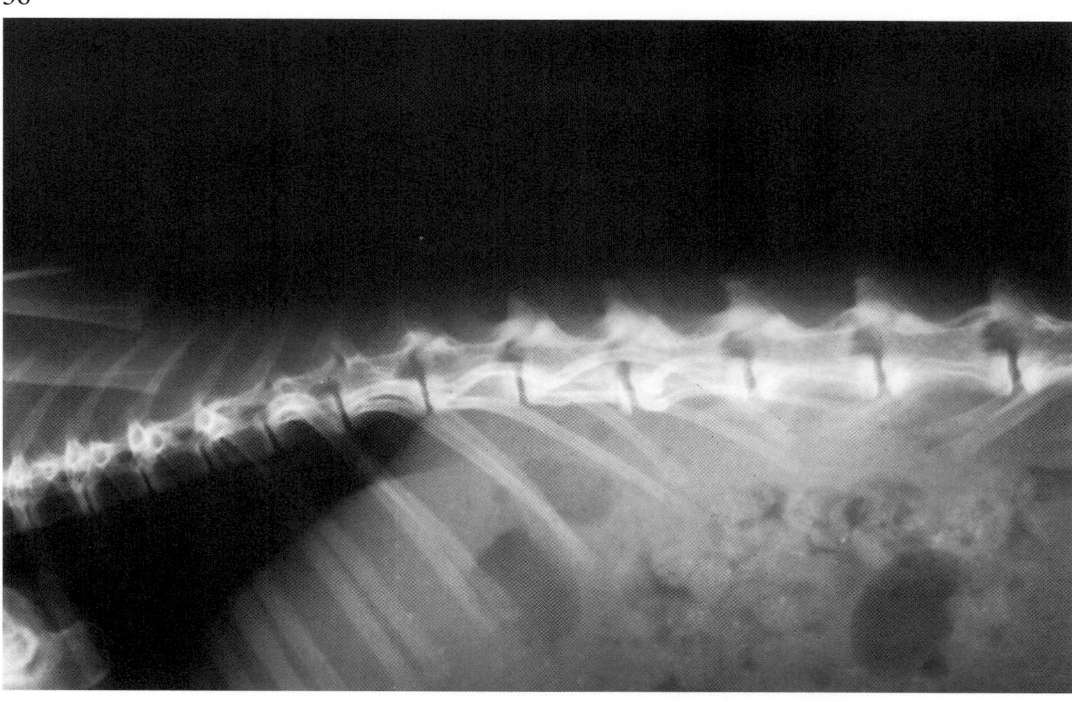

39

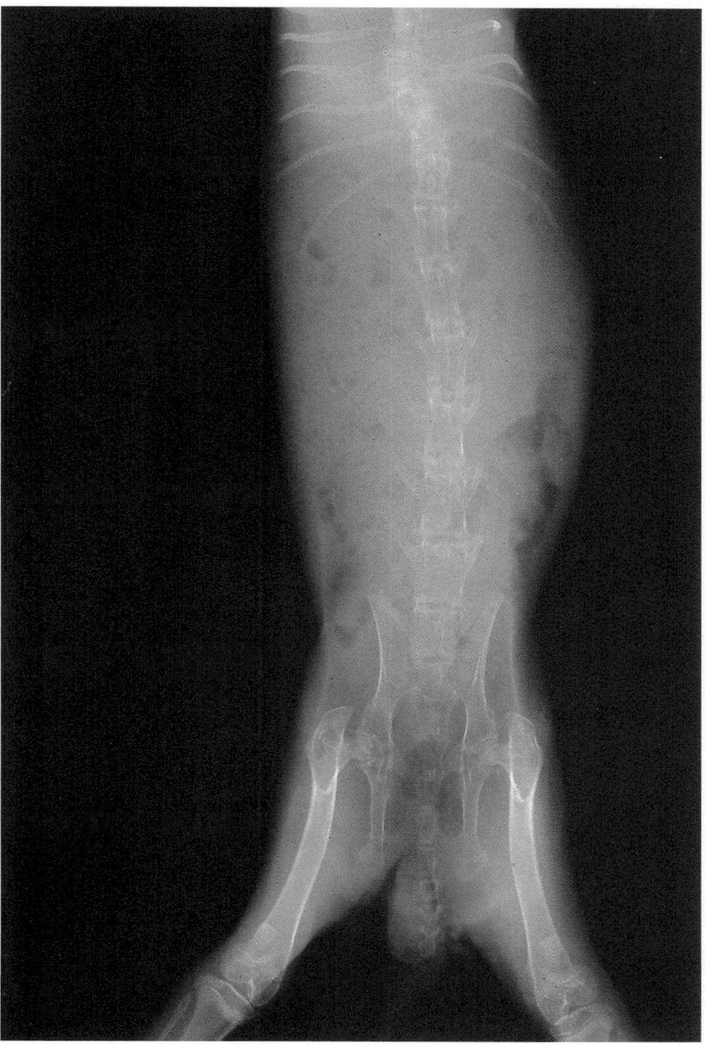

38 Vertebral Growth Plate Fracture.

Rabbit *(Oryctolagus cuniculus)*, 10 months.

The caudal epiphysis of the 12th thoracic vertebral body has slipped ventrally due to a traumatic growth plate fracture.

39 Secondary Nutritional Hyperparathyroidism.

Rabbit *(Oryctolagus cuniculus)*, juvenile, 4 months.

Generalized demineralization of the skeleton is characterized by lack of radiopacity and loss of cortical thickness of the skeletal structures. Both femurs are bowed. The vertebrae are aligned abnormally in the thoracolumbar region due to deformation of several segments.

40

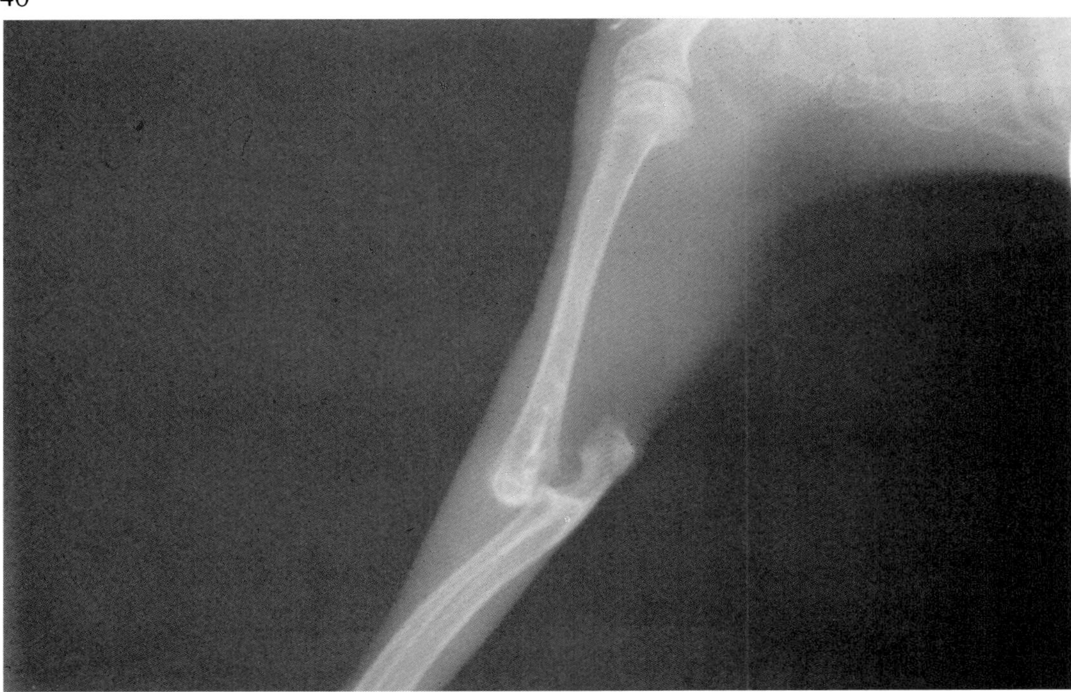

41

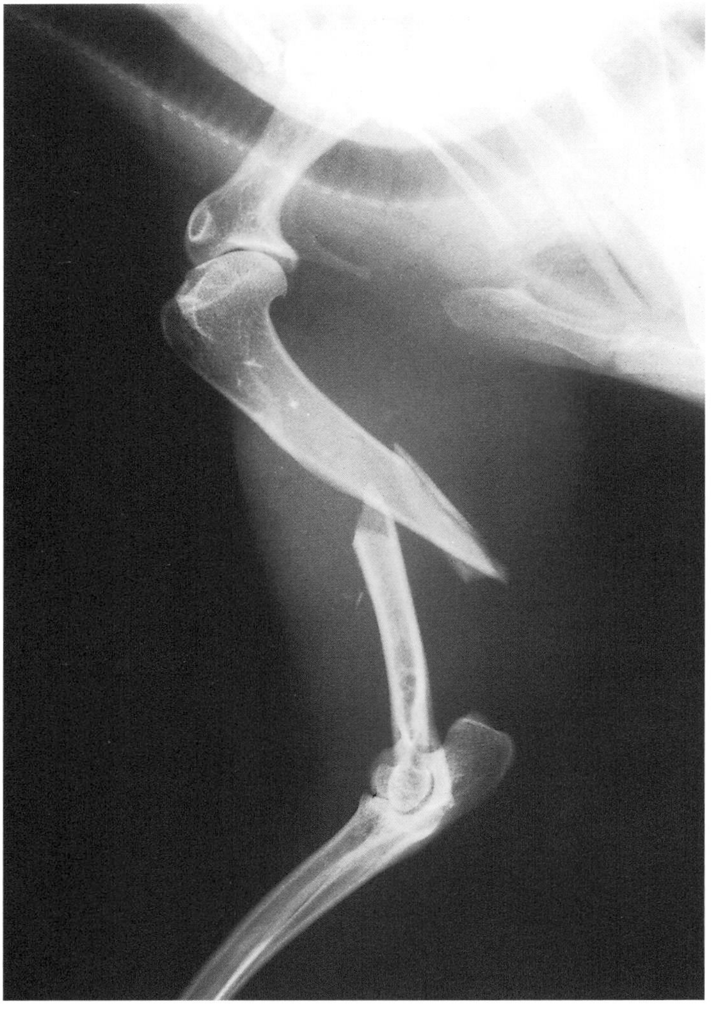

40 Elbow Luxation.

Rabbit *(Oryctolagus cuniculus)*, 4 months.

There is complete luxation of the elbow joint, with palmar and proximal displacement of the radius and ulna. There are no indications of (chip) fractures or other abnormalities.

Note: A dorsopalmar (ap) radiograph of the elbow should always be included in order not to miss any (chip)fractures.

41 Fracture of Humerus.

Rabbit *(Oryctolagus cuniculus)*, male, 5 years.

Spiral midshaft fracture of the humerus with a large butterfly fragment, dislocation and overriding of the fragments is present.

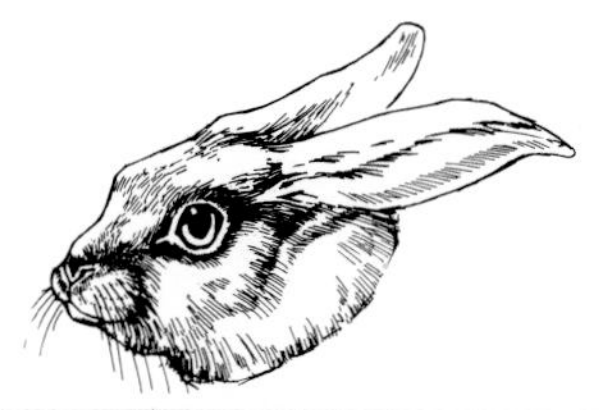

42

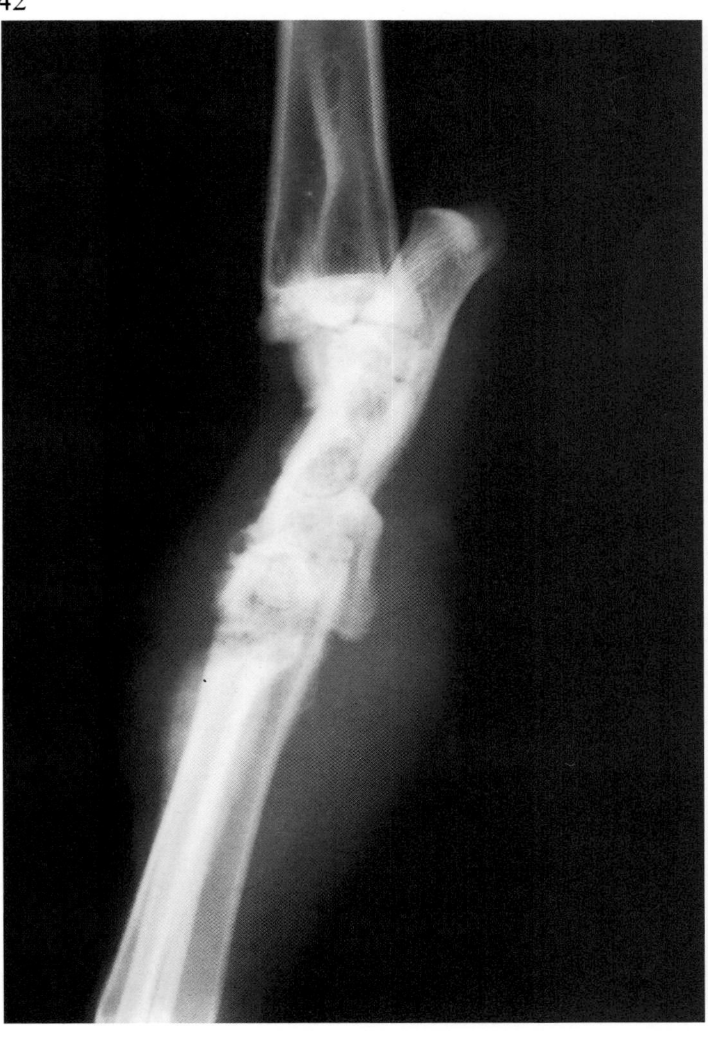

43

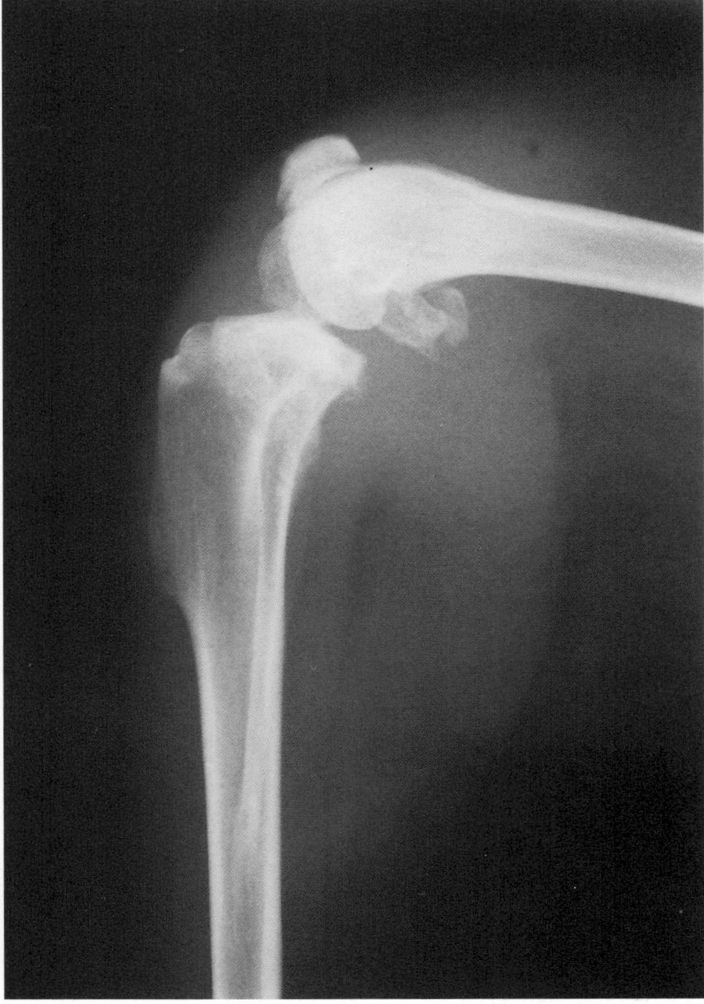

42 Septic Tarsitis.

Rabbit *(Oryctolagus cuniculus)*, adult.

Considerable soft tissue swelling is present around the tarso-metatarsal joint. In the tarso-metatarsal joint, radiographic signs of bone destruction and sequestration (small white linear bone fragments) are indicative of septic arthritis. The brushed appearance of the periosteal new bone formation at the tarsal and metatarsal bones suggests the acute stage of the infection.

43 Chronic Deformative Arthrosis.

Rabbit *(Oryctolagus cuniculus)*, female, 2 years.

Extensive periarticular soft tissue swelling and consolidated new bone formation at the patella, femoral condyles, fabellae and proximal tibia are radiographic signs of chronic arthrosis of the stifle joint (secondary joint disease of the stifle).

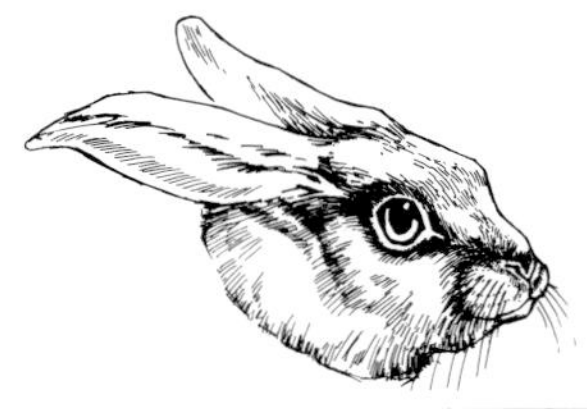

44

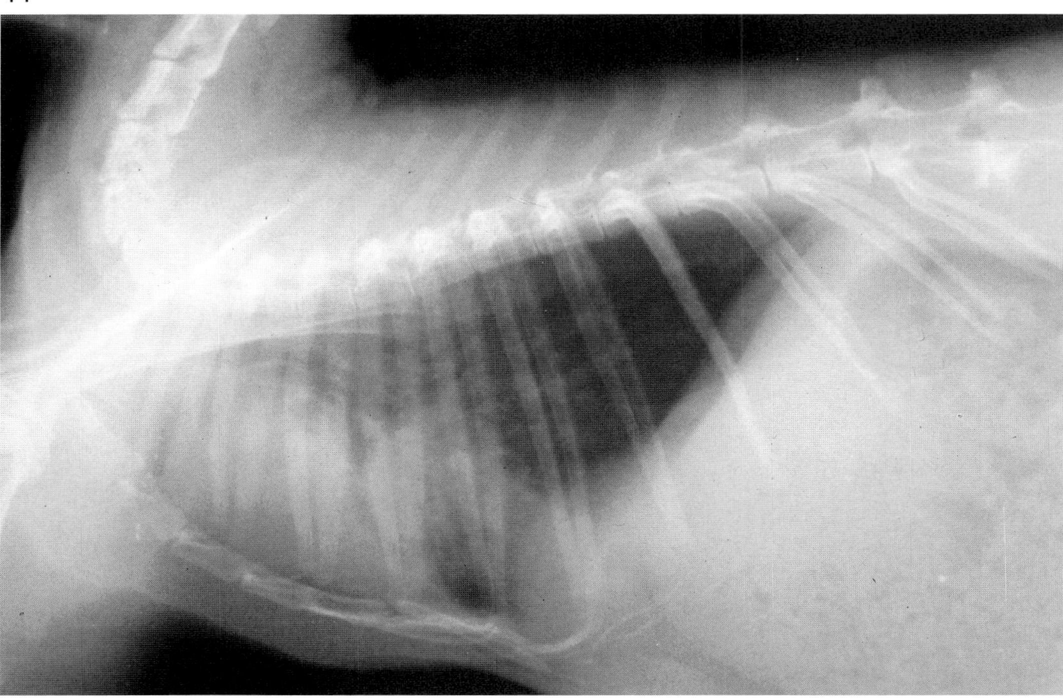

45

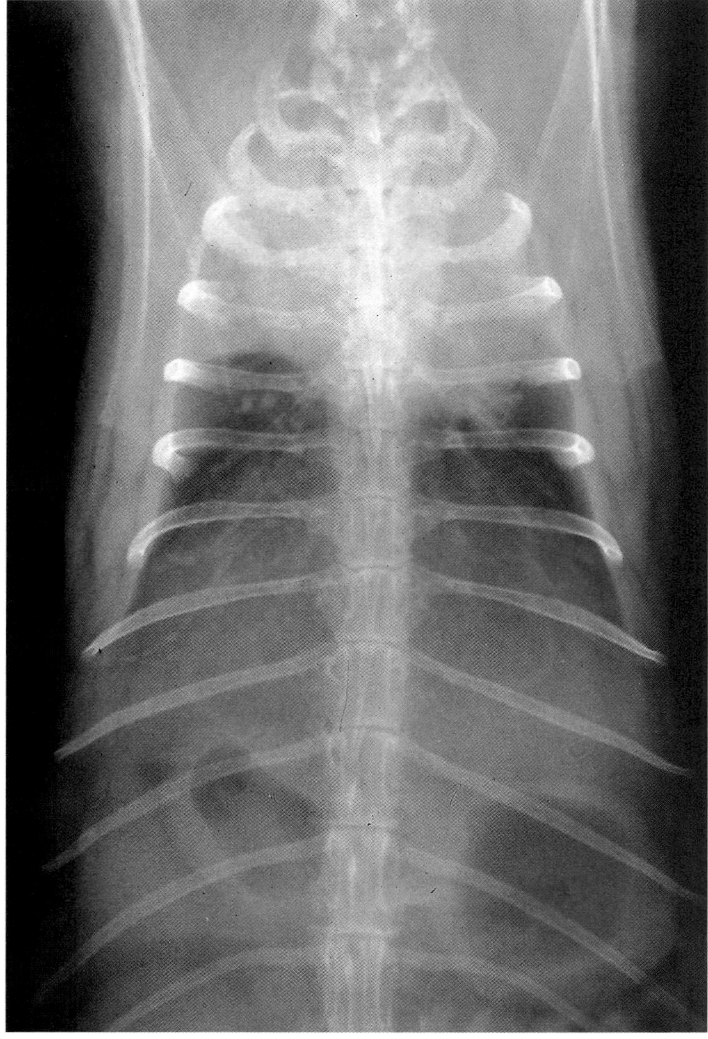

44/45 Pneumonia.

Rabbit *(Oryctolagus cuniculus)*, 5 years.

Both cranial lung lobes are consolidated, with tiny air-bronchograms extending into the consolidated pulmonary parenchyma. The cardiac shadow is partly obscured by the increased pulmonary densities.

The caudal lung lobes are well aerated dorsally, but contain alveolar changes in the ventral areas (lateral radiograph).

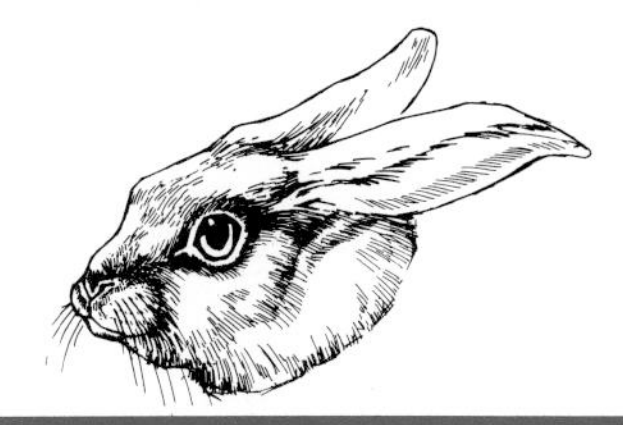

46

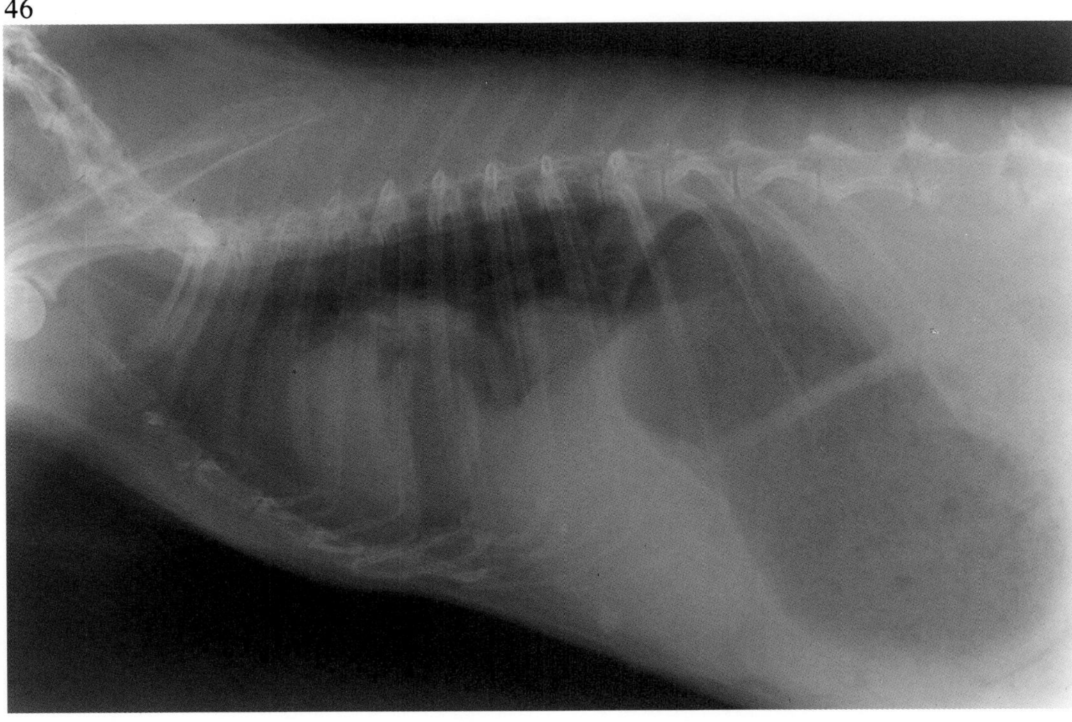

47

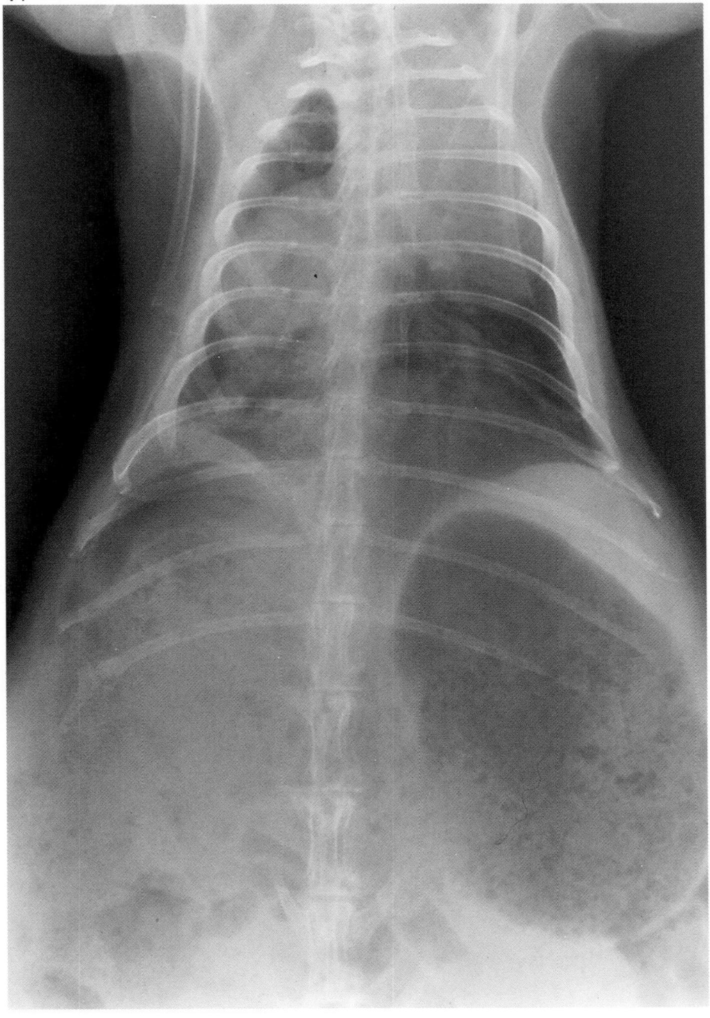

46/47 Pulmonary Abscess.

Rabbit *(Oryctolagus cuniculus)*, female, 3 years.

On the lateral film, a well-defined soft tissue mass is visible that is located ventral to the caudal vena cava between the diaphragm and the fifth pair of ribs, partly superimposing the heart. On the dorsoventral radiograph, the mass is located in the right hemithorax pushing the heart cranially and towards the left. The right caudal lung lobe also contains alveolar densities. The left lung lobes are normal. Postmortem examination revealed a large pulmonary abscess with surrounding pneumonic infiltration of the right caudal lung lobe.

48

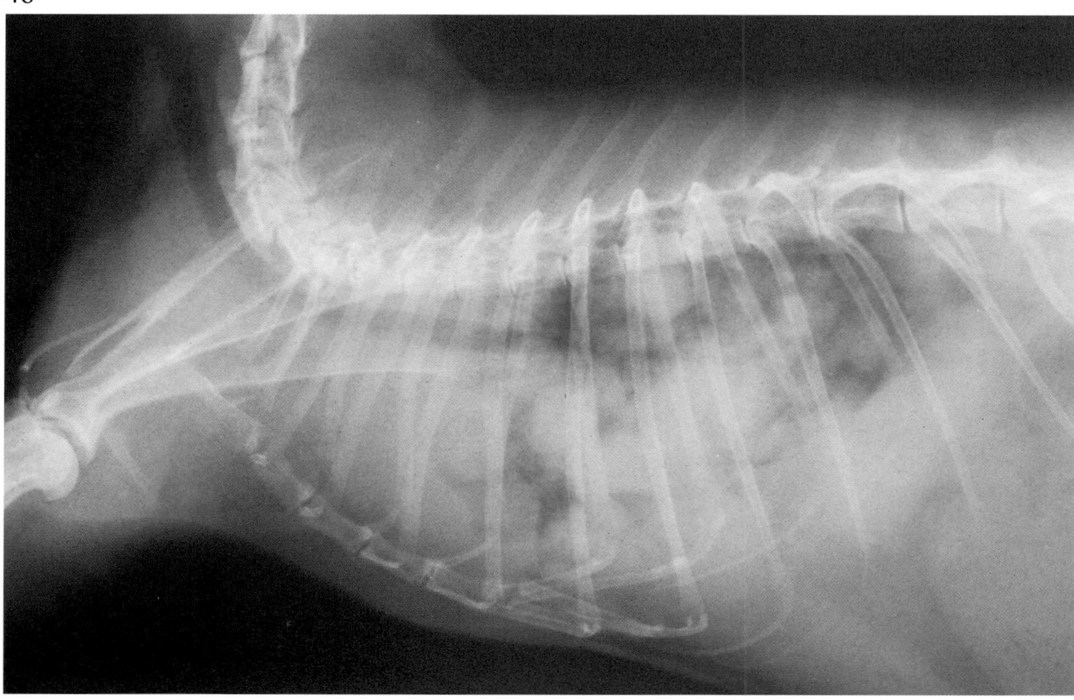

49

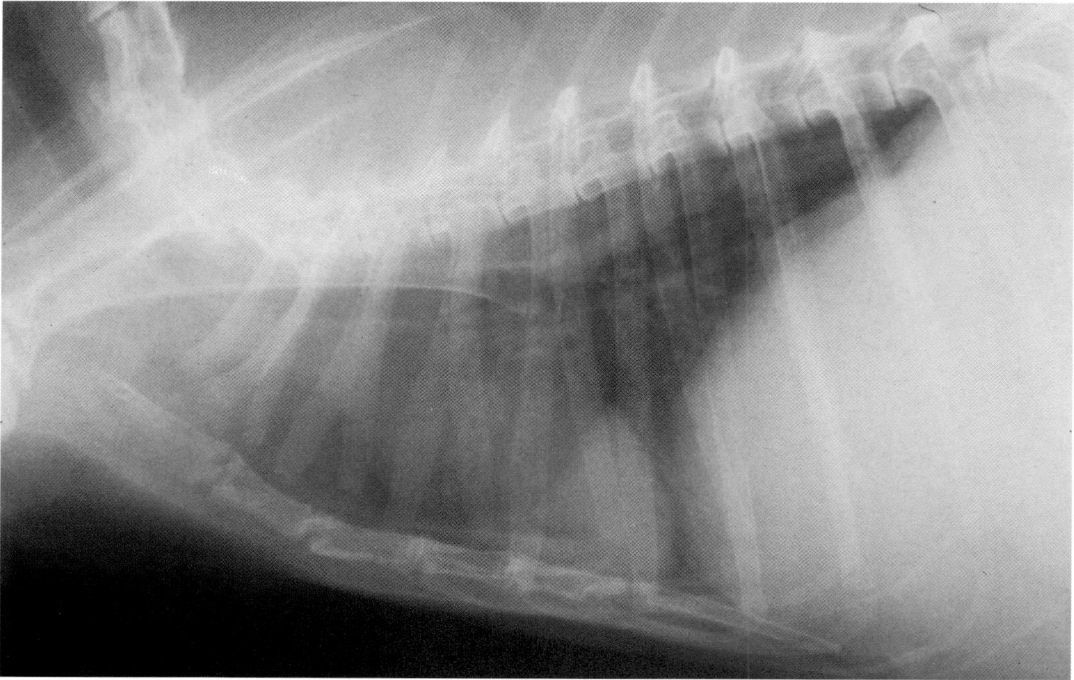

48 Metastatic Pulmonary Neoplasia.

Rabbit *(Oryctolagus cuniculus)*, adult.

In all lung lobes multiple, nodular densities are present. Some of these nodules are well-defined, others are less well-defined and tend to merge with neighbouring densities.

The cardiac and diaphragmatic outlines are blurred due to superimposition by the densities.

49 Intrathoracic Fat Deposits.

Rabbit *(Oryctolagus cuniculus)*.

In fat adult rabbits there is always a large amount of fat deposited in the thoracic cavity. On this film, the fat deposition can be recognized as a triangular shadow of low density that is superimposed over the cardiac apex. This is a normal finding.

Note: The large-sized fatty liver is also well-defined.

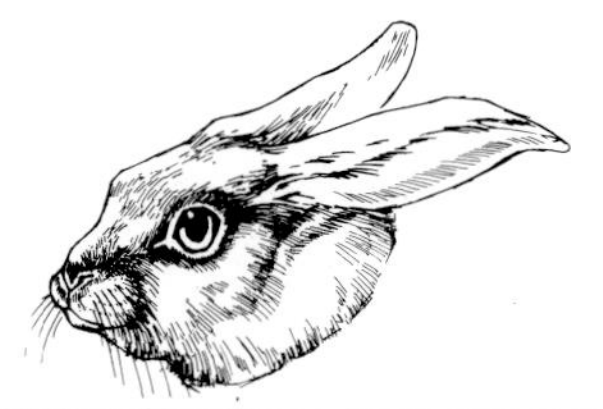

50

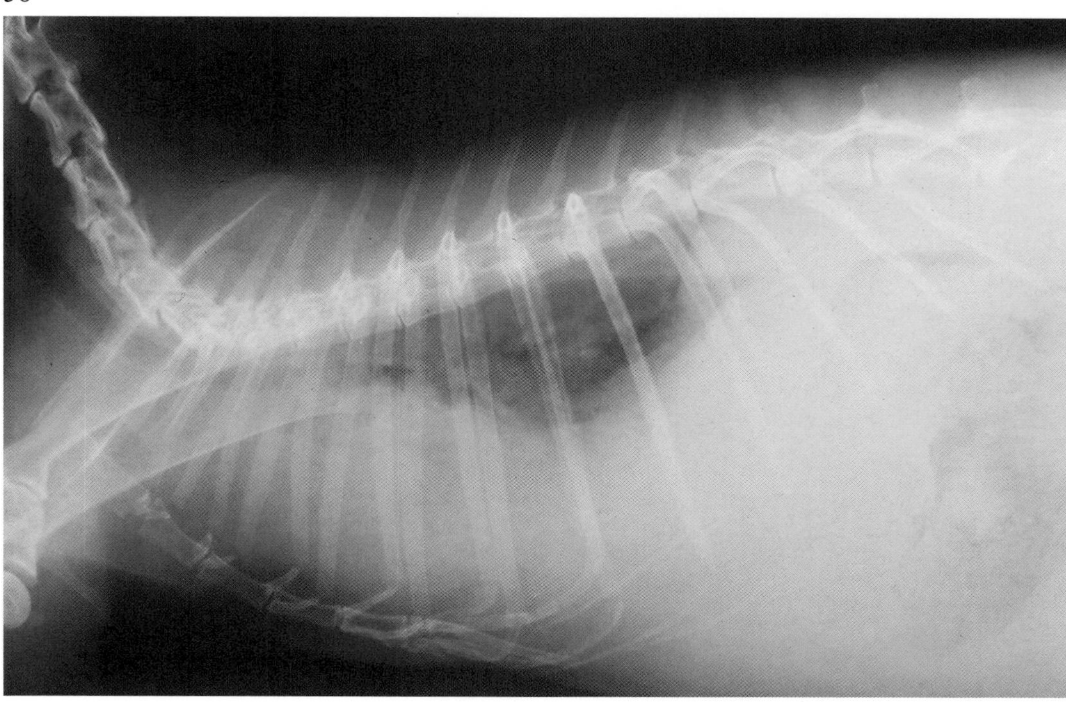

51

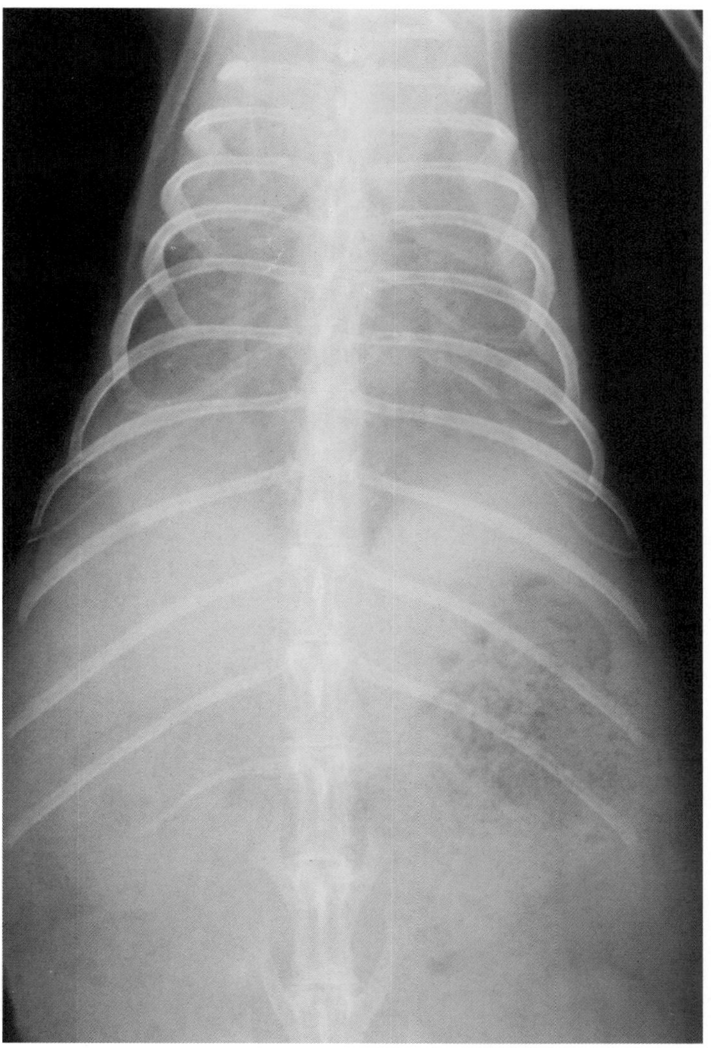

50/51 Hydrothorax (Pleural Effusion).

Rabbit *(Oryctolagus cuniculus).*

Characteristic signs of pleural effusion present on these radiographs include:

— increased hazy density of lung fields, especially in the ventral portions of the thoracic cavity obscuring the cardiac apex and ventral part of the diaphragmatic outline (lateral radiograph),

— presence of a widened, fluid-filled pleural space between the lungs and chest wall (dorsoventral radiograph),

— blunting of the costodiaphragmatic angles (both projections),

— loss of the well-defined borders of the cardiac silhouette (dorsoventral radiograph).

52

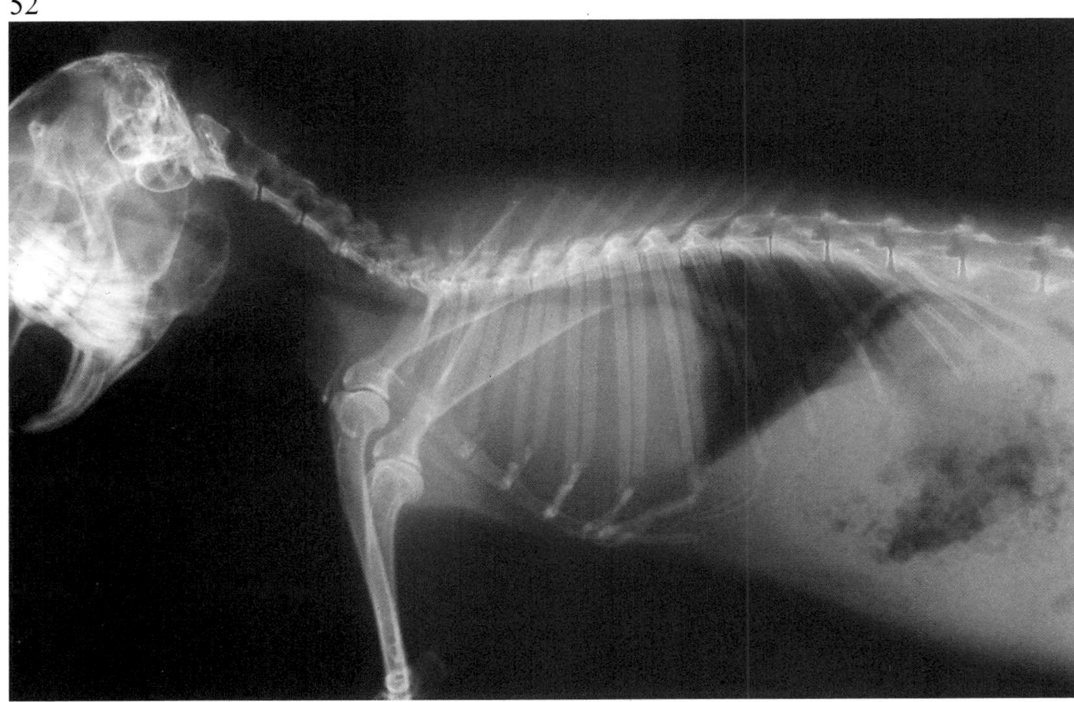

53

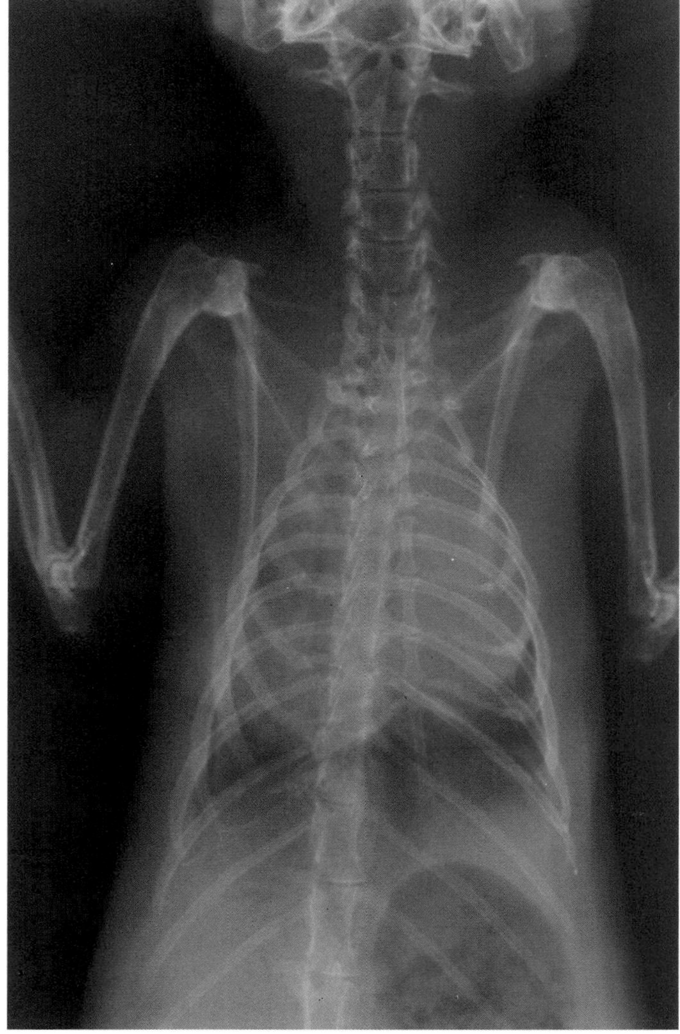

52/53 Mediastinal Mass.

Rabbit *(Oryctolagus cuniculus)*, 5 years.

The cranial half of the thoracic cavity is occupied by a soft tissue mass that presents a positive silhouette sign with the heart. The latter indicates that the mass lies in close contact with the heart. The trachea is elevated. The cranial lung lobes are not inflated, probably due to compression atelectasis. The caudal lung lobes are well inflated. The mediastinal mass proved to be a thymic lymphosarcoma.

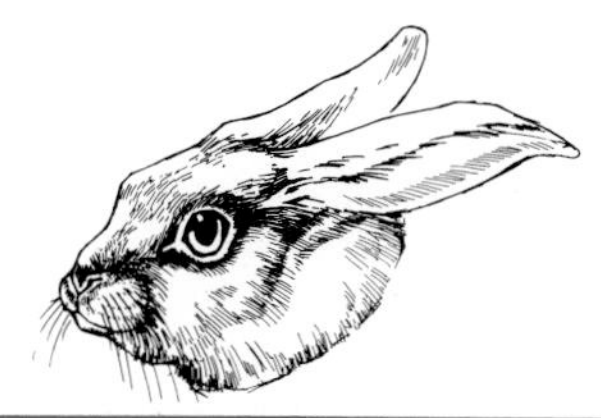

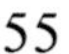

54

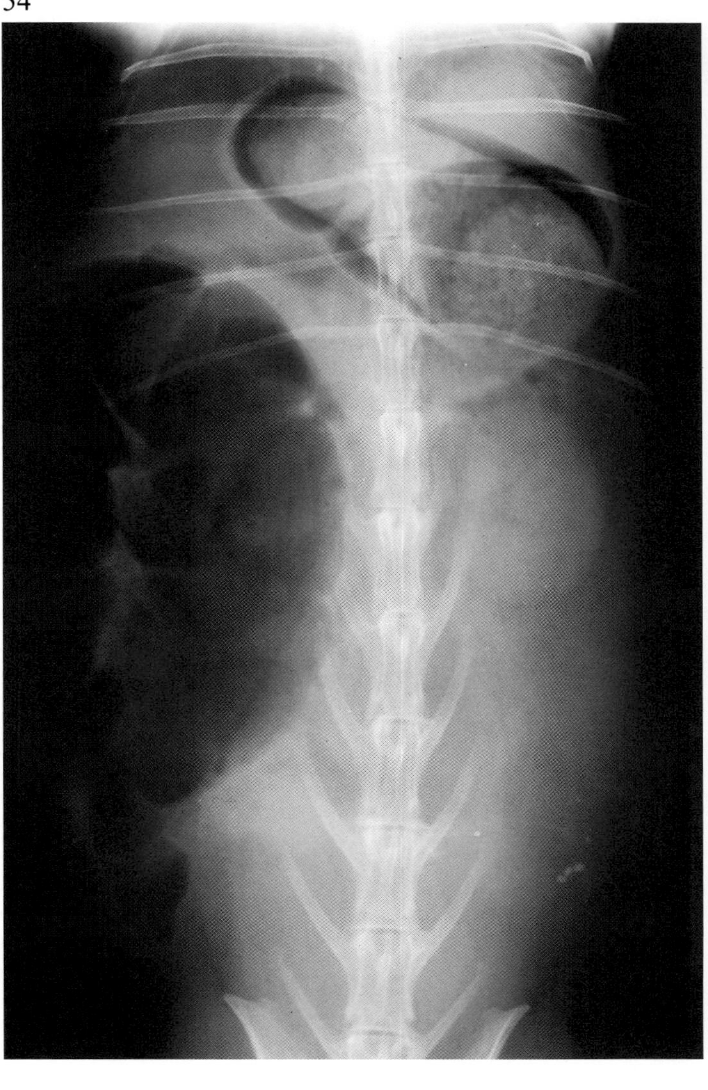

55

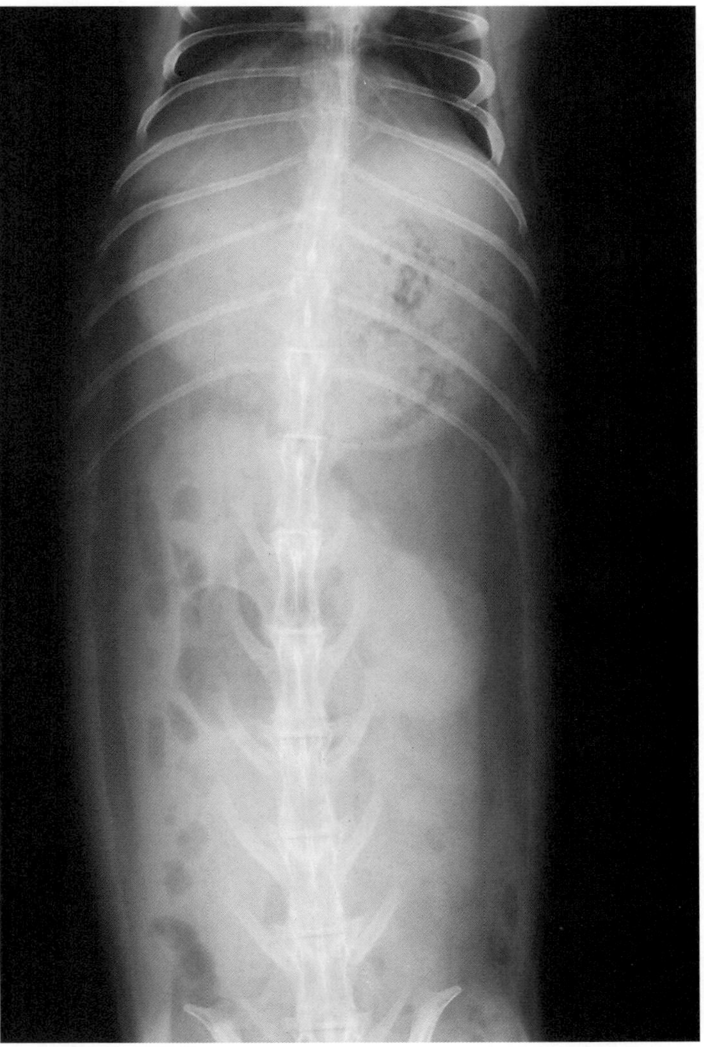

54 Gastric Hairball (Trichobezoar).

Rabbit *(Oryctolagus cuniculus)*, male, 2 years.

The stomach of this animal contains a well-delineated homogeneous mass in the gastric antrum that is outlined by air. This mass represents a gastric hairball or trichobezoar.

The granular material in the gastric fundus is food. The right side of the peritoneal cavity is occupied by the gas-distended cecum.

55 Gastric Hairball (Trichobezoar).

Rabbit *(Oryctolagus cuniculus)*, male, 2 years.

When the stomach is filled with food the presence of a hairball is easily concealed by the superimposed granular density of the ingested food. However, fasting of the animal will permit radiographic confirmation of a solid hairball (see FIG. **54**).

56

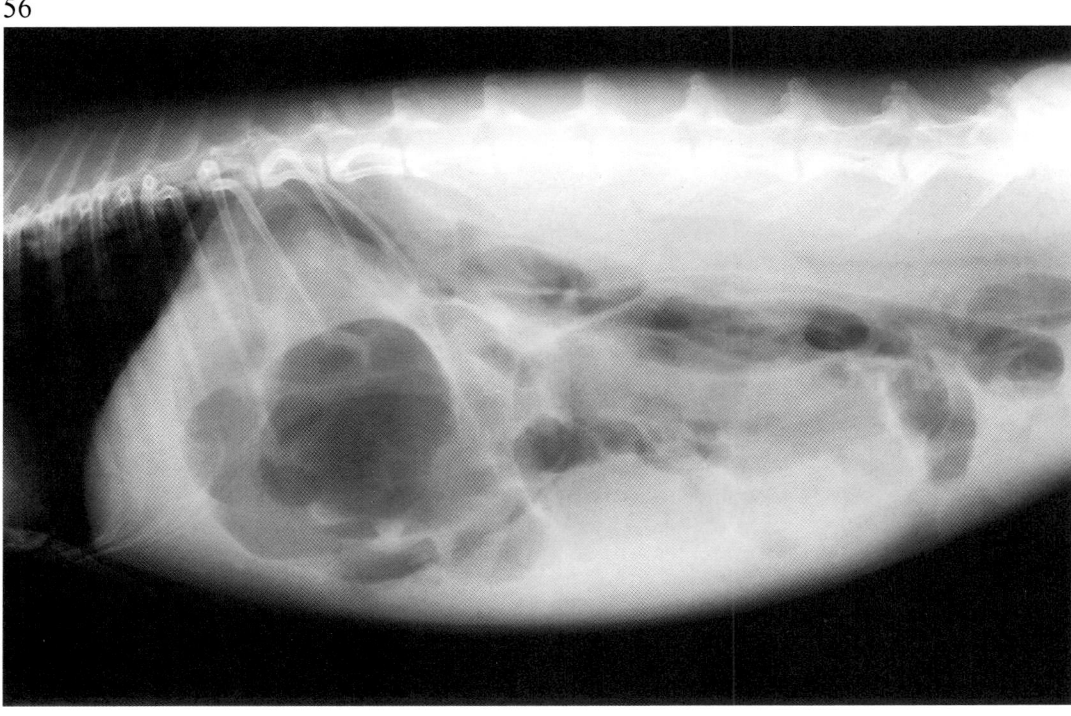

57

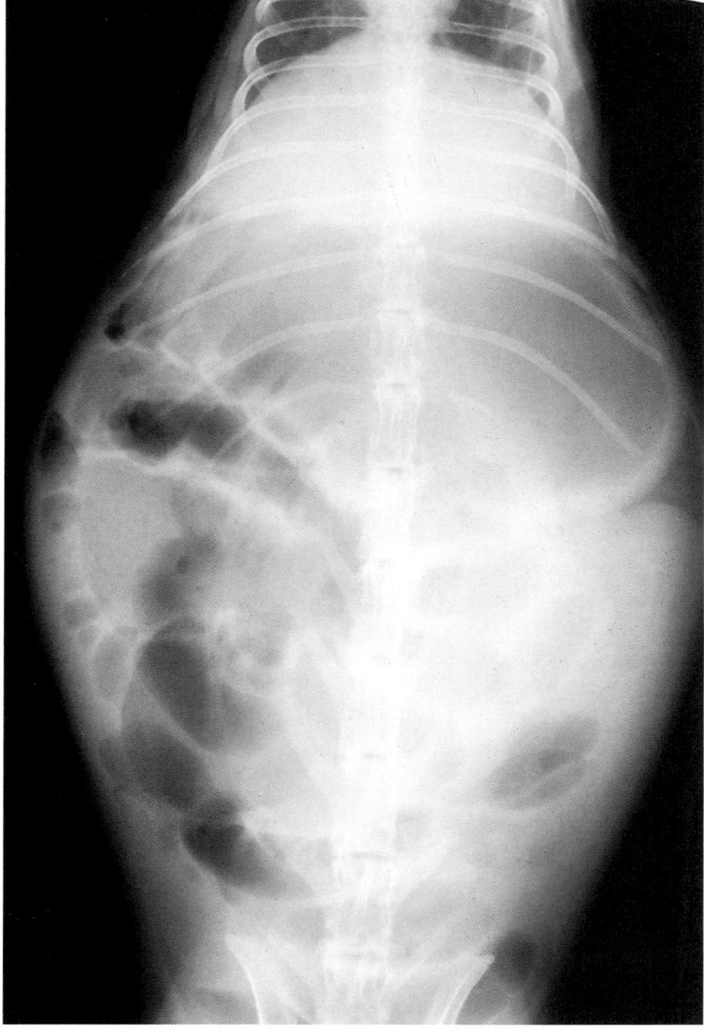

56/57 Mucoid Enteritis.

Rabbit *(Oryctolagus cuniculus)*, 1 year.

The radiographic presentation of this disease is dominated by the presence of large amounts of gas and fluid contents in the gastrointestinal tract.

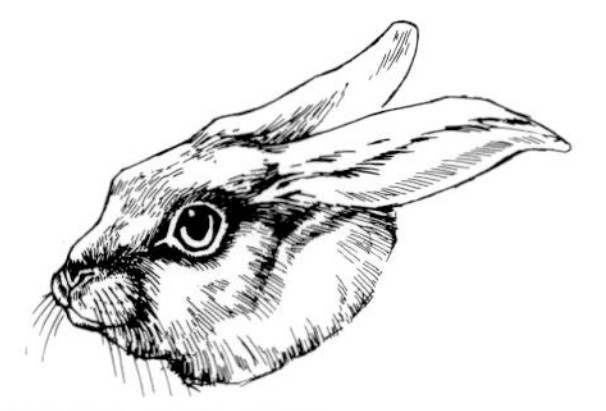

58

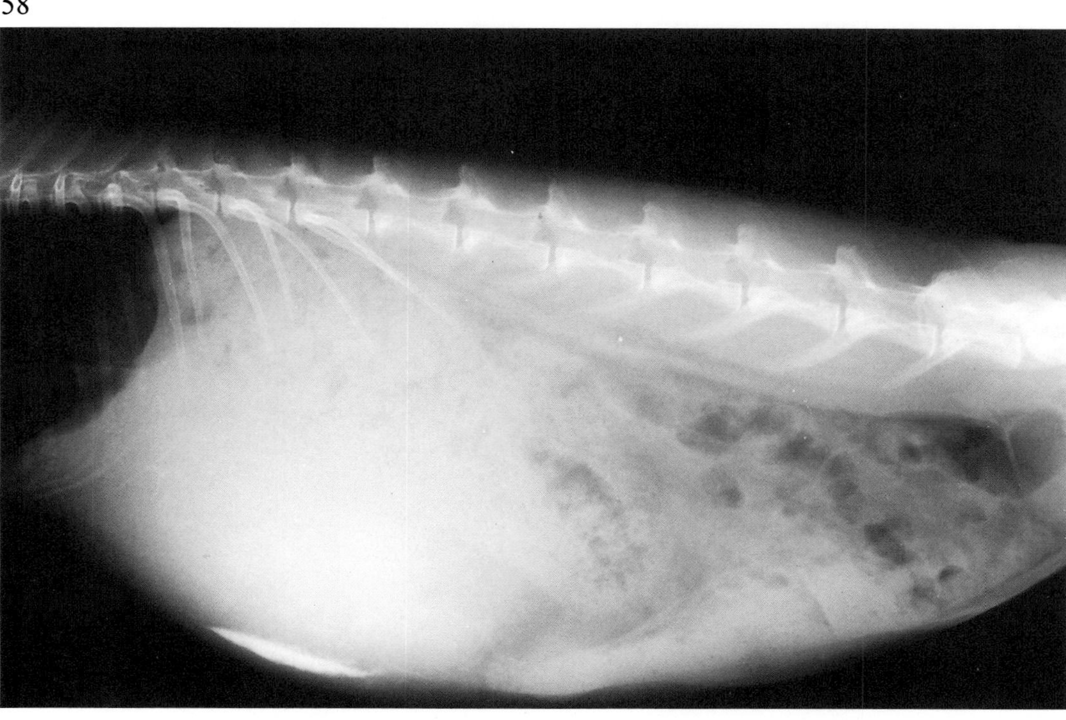

59

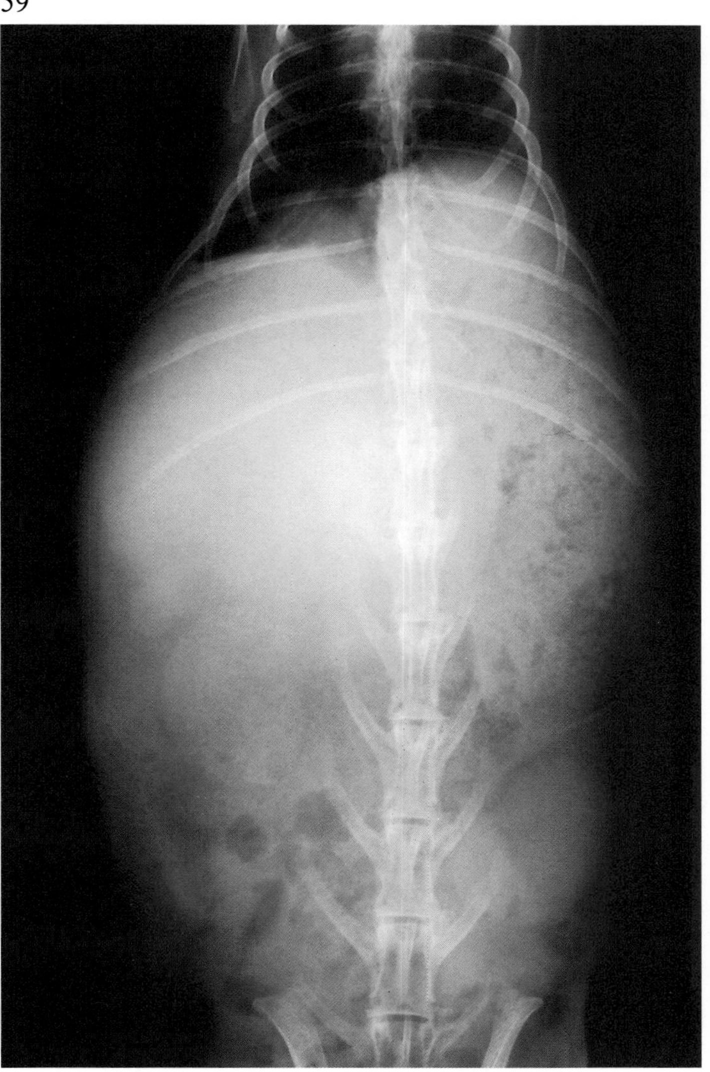

58/59 Liver Abscess.

Rabbit *(Oryctolagus cuniculus)*, adult.

A large, well-defined soft tissue mass is present in the right cranial section of the abdomen and extends from the diaphragm halfway into the abdominal cavity. The mass displaces the stomach dorsally and to the left, while both kidneys are located far caudally.

These findings indicate marked enlargement of the liver. The radiographic texture of the liver mass is homogeneous without patterns of calcification. However, on the lateral film a dense line is present at the bottom of the mass suggesting a radiopaque sediment collection at the bottom of a fluid-filled cavity.

The mass proved to be a large liver abscess containing some calcified, crystalline material.

60

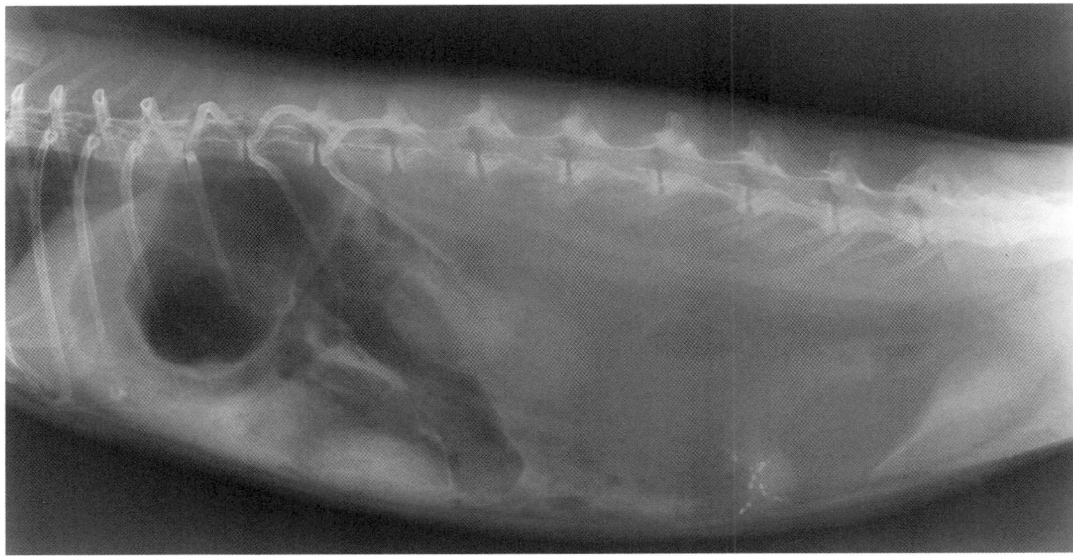

61

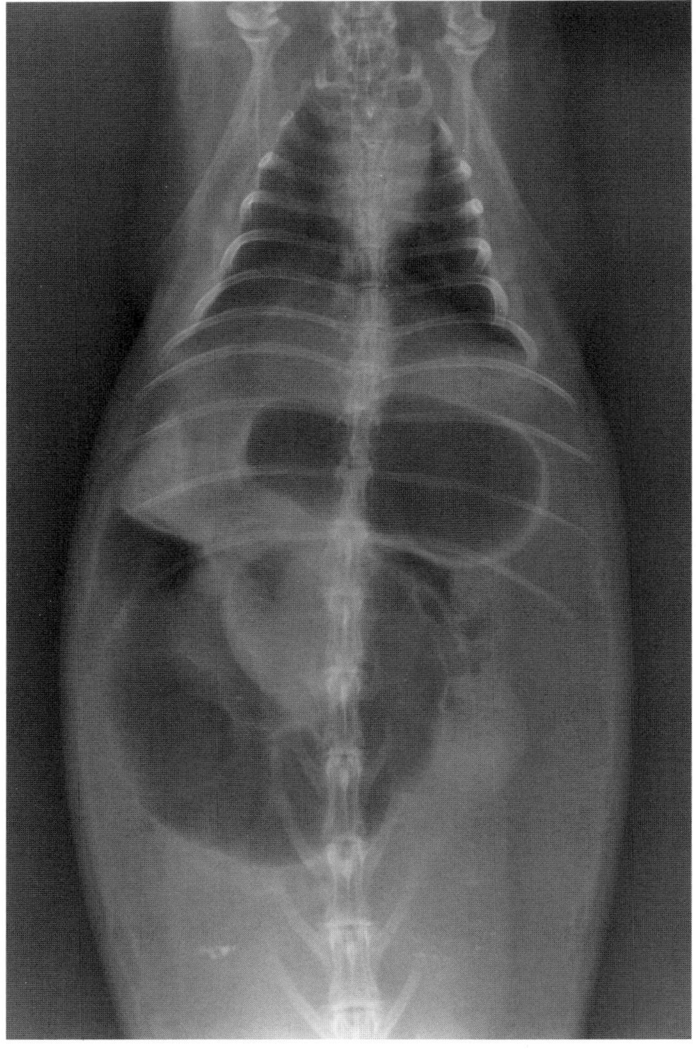

60/61 Calcified Ovaries.

Rabbit *(Oryctolagus cuniculus)*, female, adult.

In the mid-abdominal region, between the bladder and the kidneys, a ventrally curved, looplike soft tissue density is seen surrounded by large amounts of fat deposits. This is the uterus that extends to the ovaries which are located near the ventral abdominal wall. The ovaries can be recognized due to the presence of irregular calcifications.

The urinary bladder is slightly opacified as a result of the high concentration of radiodense urinary crystals.

The ventrodorsal radiograph shows both ovaries located on both sides of L_4-L_5. Both kidneys are also clearly visible due to the large amount of perirenal fat.

The gastrointestinal tract is empty except for a few gaspockets.

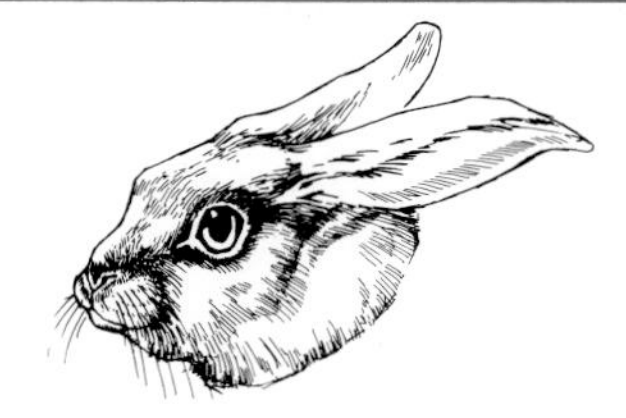

62

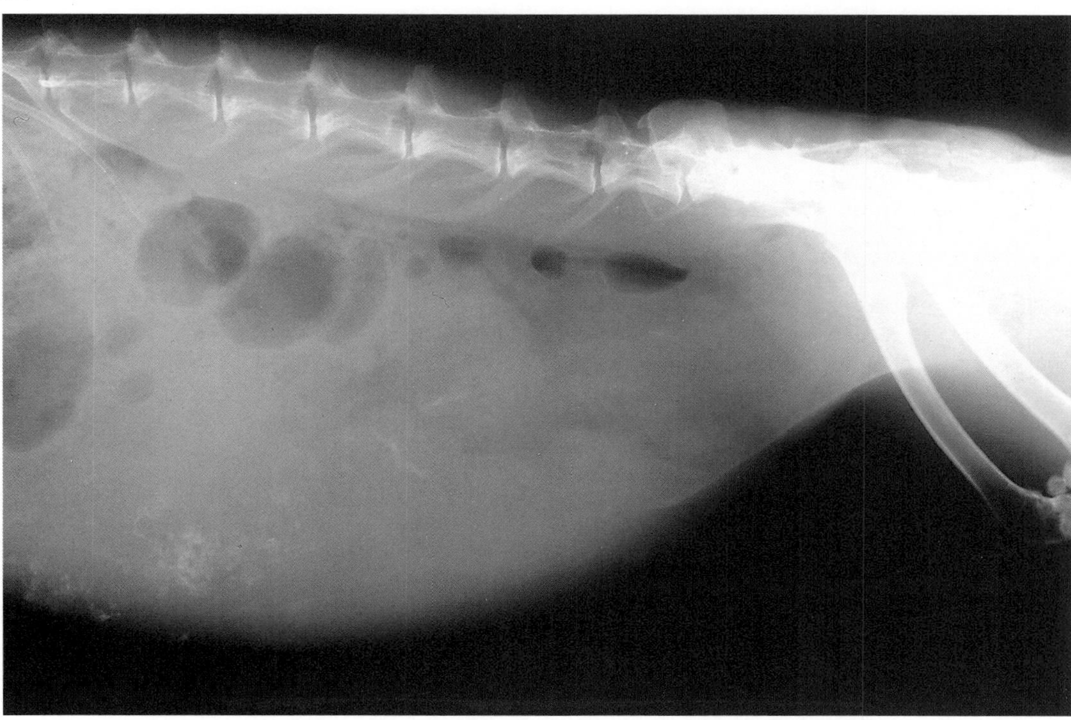

63

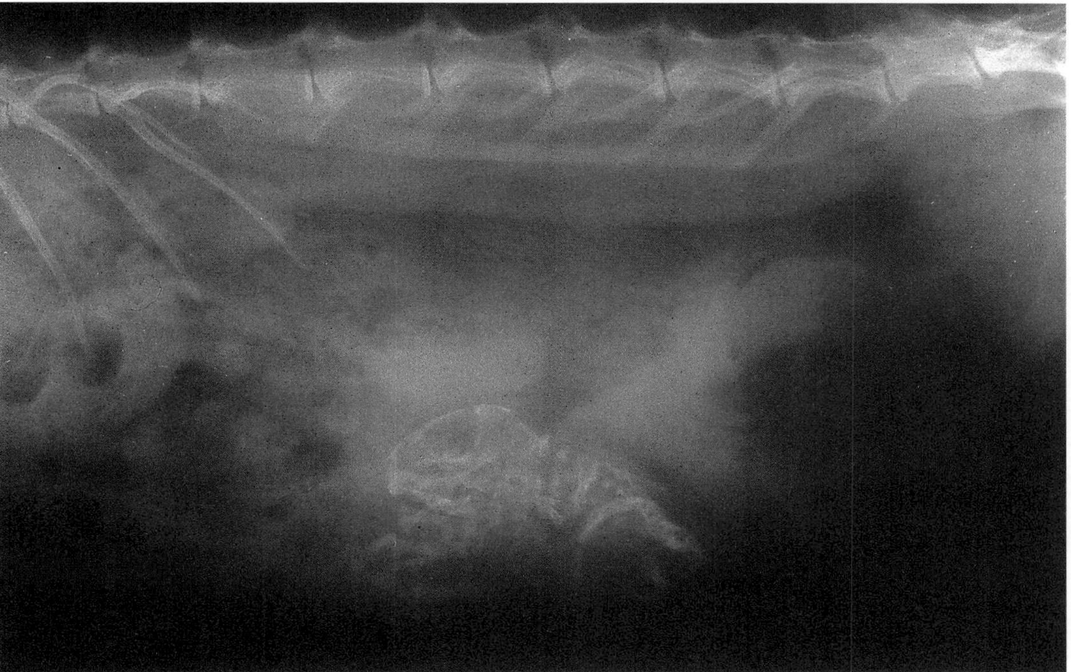

62 Pyometra.

Rabbit *(Oryctolagus cuniculus)*, female, 2 years.

The ventral abdominal cavity contains a large fluid-dense elongated structure with irregular calcifications. The intestines are positioned dorsal and cranial to the density. The structures proved to be a pyometra.

63 Fetal Mummification.

Rabbit *(Oryctolagus cuniculus)*, female, adult.

The irregularly-arranged calcified skeletal structures in the ventral abdomen represent the remnants of a mummified fetus.

64

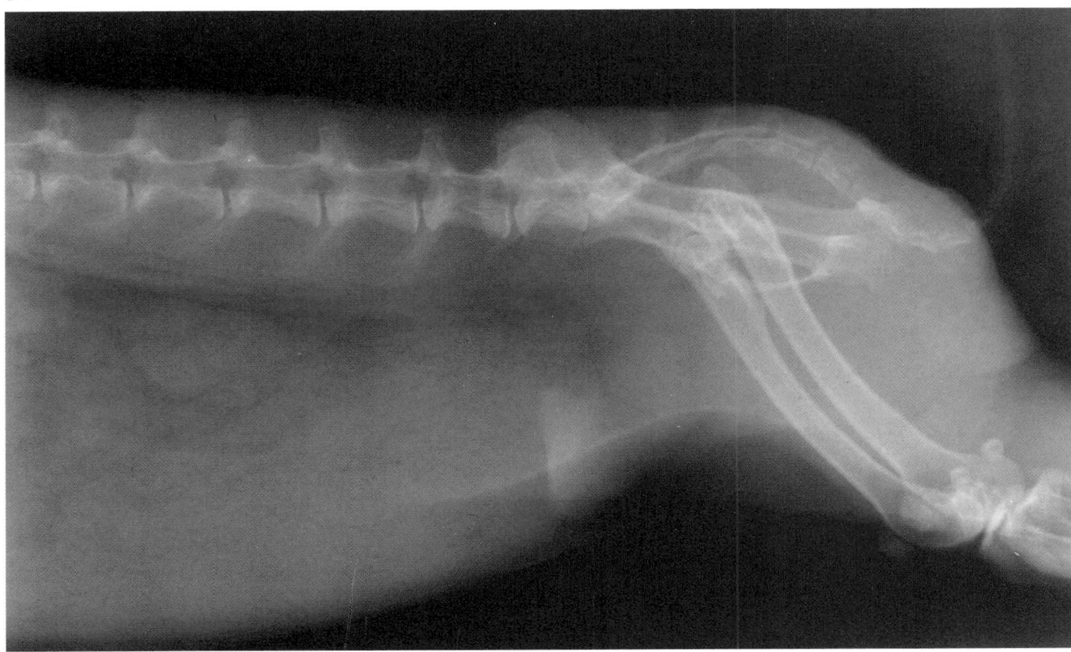

65

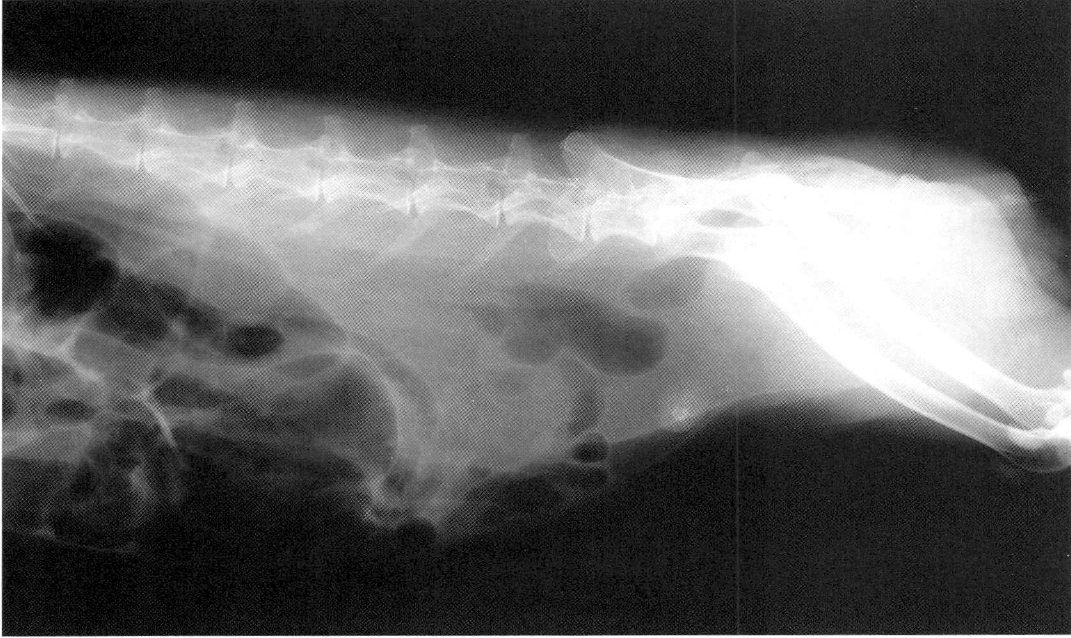

64 Opacification of the Urinary Bladder.

Rabbit *(Oryctolagus cuniculus)*, 3 years.

The radiographic opacity of the urinary bladder is due to the high concentration of crystals in the residual urine.

Note: The urinary bladder is indented cranially by the food-filled cecum.

65 Urolithiasis.

Rabbit *(Oryctolagus cuniculus)*, female, 4 years.

The urinary bladder contains a single layered calculus.

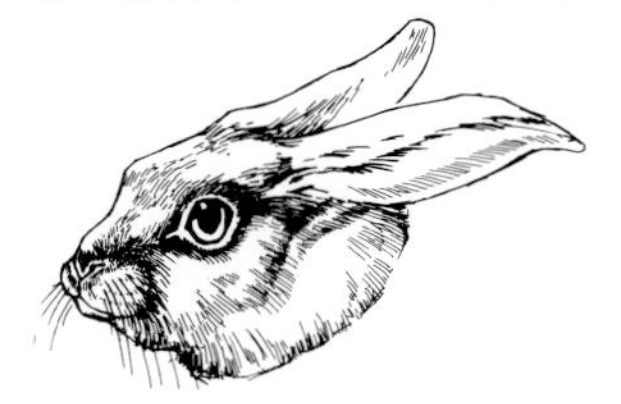

66

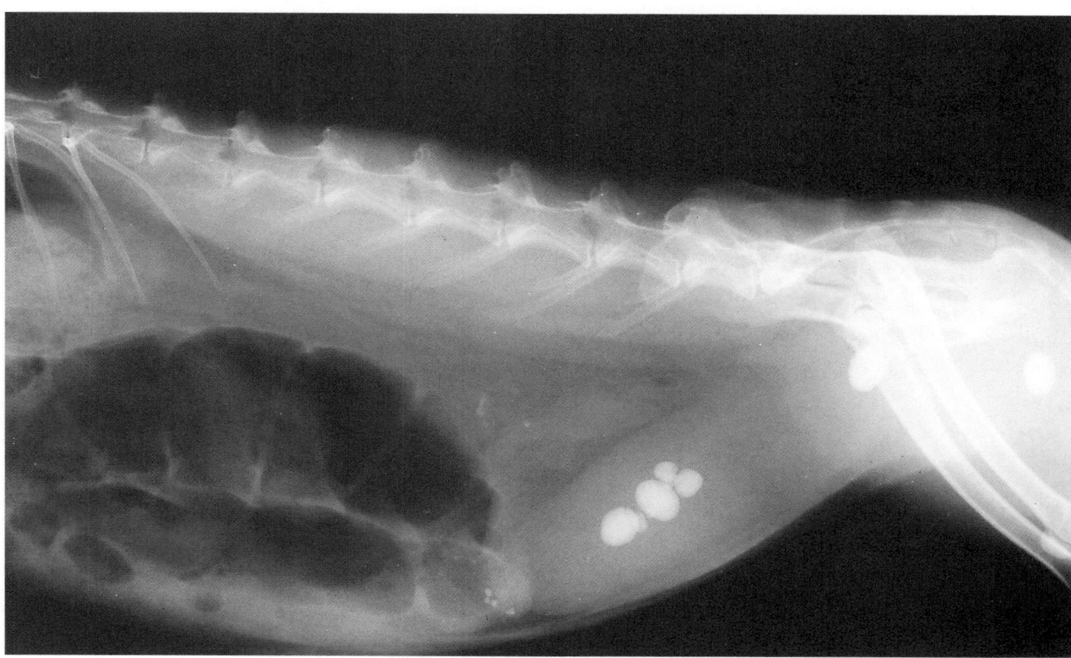

67

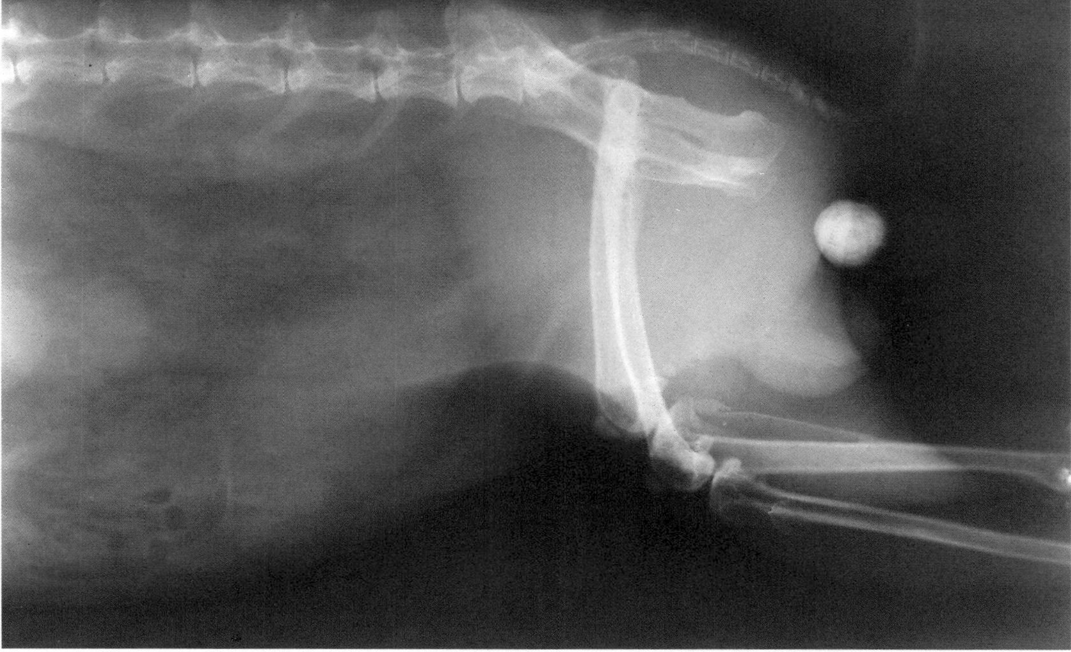

66 Urolithiasis.

Rabbit *(Oryctolagus cuniculus)*, adult.

The well-filled urinary bladder contains several rounded calculi. Outside of the bladder two more calculi are visible, one calculus is lodged in the neck of the bladder (trigon area), and the other is lodged more distally in the urethra.

Note: Dorsal to the bladder the uterus can be seen. And cranial to the urinary bladder the calcified ovaries are visible. The cecum contains large amounts of gas.

67 Urolithiasis.

Rabbit *(Oryctolagus cuniculus)*, female, 4 years.

In the most distal portion of the urethra, a single urinary calculus with characteristic concentric layering is lodged.

68

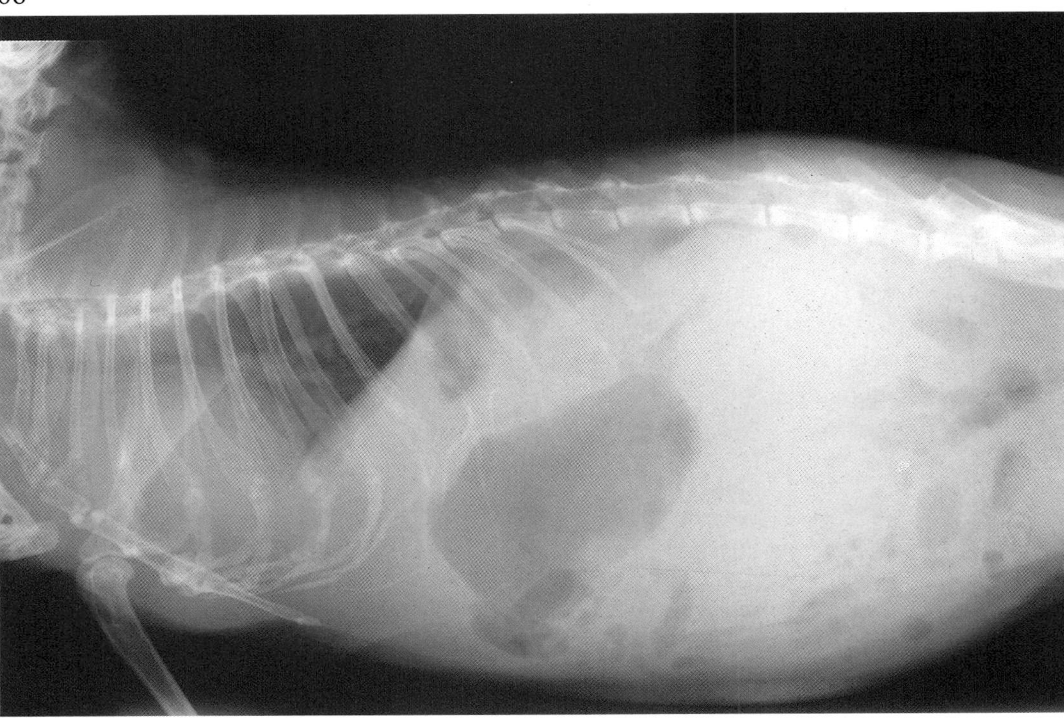

69

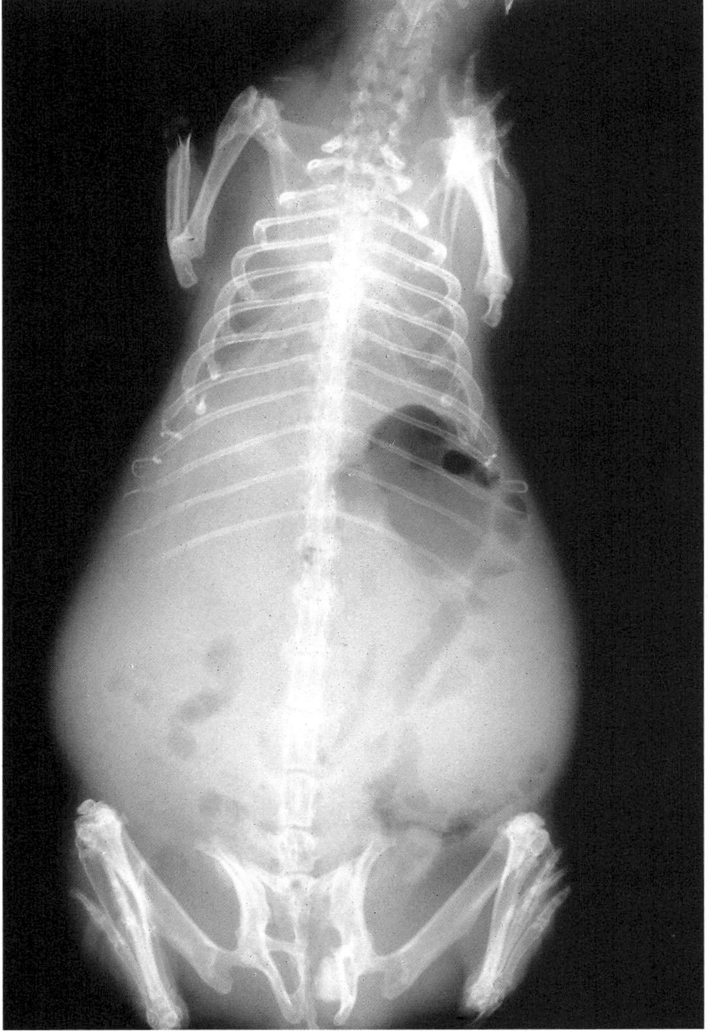

68/69 Hydrops Ascites.

Rabbit *(Oryctolagus cuniculus)*, female, 6 years.

There is a generalized increased density with loss of visceral detail in the distended abdominal cavity, characteristic of peritoneal fluid accumulation. Gas shadows are seen in the stomach and several small bowel loops.

The cardiac silhouette is greatly enlarged and the caudal vena cava is congested. Both signs are indicative of right heart failure causing ascites.

Note: Radiographically it is not possible to determine the character and type of the ascitic fluid in the peritoneal cavity.

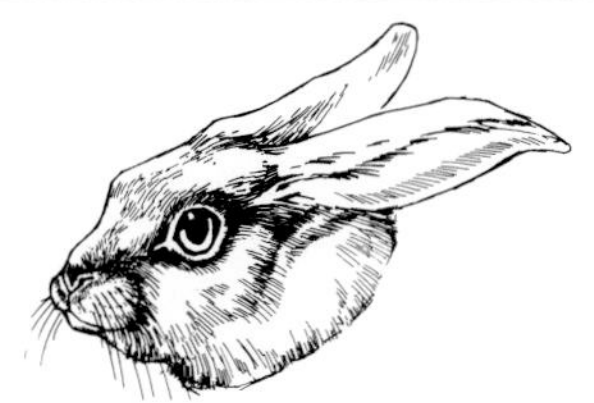

70

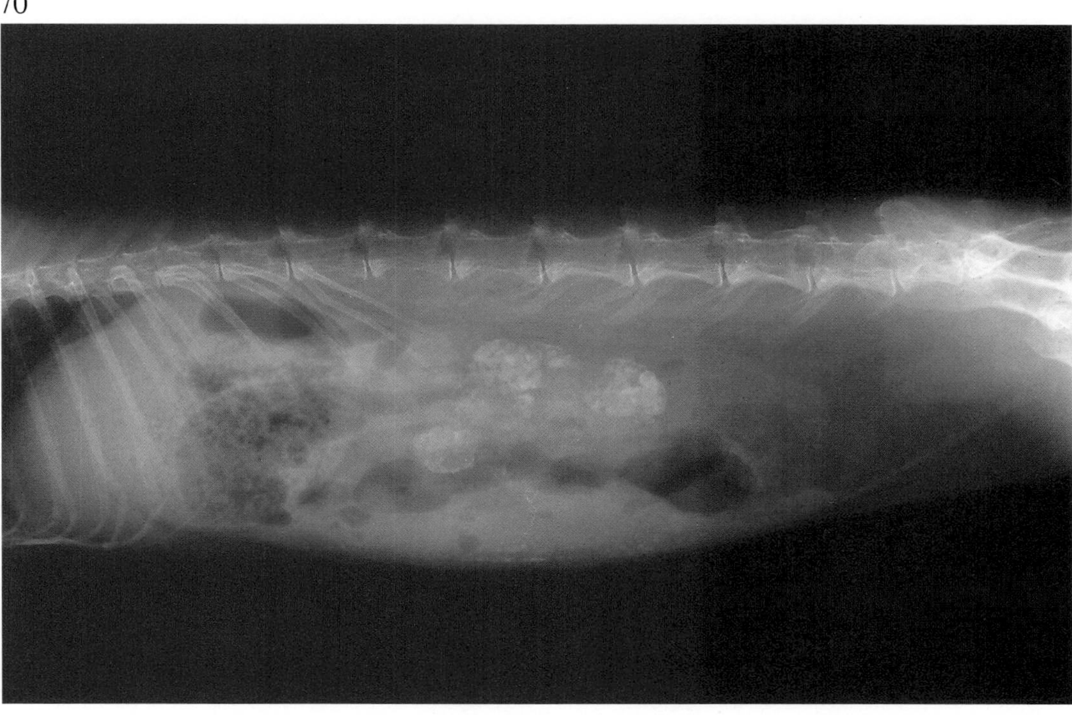

71

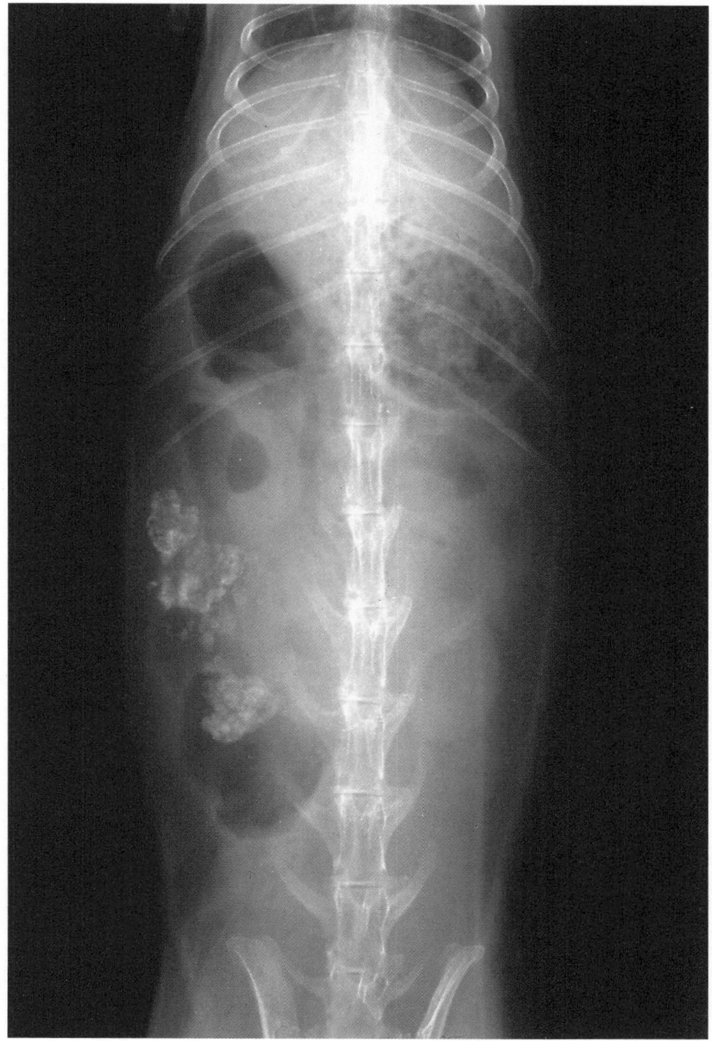

70/71 Fat Necrosis.

Rabbit *(Oryctolagus cuniculus)*, 1 year.

The irregular calcifications in the right mid-abdominal area are due to localized chronic inflammation of fatty tissue with subsequent necrosis and dystrophic calcification.

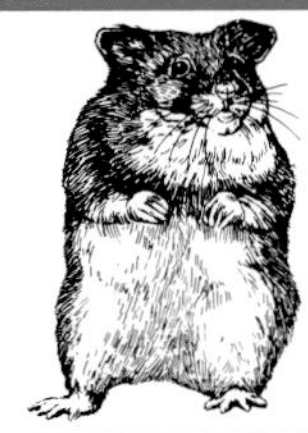

Small Mammals: Hamster

Radiographic Anatomy

72

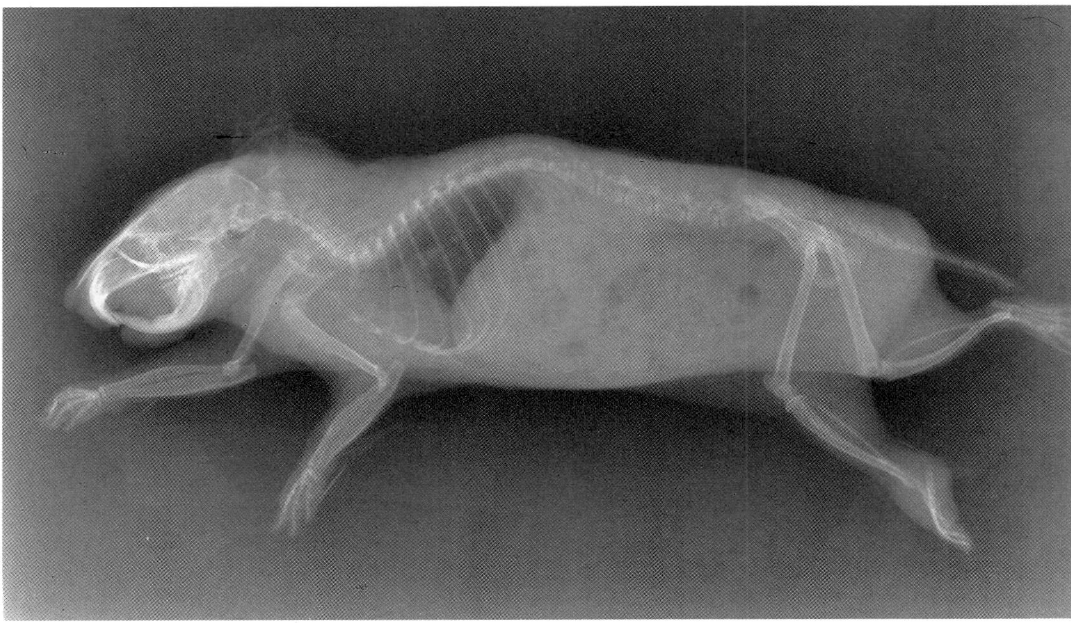

73

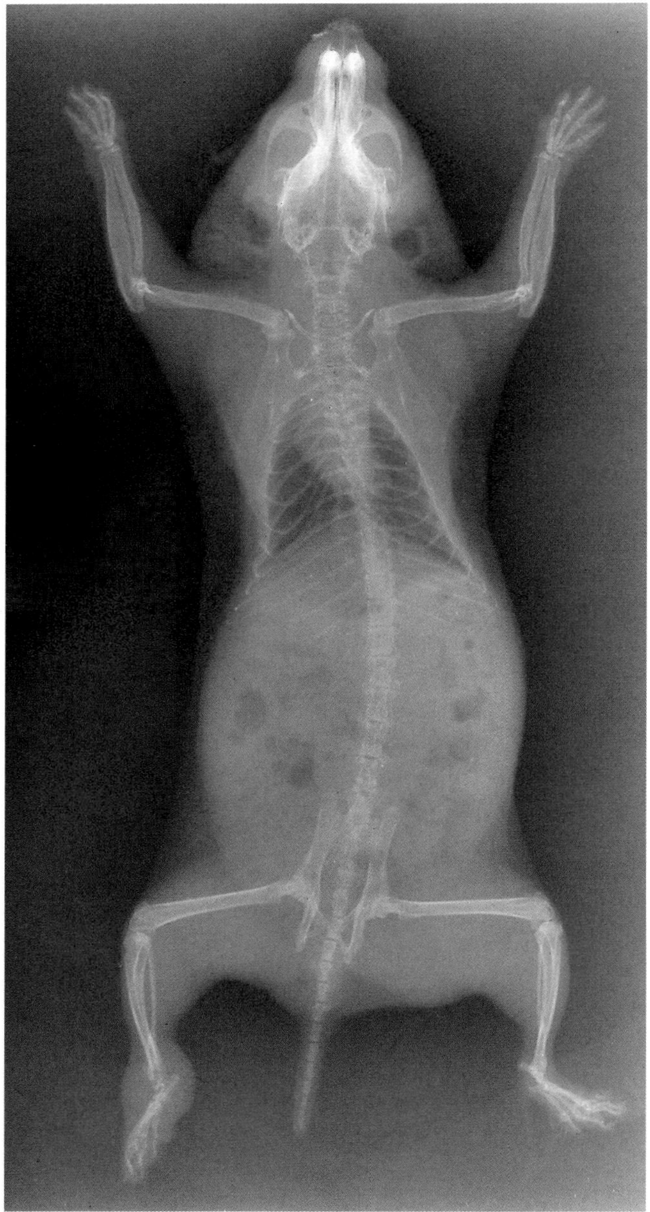

72/73 Normal Radiographic Appearance, lateral and ventrodorsal.

Golden hamster *(Mesocricetus auratus),* female, adult.

The heart is visible inside the thorax, with the apex pointing caudolaterally to the left.

In the golden hamster as well as in other small pet mammals, the abdomen is relatively large in comparison to the thorax. The voluminous gastrointestinal tract shows lack of contrast, as in many omnivorous rodents. Gas shadows are distributed throughout the entire intestinal tract.

The kidneys are situated dorsally near the first lumbar vertebral body and are faintly visible on the lateral radiograph.

Small Mammals: Hamster

Radiographic Anatomy

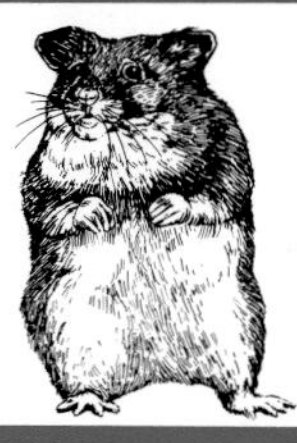

72 A

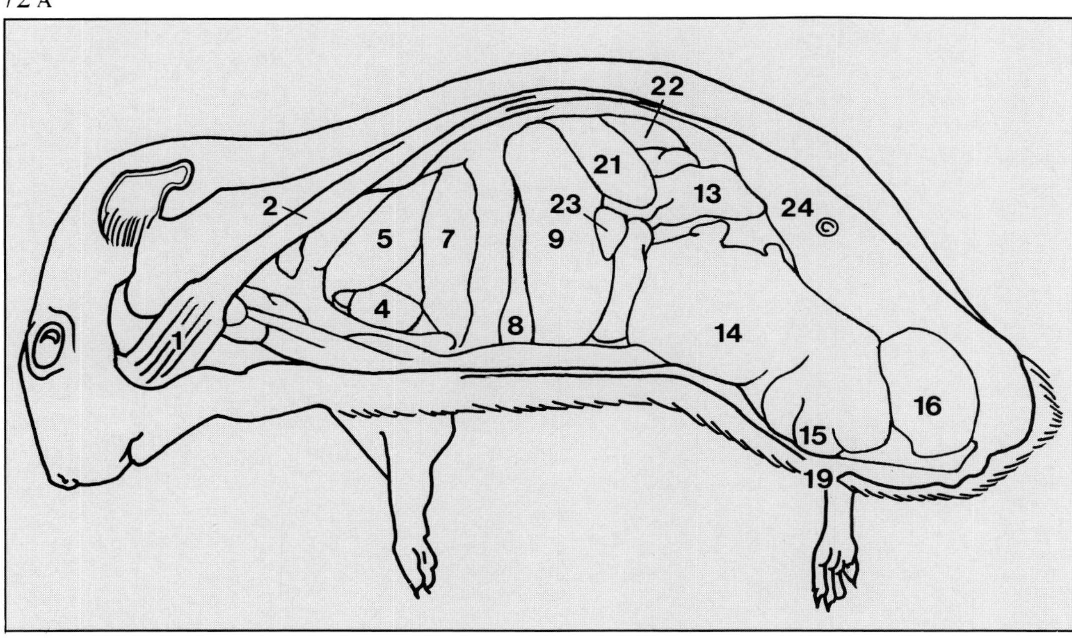

73 A

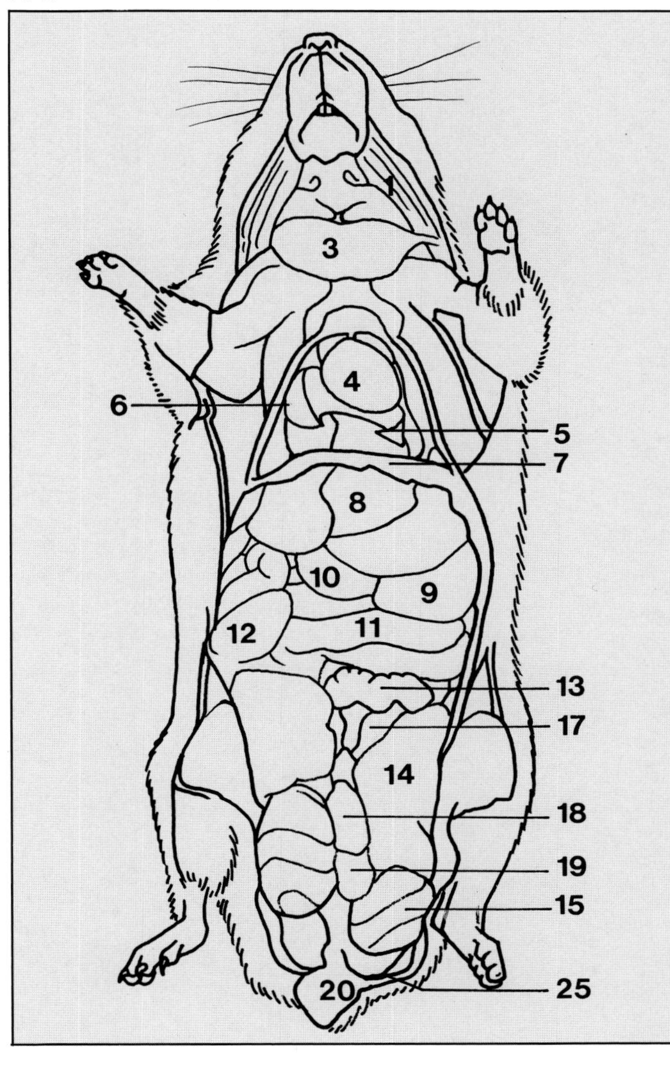

Because individual organs are poorly defined on radiographs, an anatomic drawing with size, shape and location of these organs in an adult male animal is presented.

72A/73A Anatomical Drawing,

lateral and ventrodorsal.

Chinese striped-back hamster *(Cricetulus griseus)*, male, adult.

Cheek pouch, bursa buccalis (**1**), m. retractor bursae buccalis (**2**), fat pad (**3**), heart (**4**), left lung (**5**), right lung (**6**), diaphragm (**7**), liver (**8**), proventriculus (**9**), glandular stomach (**10**), jejunum (**11**), cecum (**12**), vesicular gland (**13**), fat pad and head of epidymidis (**14**), testes (**15**), tail of epidymidis (**16**), bladder (**17**), penis (**18**), preputial orifice (**19**), anus (**20**), spleen (**21**), kidneys (**22**), pancreas (**23**), acetabulum (**24**), scrotum (**25**).

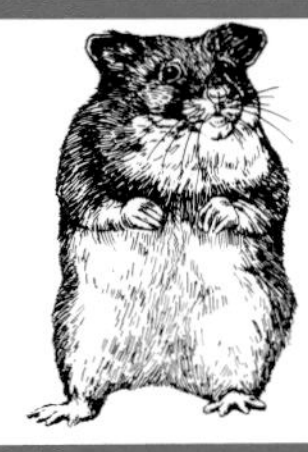

Small Mammals: Hamster

Radiographic Abnormalities

74

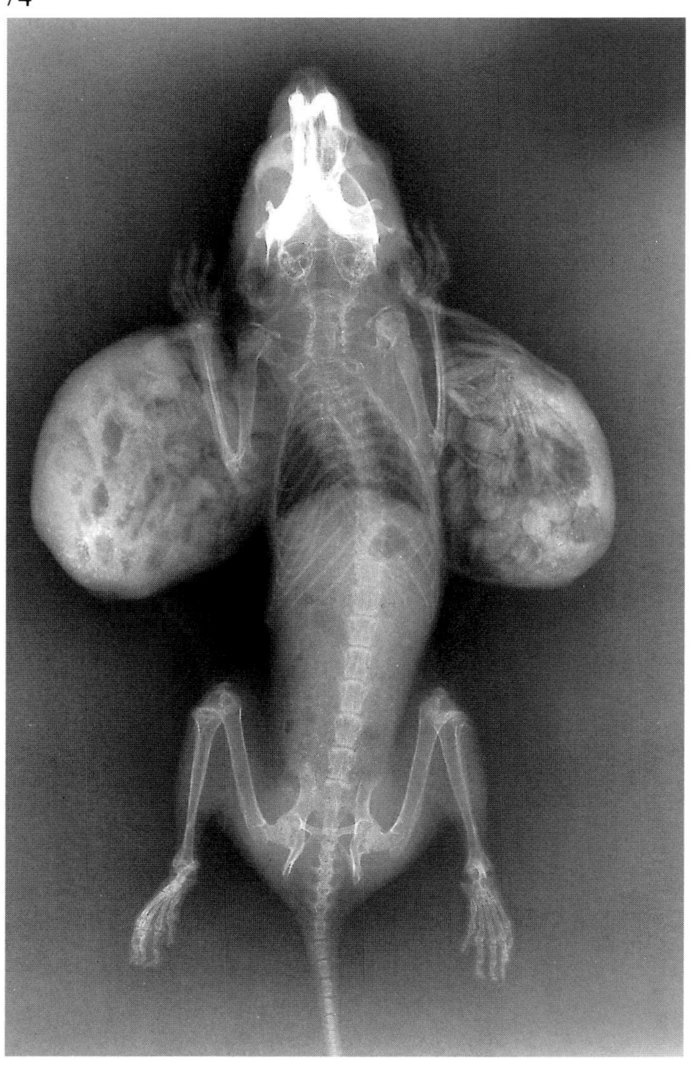

75

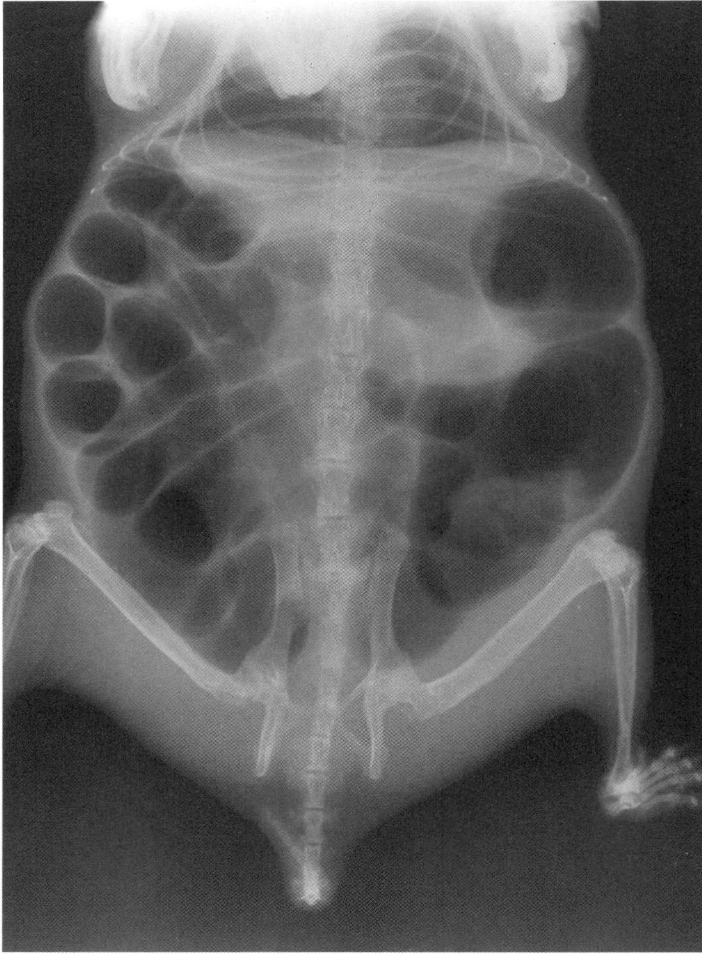

74 Impaction of the Cheek Pouch.

Golden hamster *(Mesocricetus auratus)*, adult.

Both cheek pouches are severely dilated. When extremely full they extend far caudally.

75 Tympany.

Golden hamster *(Mesocricetus auratus)*, adult.

There is extreme gaseous distension of all the intestinal loops due to a rectal prolapse inducing intestinal obstruction.

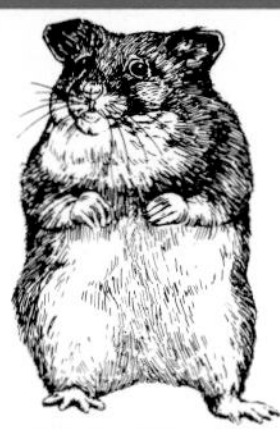

76

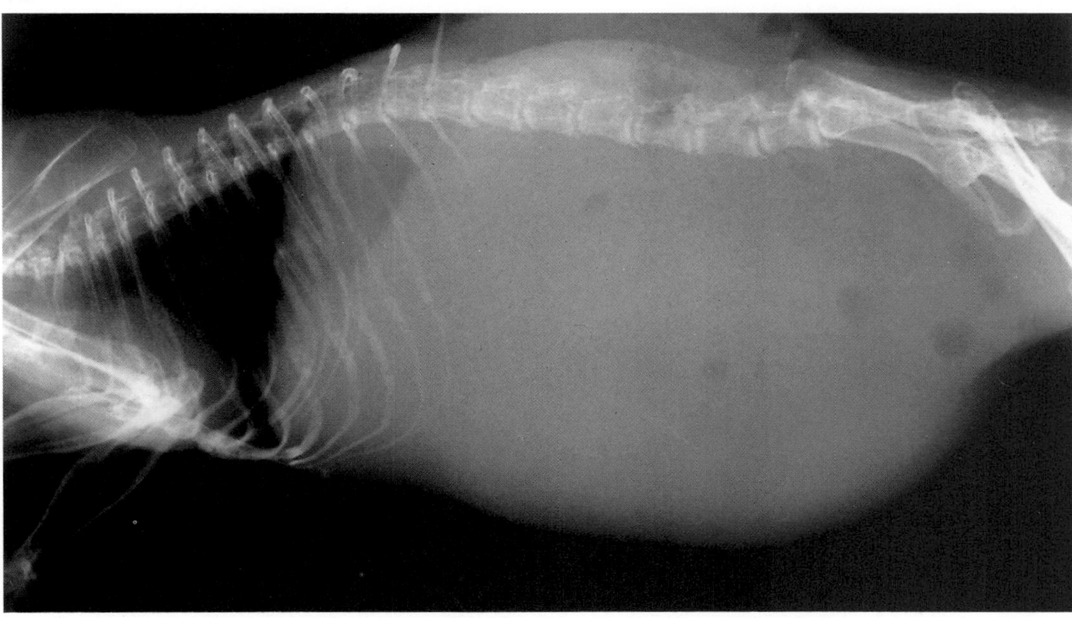

77

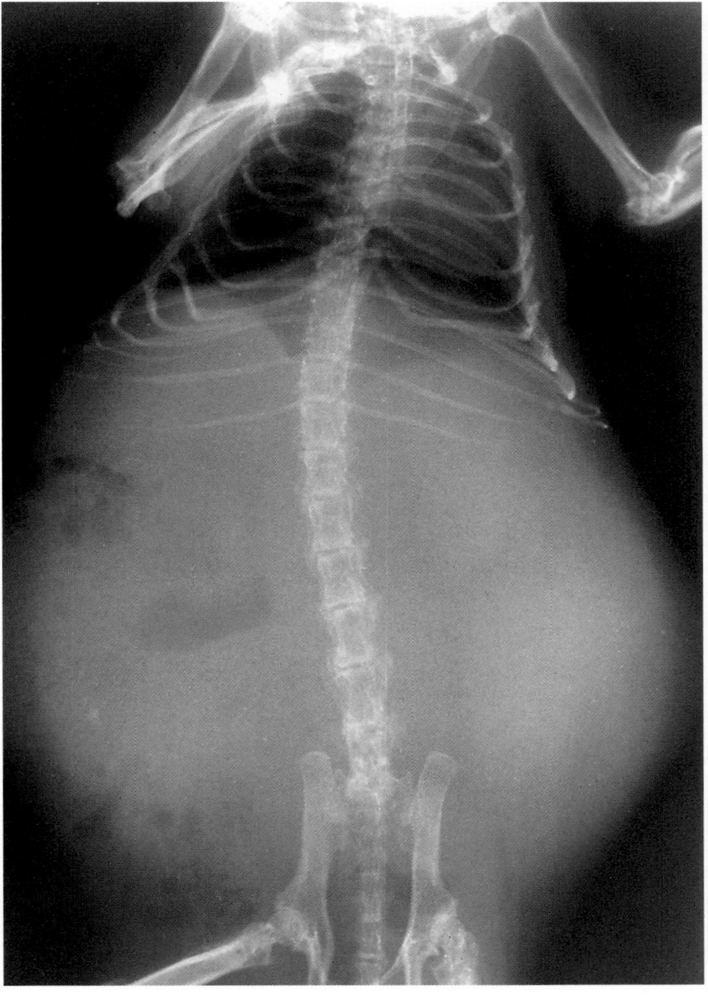

76/77 Mass in the Left Abdomen.

Golden hamster *(Mesocricetus auratus)*, adult.

The abdomen is distended and has a generalized fluid density. The intestinal loops are displaced dorsally and to the right due to a soft tissue structure in the left abdomen. The abdominal viscera cannot be defined. At necropsy, the mass proved to be a liver tumor.

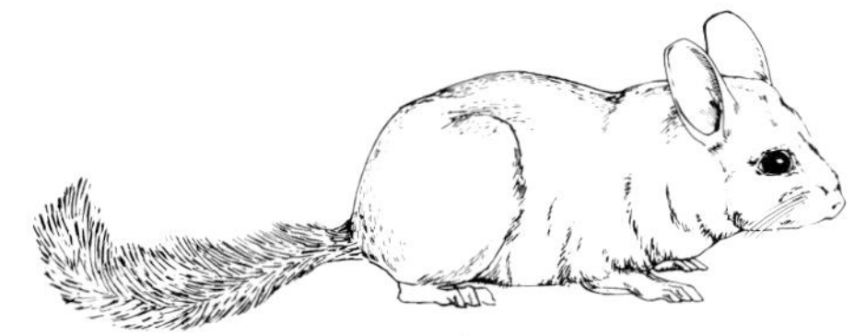

Small Mammals: Chinchilla

Radiographic Anatomy

78

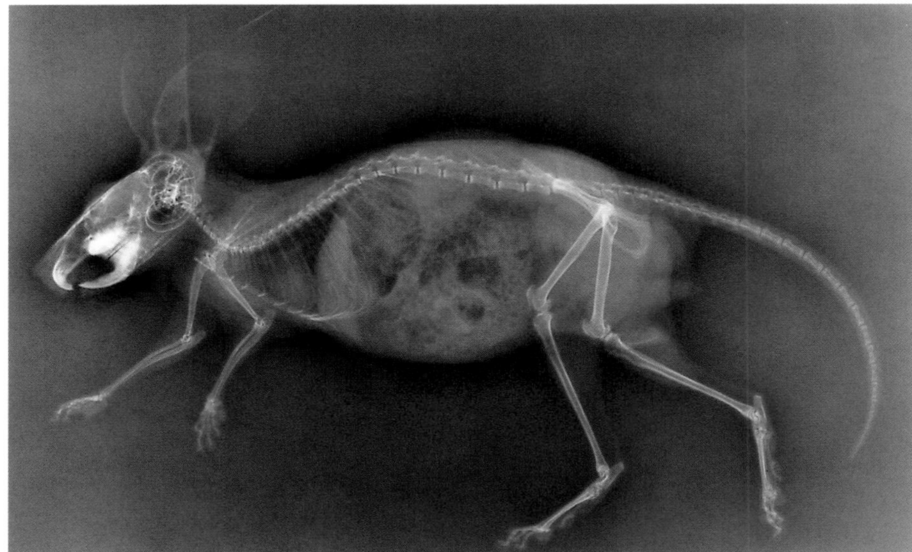

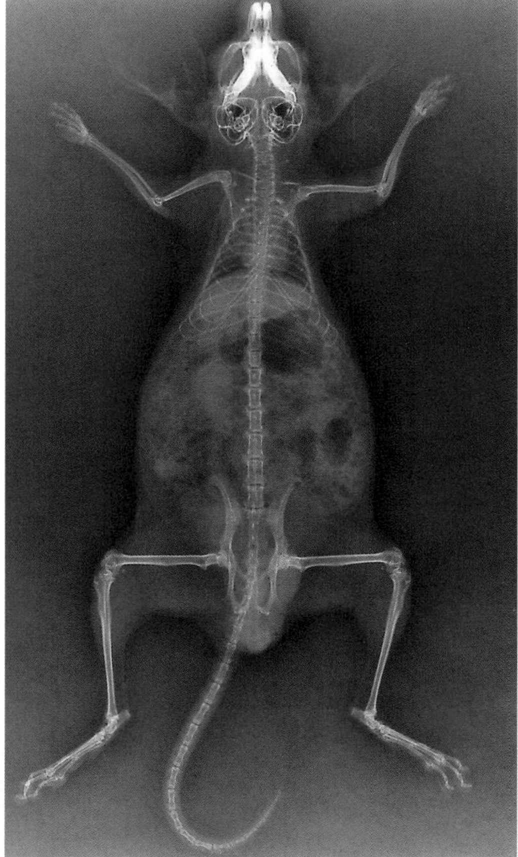

78 A

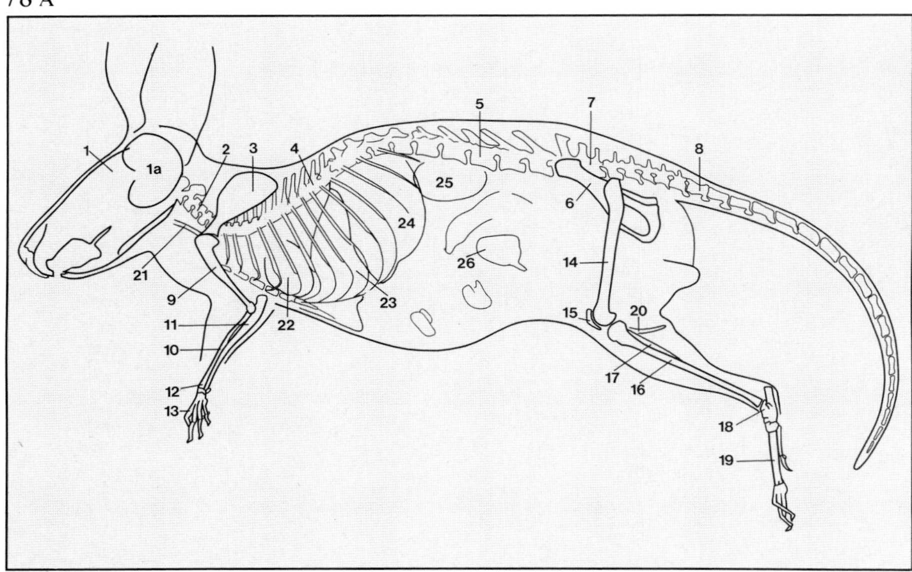

78/78A/79 Normal Radiographic Appearance,
lateral and ventrodorsal.

Chinchilla *(Chinchilla lanigera)*, male, adult.

The thorax is very small in comparison to the abdomen. The heart is clearly defined. In the abdomen, the liver is clearly outlined by the air-filled stomach. The intestinal loops have a finely granular appearance due to the presence of food particles and small gas bubbles.

The right kidney is visible at the level of the second and third lumbar vertebrae. The left kidney is located more medially and is difficult to distinguish.

Cranium (**1**) and bullae tympani (**1a**); v. cervicales (**2**); scapula (**3**); v. thoracicae (**4**); v. lumbales (**5**); pelvis (**6**); v. sacrales (**7**); v. caudales (**8**); humerus (**9**); radius (**10**); ulna (**11**); metacarpus (**12**); phalanges (**13**); femur (**14**); patella (**15**); tibia (**16**); fibula (**17**); tarsus (**18**); metatarsus (**19**); os penis (**20**); trachea (**21**); heart (**22**); liver (**23**); stomach (**24**); right kidney (**25**); intestines (**26**).

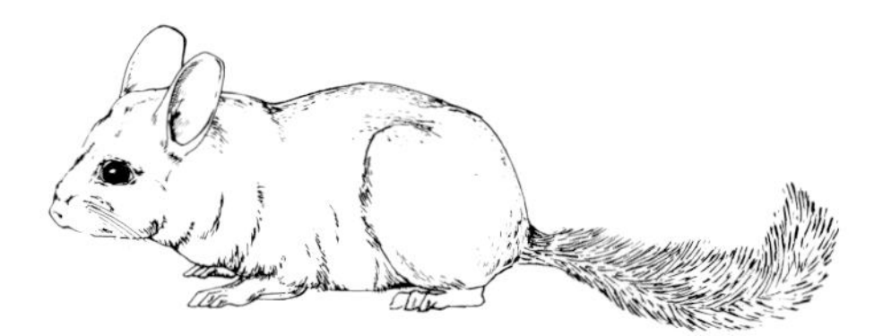

80

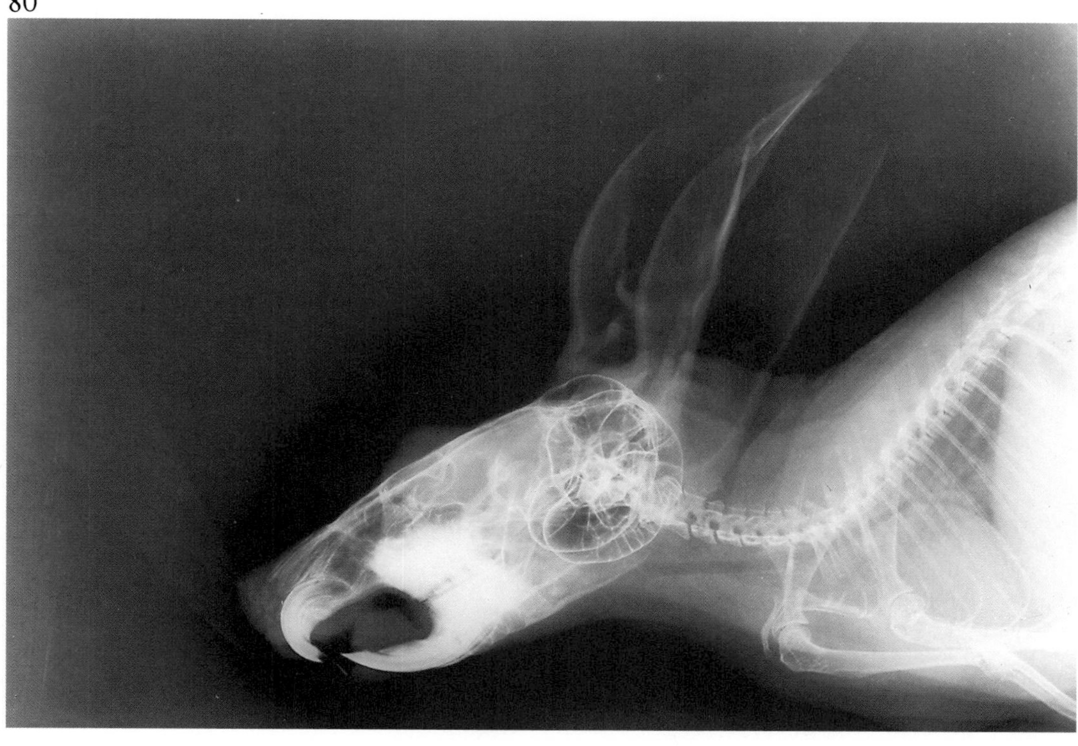

81

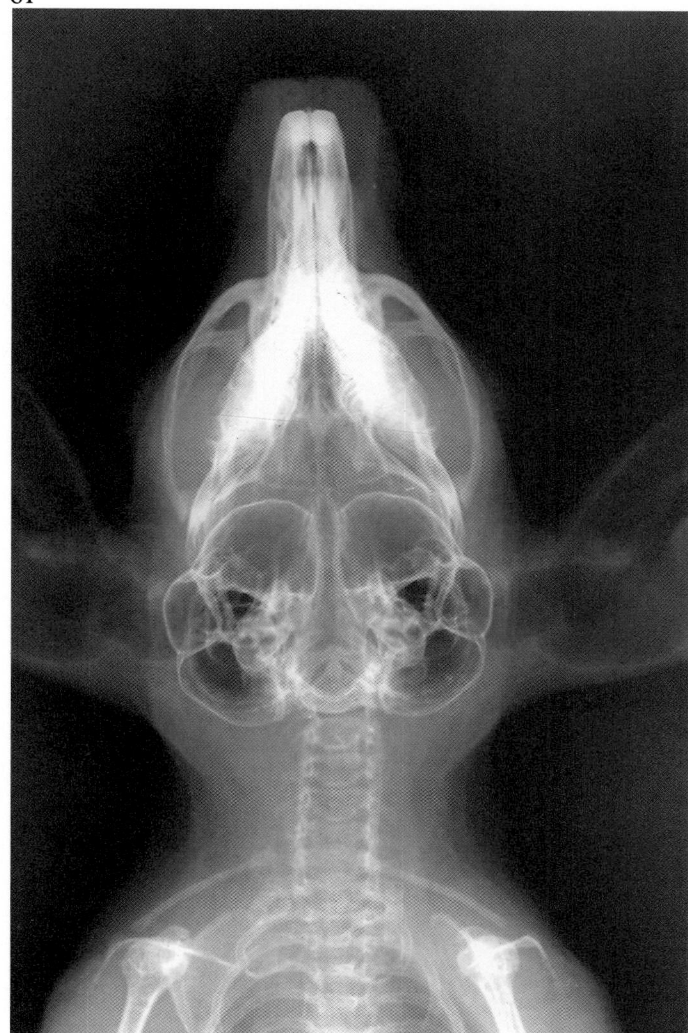

80/81 Skull: Normal Radiographic Appearance, lateral and dorsoventral.

Chinchilla (*Chinchilla lanigera*), male, adult.

The nocturnal and diurnal chinchilla has especially well-developed senses. Radiographically, the large bullae tympani are evident.

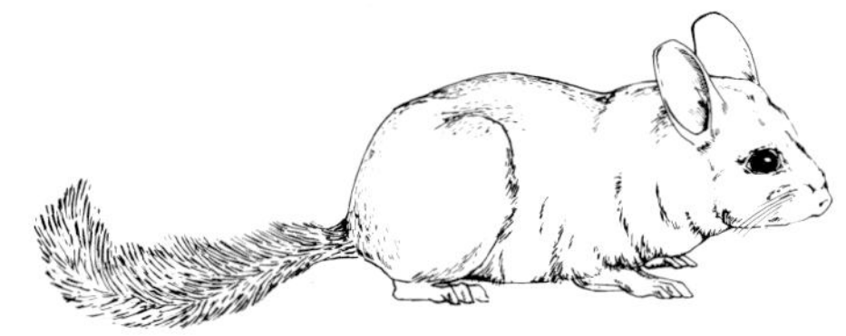

82

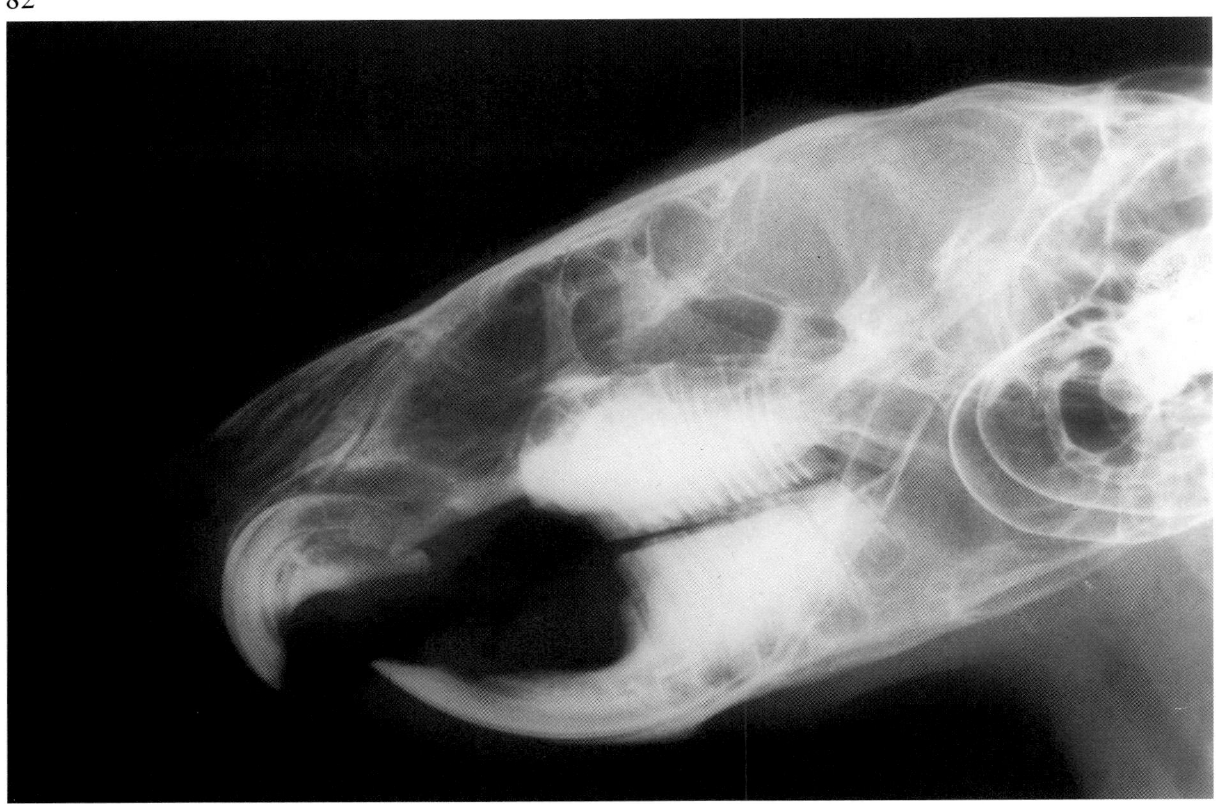

82 Fracture of the Os palatinum.

Chinchilla *(Chinchilla lanigera)*, adult.

The bony palate is fractured. The minor dislocation results in a malocclusion.

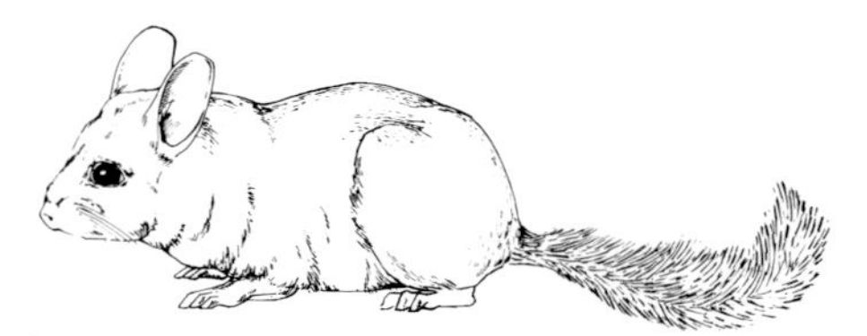

83

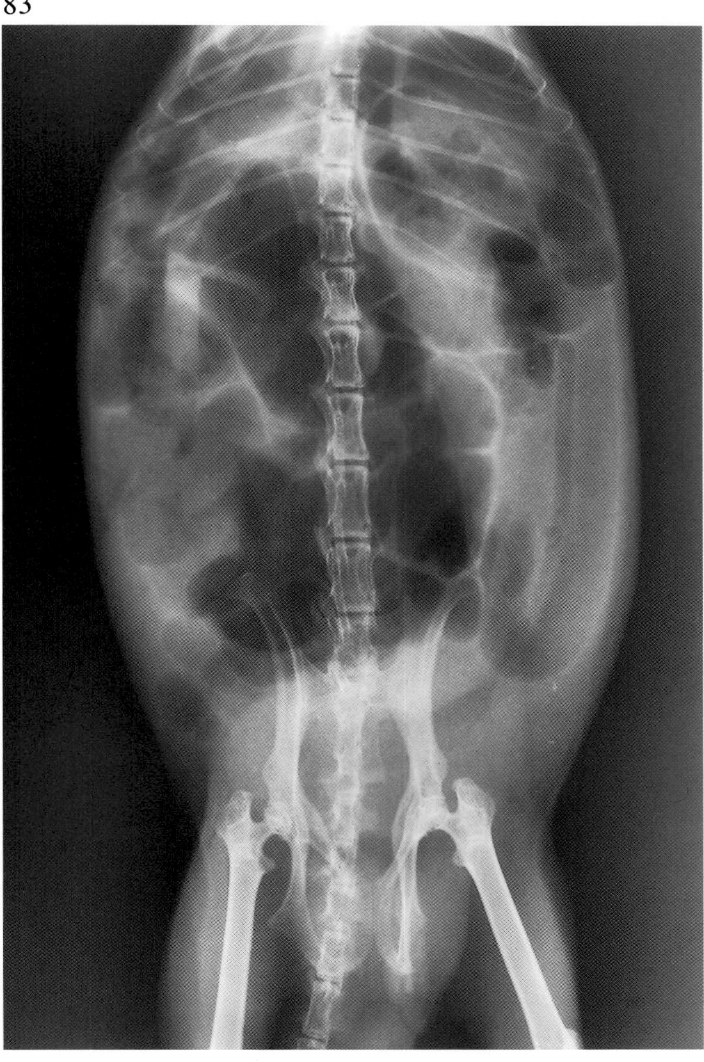

84

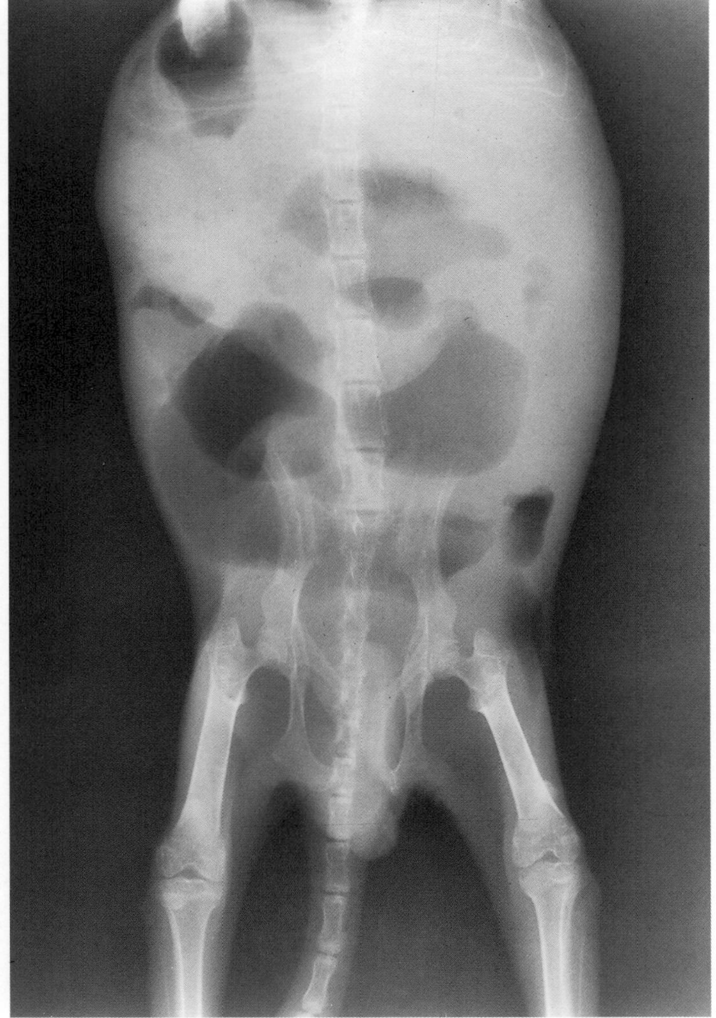

83 Ileus.

Chinchilla *(Chinchilla lanigera)*, male, adult.

Severely distended and gas-filled intestinal loops are compatible with ileus. This was caused by an abscess in the mesenteric region.

84 Ileus.

Chinchilla *(Chinchilla lanigera)*, male, adult.

Some of the small intestinal loops are severely dilated by gas and food. In this case, the ileus was caused by food impaction in one of the proximal jejunal loops.

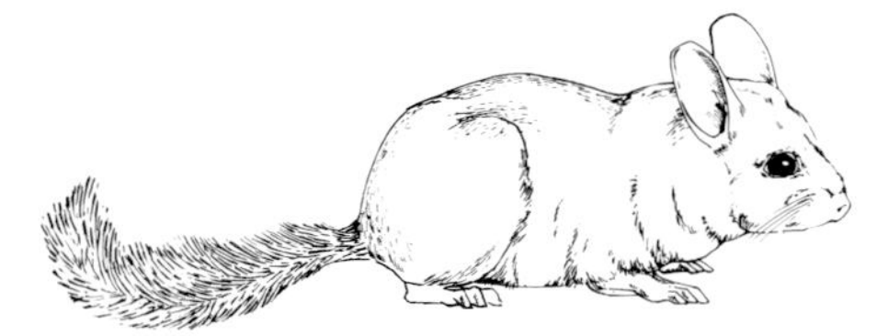

Small Mammals: Chinchilla

Radiographic Abnormalities

85

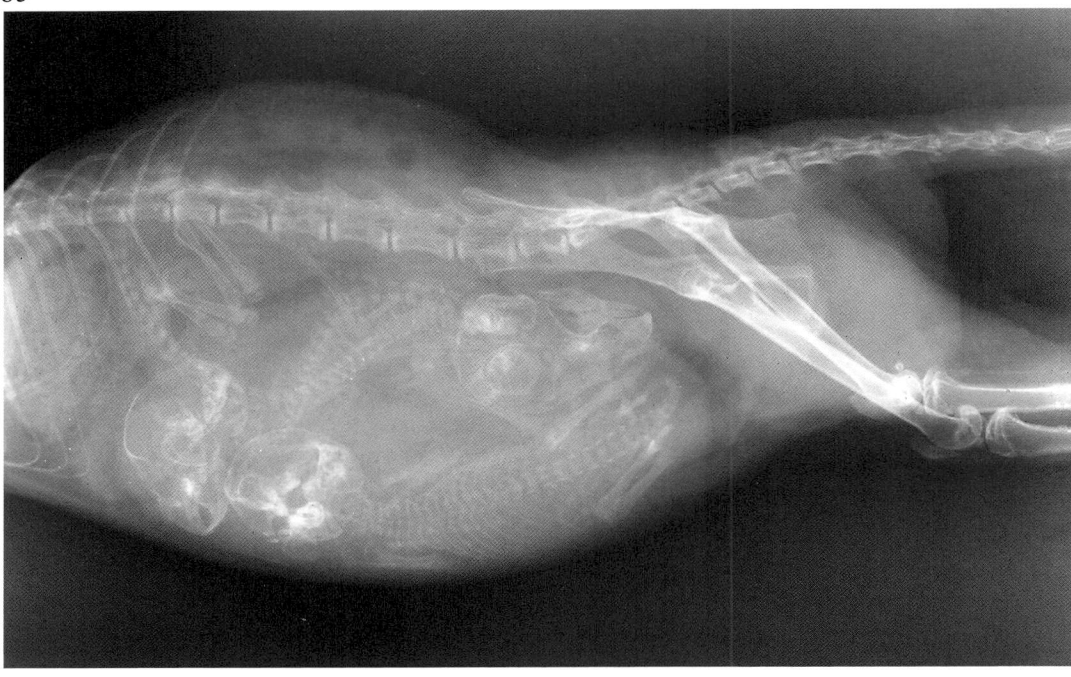

86

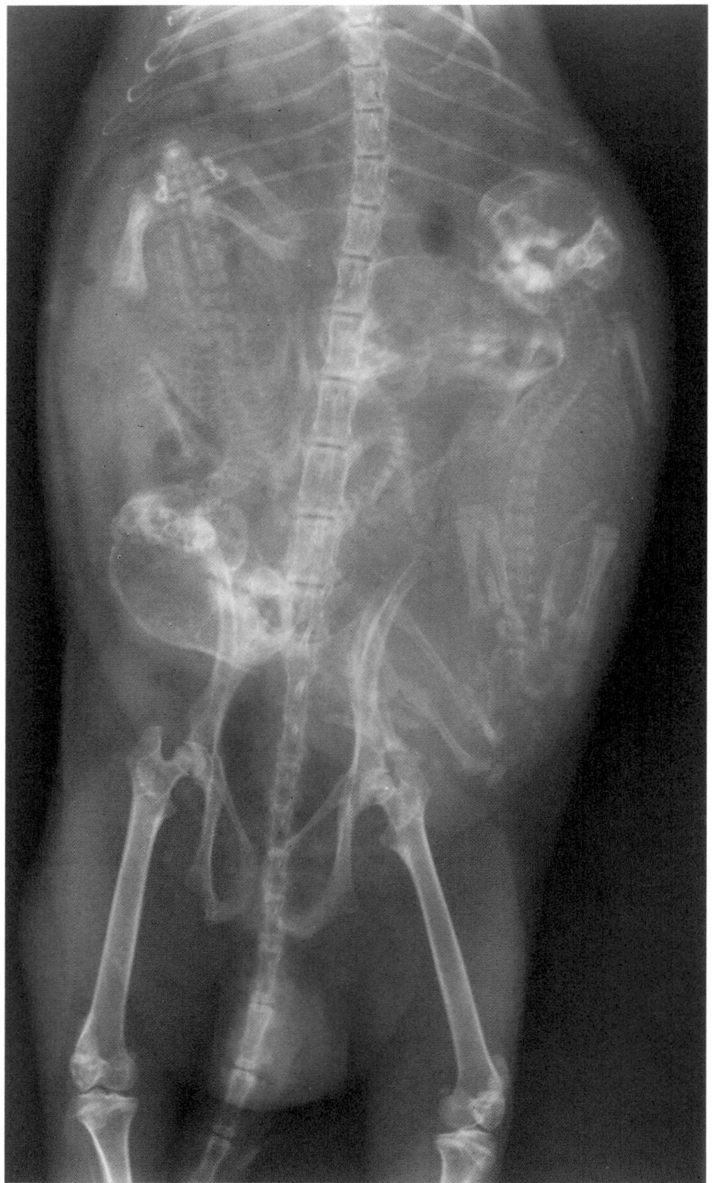

85/86 Protracted Birth.

Chinchilla *(Chinchilla lanigera)*, female, adult.

The skeletons of 3 mature fetuses are clearly visible. The pelvic symphysis (ventrodorsal view) is only slightly widened. The most caudal fetus is not correctly aligned with the birth canal.

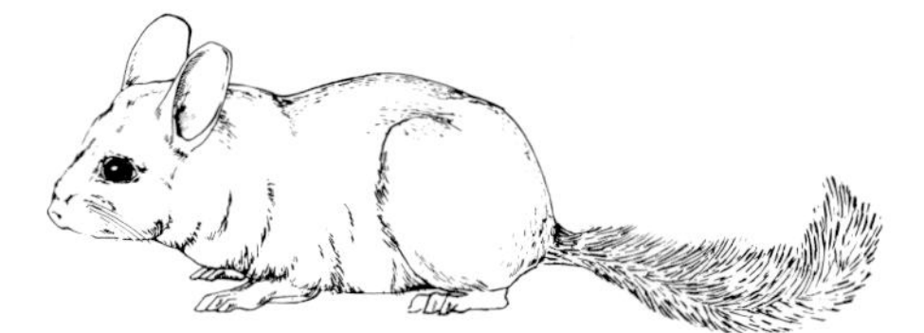

87

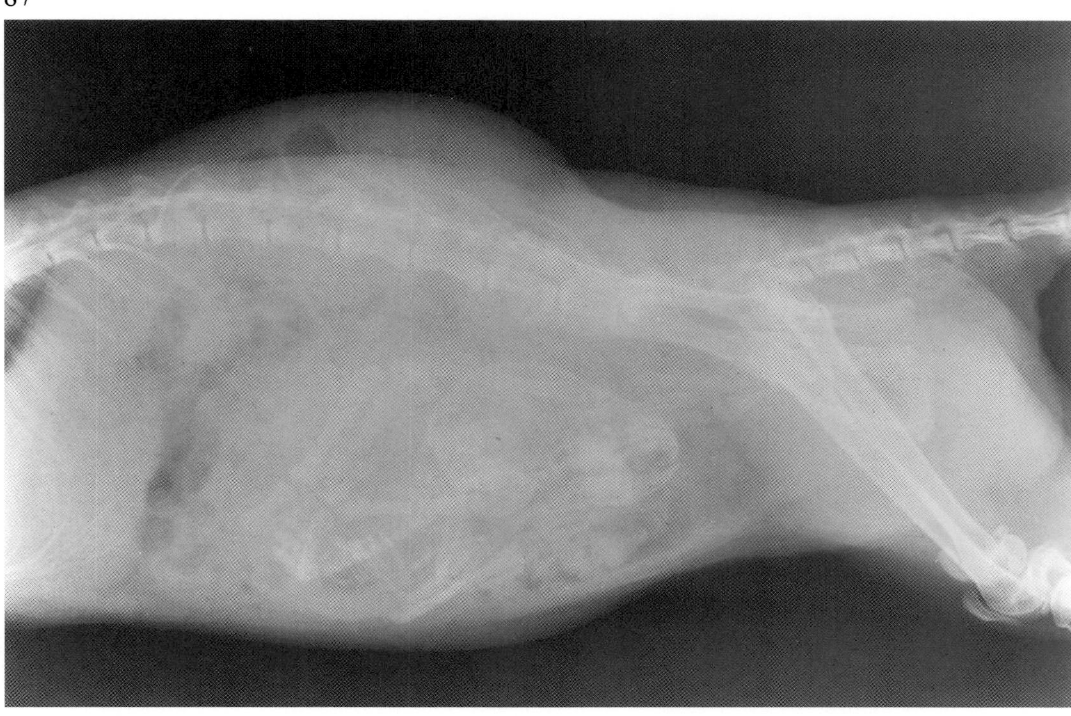

88

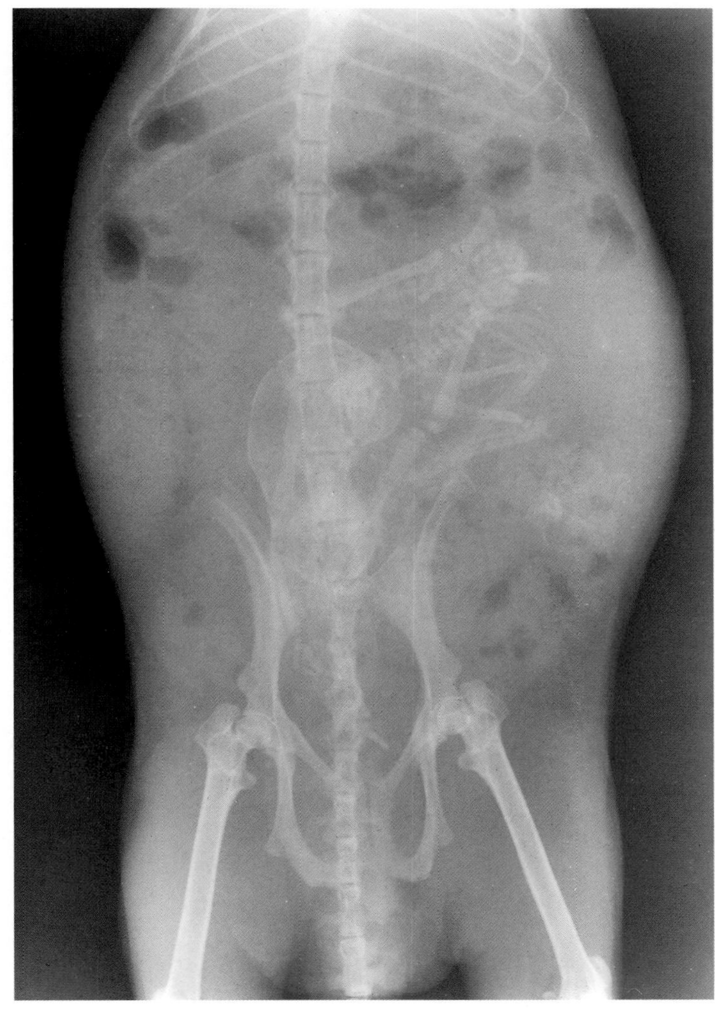

87/88 Fetal Malformation.

Chinchilla *(Chinchilla lanigera)*, female, adult.

The skeleton of a mature fetus can be seen. The vertebral column is abnormally curved, which is visible in both projections and therefore allows a radiographic diagnosis of schistosoma reflexum.

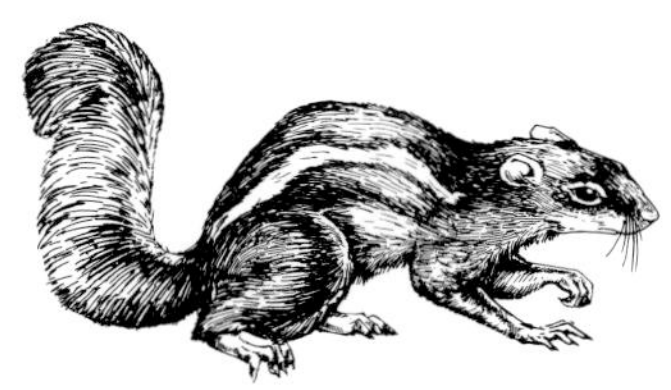

Small Mammals: Chipmunk

Radiographic Anatomy

89

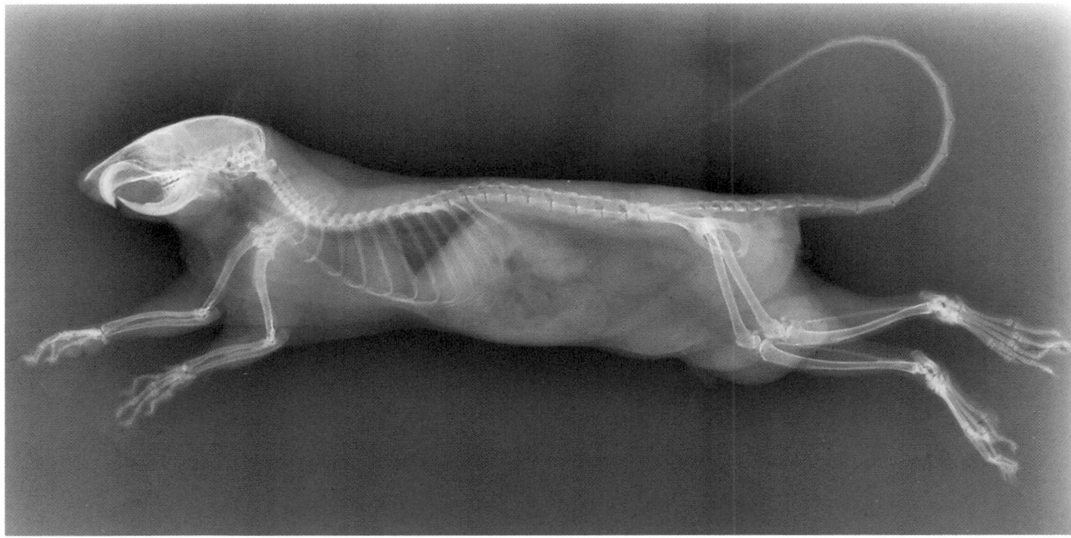

90

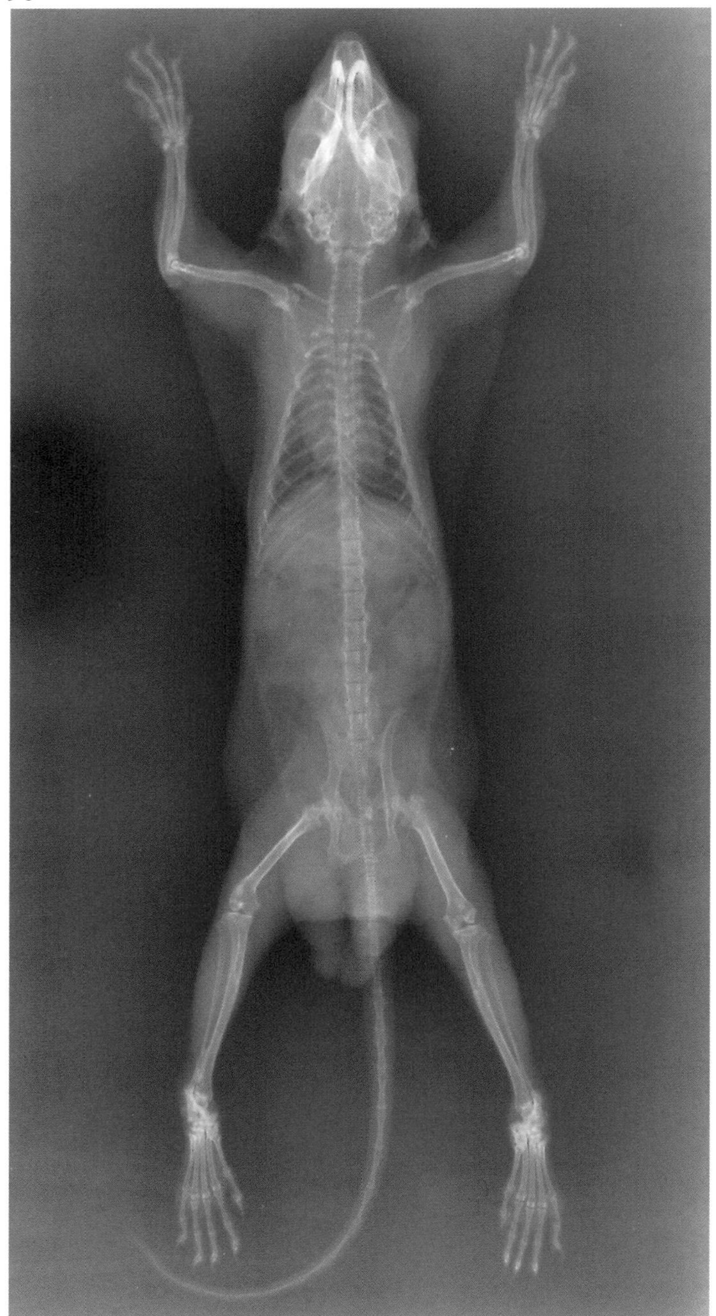

89/90 Normal Radiographic Appearance, lateral and ventrodorsal.

Asiatic Chipmunk *(Eutamias sibiricus)*, male, adult.

The abdomen is voluminous in comparison to the thorax. The heart of the chipmunk has relatively large auricles and a blunted conical shape. The cardiac apex points towards the left.

The liver is the most radiodense organ in the abdomen. It is situated entirely under the costal arch.

On the lateral radiograph, the kidneys can be seen in the lumbar region directly caudal to the costal arch.

The os penis is visible on the lateral radiograph. The testes are easily recognized due to seasonal increase in size.

In some animals, the tibia and fibula are not united.

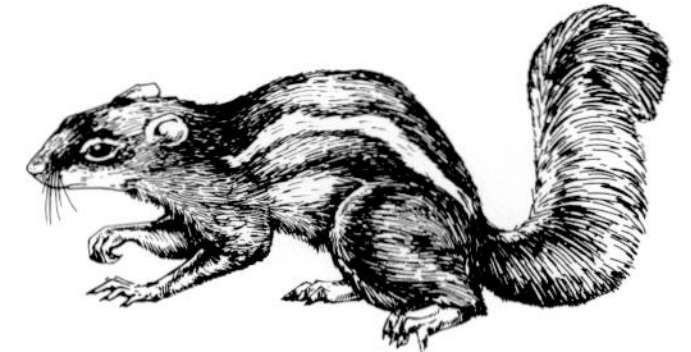

91

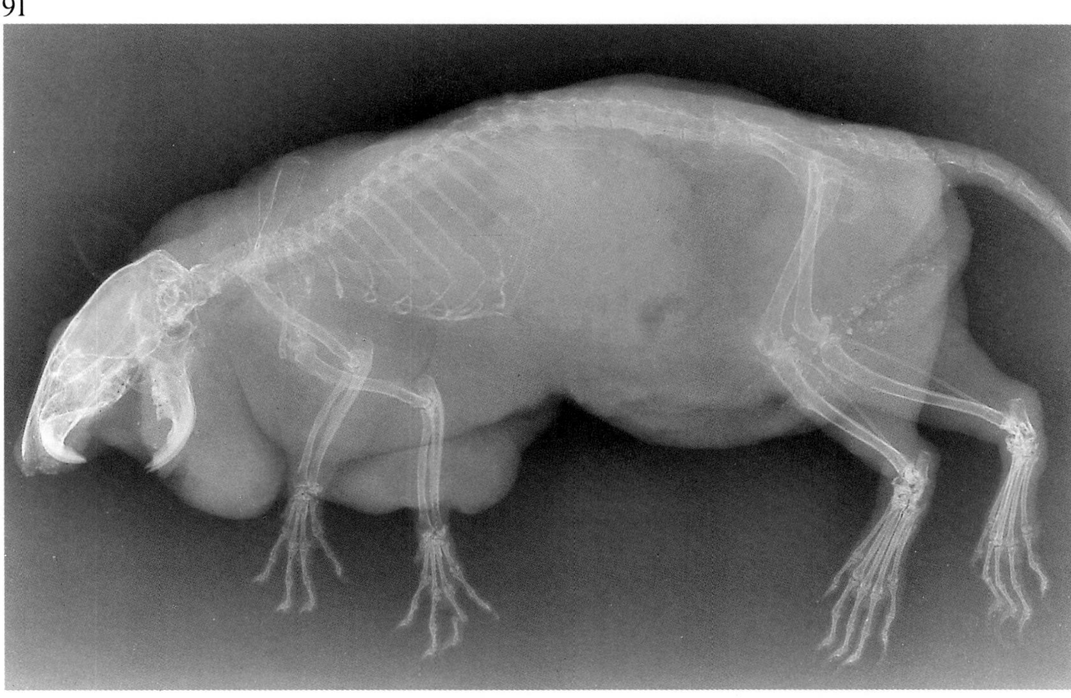

92

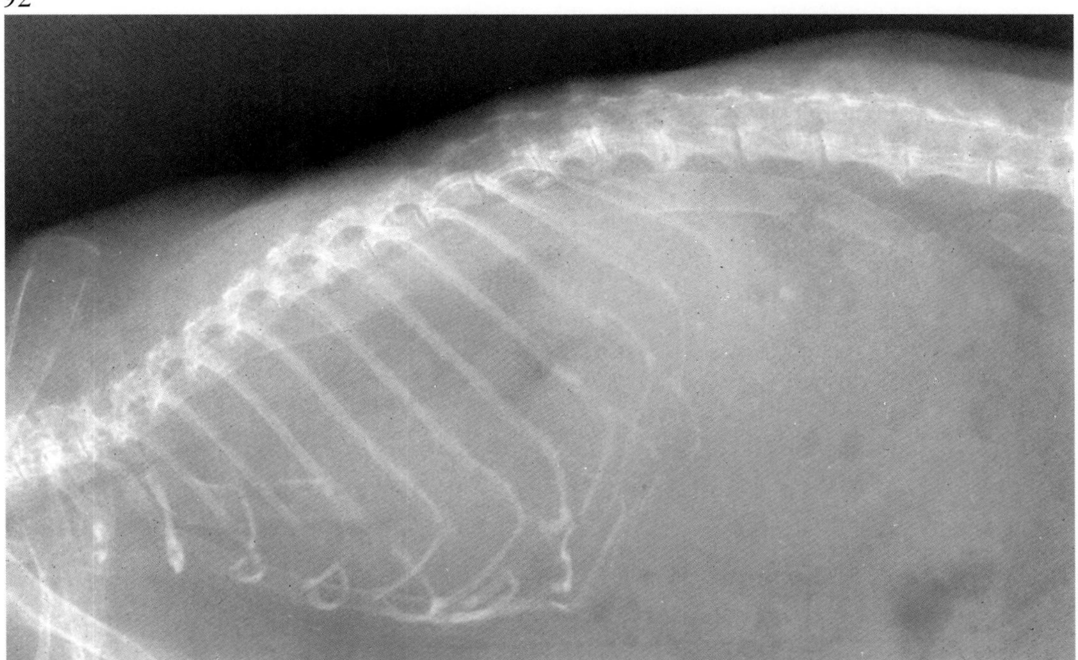

91/92 Calcification of the Aortic Wall.

Asiatic Chipmunk *(Eutamias sibiricus)*, female, adult.

The animal is very obese. Due to pulmonary congestion of this dying animal, the lungs are not fully aerated. Dorsal to the heart, the calcified aorta can be followed all the way to the pelvic region.

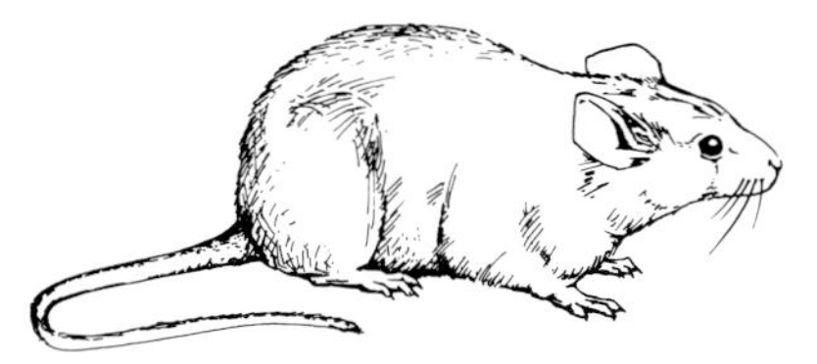

Small Mammals: Mouse

Radiographic Anatomy

93

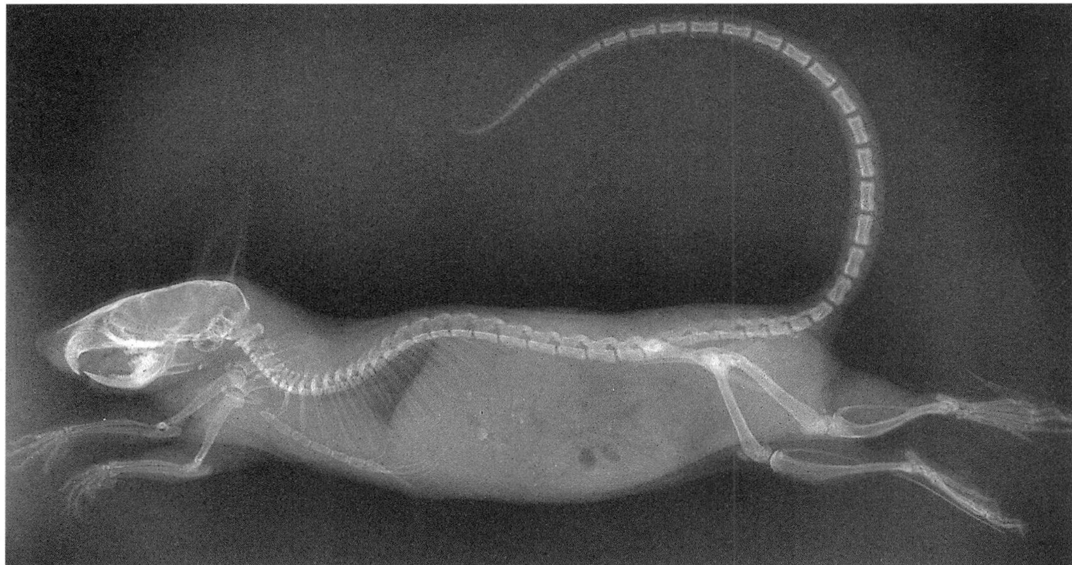

94

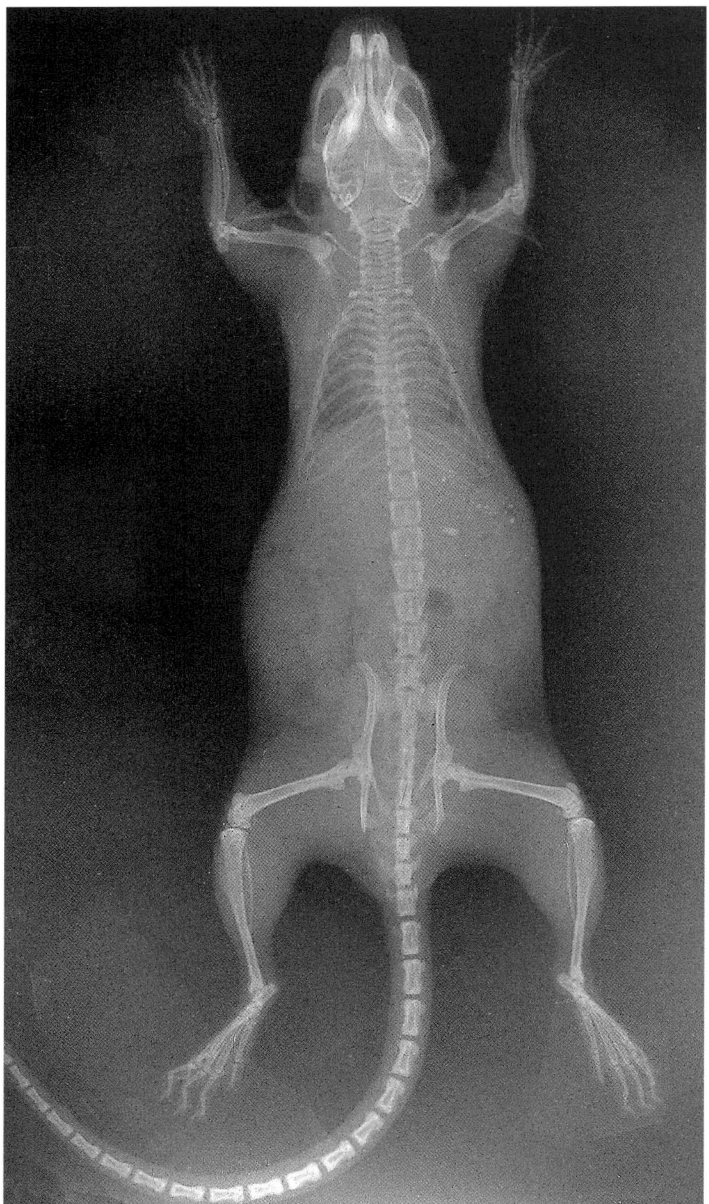

93/94 Normal Radiographic Appearance, lateral and ventrodorsal.

House Mouse *(Mus musculus)*, female, adult.

In the thorax, only the caudal lunglobes and the heart can be distinguished.

The abdominal organs are not well-defined. Food particles and small gas bubbles are visible in the gastrointestinal tract.

In the mouse, the incisors are not as deeply imbedded in the mandible and maxilla as in the guinea pig or hamster.

Small Mammals: Rat

Radiographic Anatomy

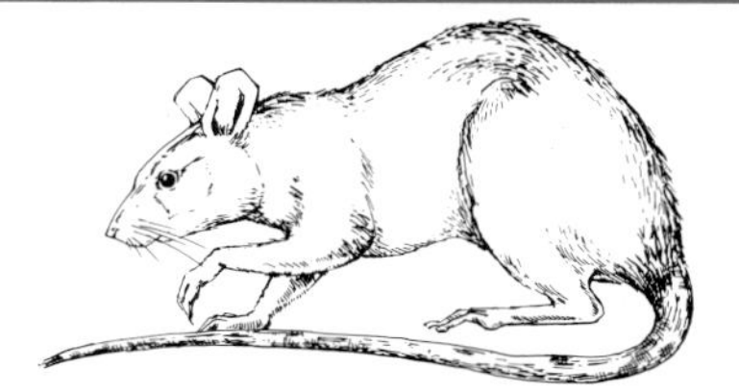

95

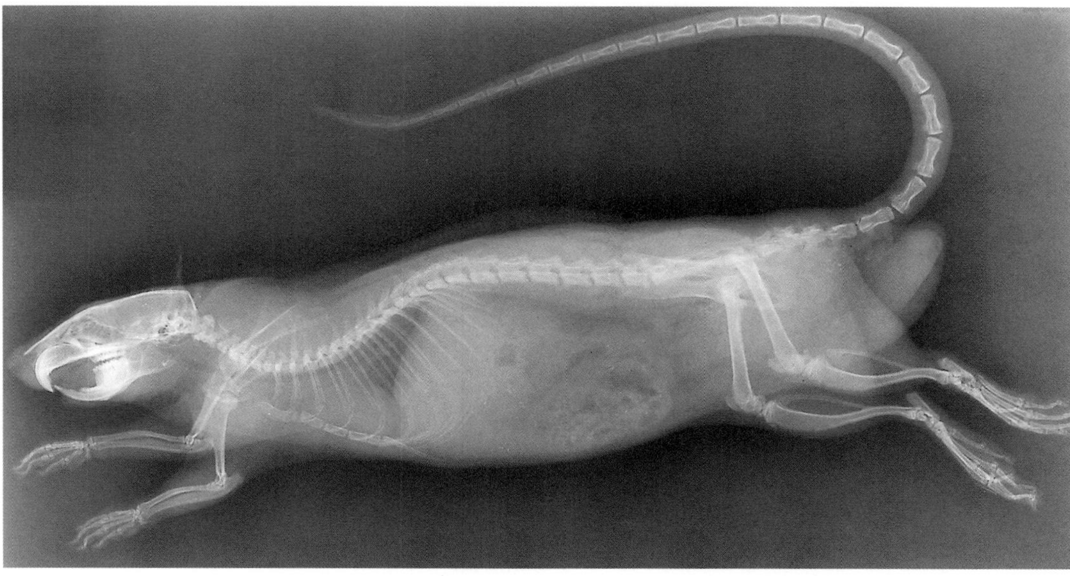

96

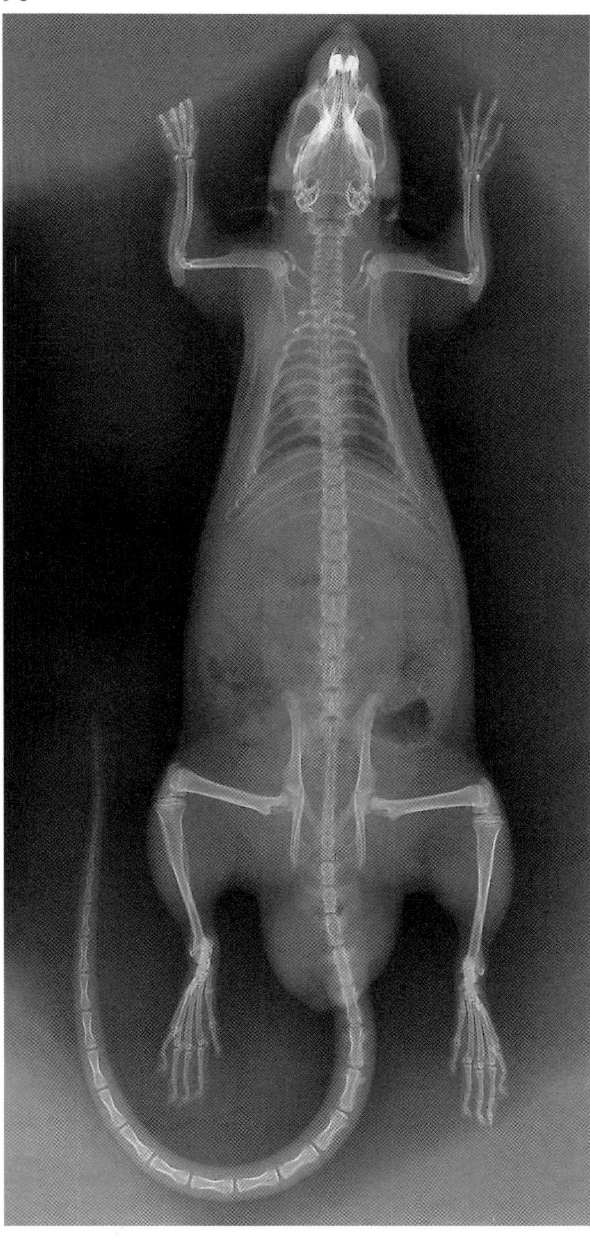

95/96 Normal Radiographic Appearance, lateral and ventrodorsal.

Rat *(Rattus norvegicus)*, male, adult.

In the thorax, the heart and caudal lung lobes can be distinguished. The abdominal organs are clearly defined. The liver is located entirely within the costal region. The kidneys are located directly posterior to the costal arches in a paramedian plane. Food masses are present in the colon and rectum. Small intestinal loops in the ventral abdomen contain gas.

In the caudal abdomen, the testes and fat pads are visible.

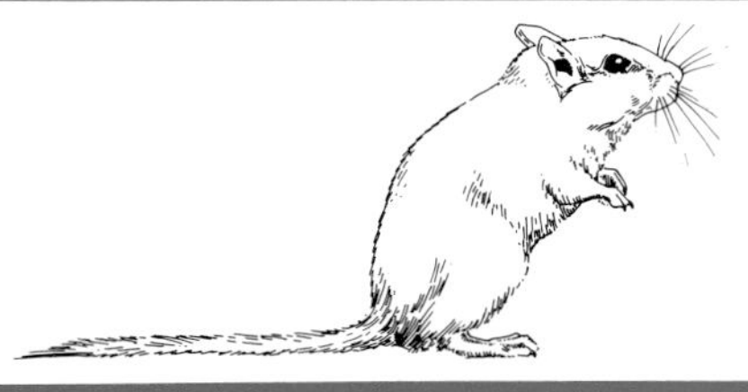

Small Mammals: Gerbil

Radiographic Anatomy

97

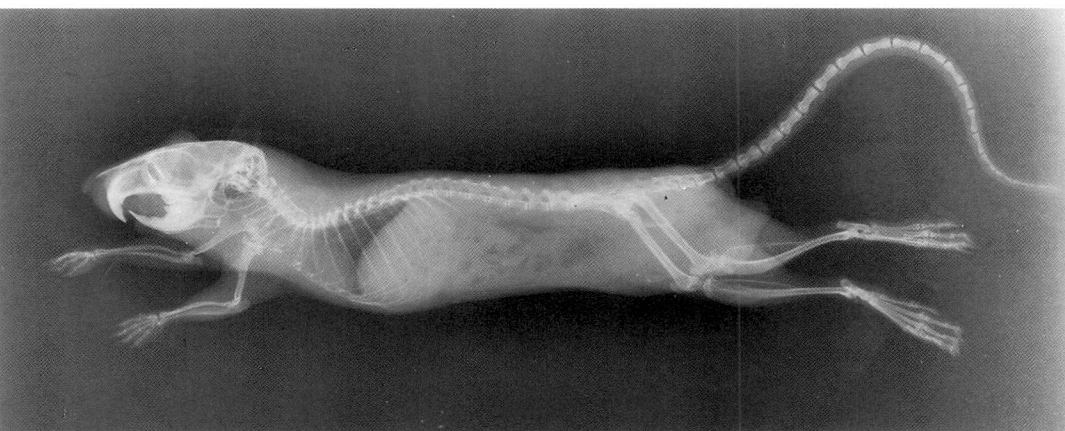

98

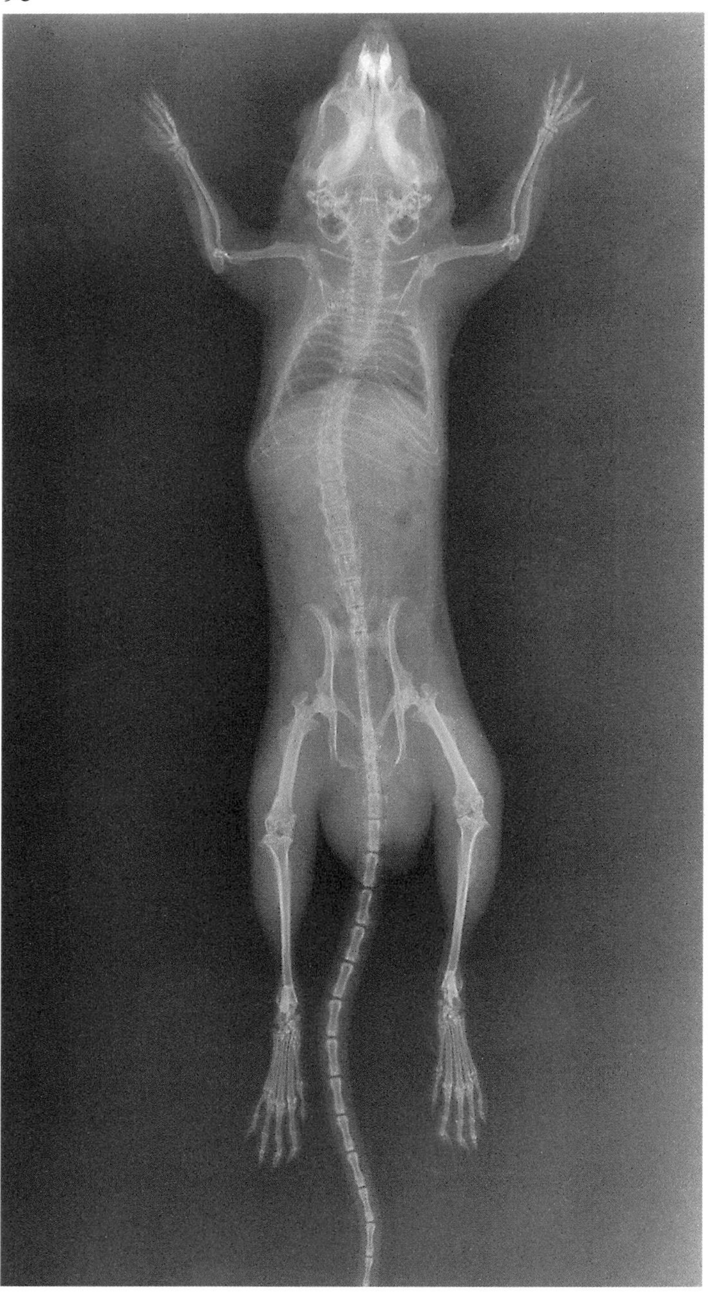

97/98 Normal Radiographic Appearance, lateral and ventrodorsal.

Mongolian Gerbil *(Meriones unguiculatus)*, male, adult.

The thorax is relatively spacious. The liver and gastrointestinal tract show no special features; they are located in the cranial abdomen due to the space-occupying, well-developed scrotal fat pads. These fat pads extend from the os penis to the umbilical region.

Small Mammals: Gerbil

Radiographic Anatomy

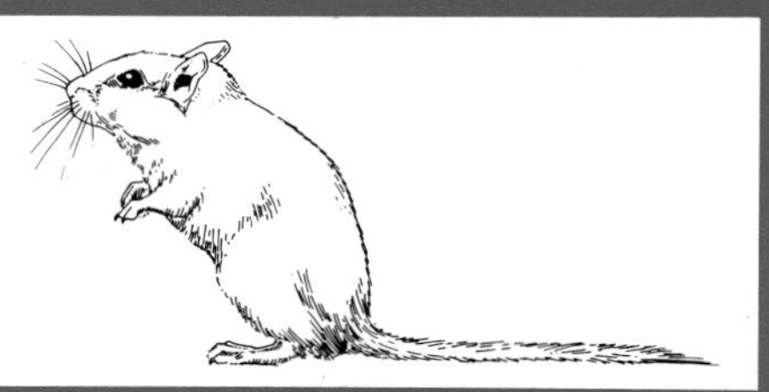

97 A

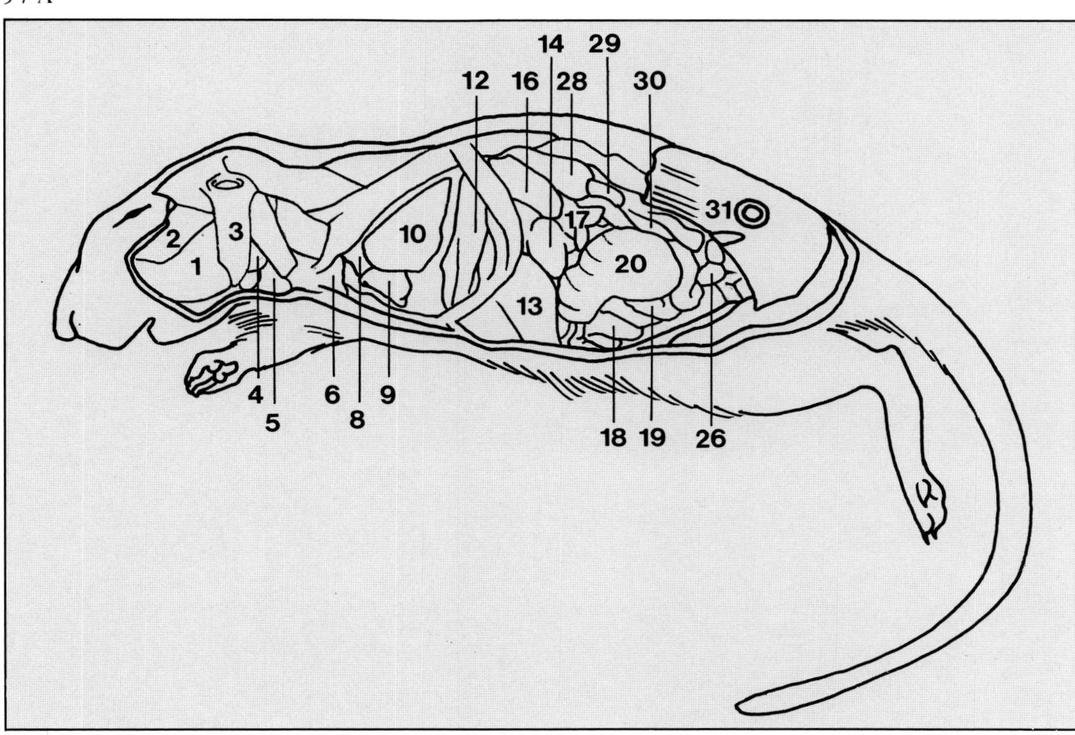

98 A

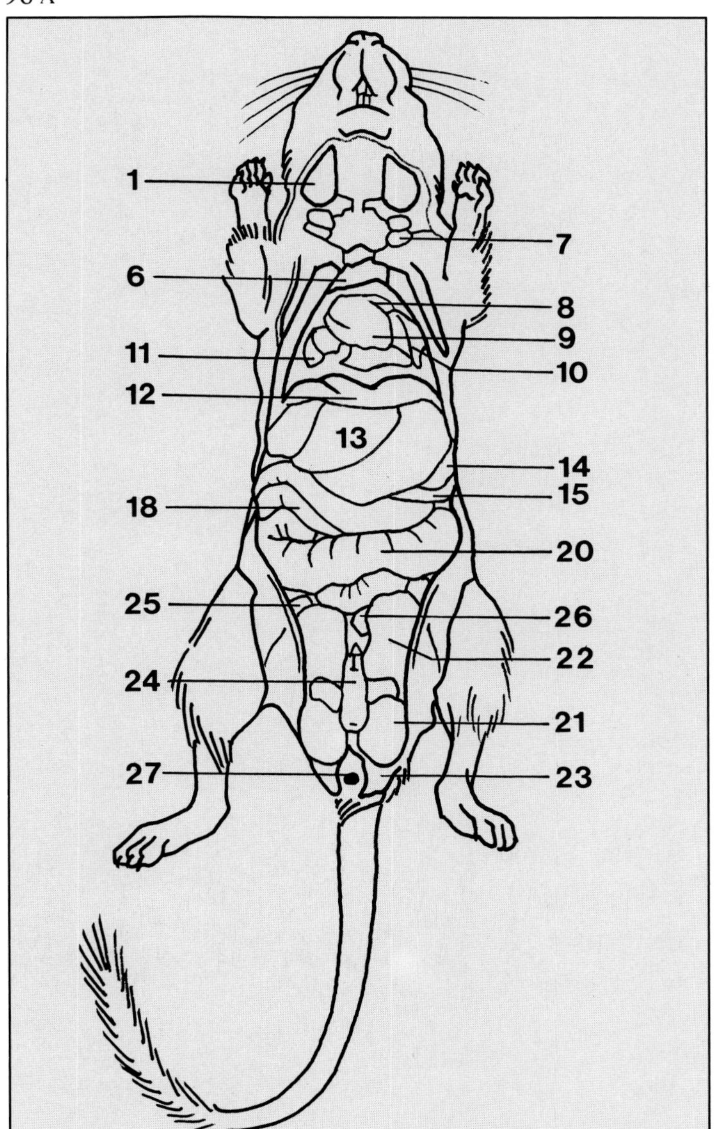

As a guide to the location and size of the organs in the mongolian gerbil, drawings of the anatomy of a female (lateral) and male (ventrodorsal) animal are shown.

97A Anatomical Drawing, lateral.

Mongolian Gerbil *(Meriones unguiculatus)*, female.

M. masseter (**1**); facial nerve (**2**); parotid gland (**3**); mandibular lymph nodes (**4**); mandibular salivary gland (**5**); thymus (**6**); left atrium (**8**); left ventricle (**9**); lungs (**10**); diaphragm (**12**); liver (**13**); stomach (**14**); spleen (**16**); pancreas (**17**); jejunum (**18**); ileum (**19**); cecum (**20**); bladder (**26**); left kidney (**28**); ovary (**29**); uterus (**30**); acetabulum (**31**).

98A Anatomical Drawing, ventrodorsal.

Mongolian Gerbil *(Meriones unguiculatus)*, male.

M. masseter (**1**); thymus (**6**); clavicle (**7**); left auricle (**8**); left ventricle (**9**); left lung (**10**); right lung (**11**); diaphragm (**12**); liver (**13**); stomach (**14**); greater omentum (**15**); jejunum (**18**); cecum (**20**); testes (**21**); fat pad and head of epidymidis (**22**); tail of epidymidis (**23**); penis (**24**); vesicular gland (**25**); bladder (**26**); anus (**27**).

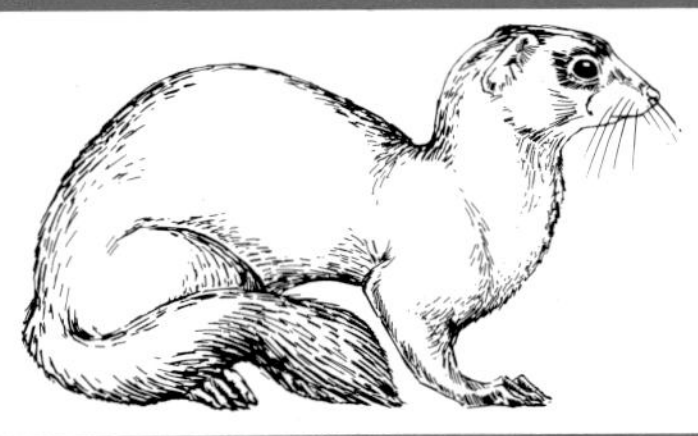

Small Mammals: Ferret

Radiographic Anatomy

99

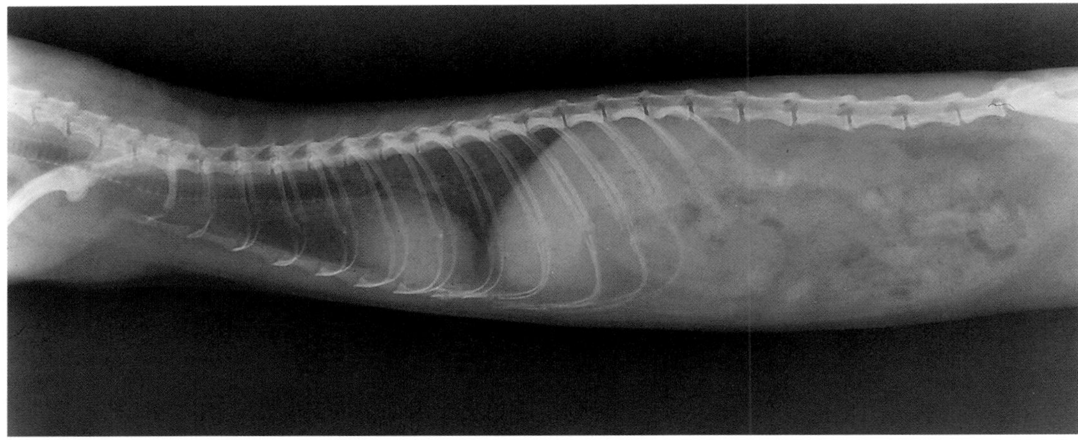

99 A

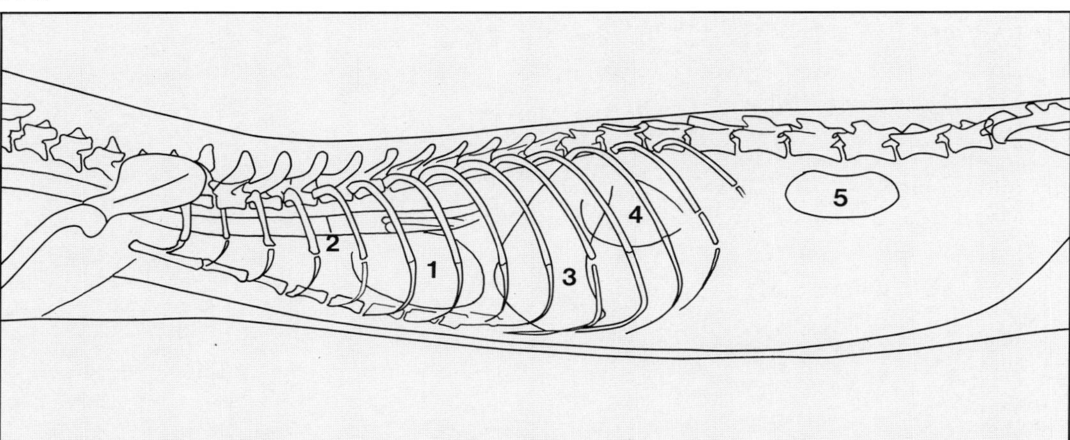

100

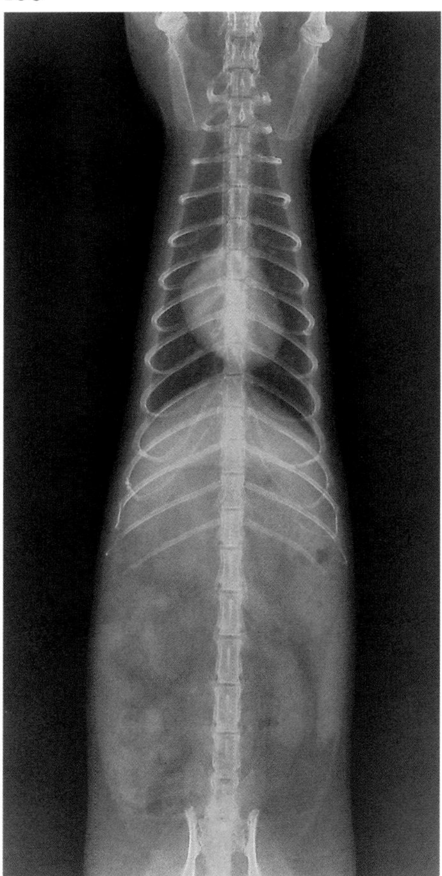

99/99A/100 Normal Radiographic Appearance, lateral and ventrodorsal.

Ferret *(Mustela putorius f. furo)*, female, adult.

In the elongated thorax, the heart (**1**), trachea (**2**) and lungs are clearly defined. The liver (**3**) is demarcated by the food-filled stomach (**4**) and by the diaphragm. The spleen is clearly defined on the left side in the ventrodorsal view. The left kidney (**5**) is present at the level of the third and fourth lumbar vertebrae. The right kidney is visible at the level of the first and third lumbar vertebrae and can only be defined on the ventrodorsal radiograph. Intestinal loops are filled with food.

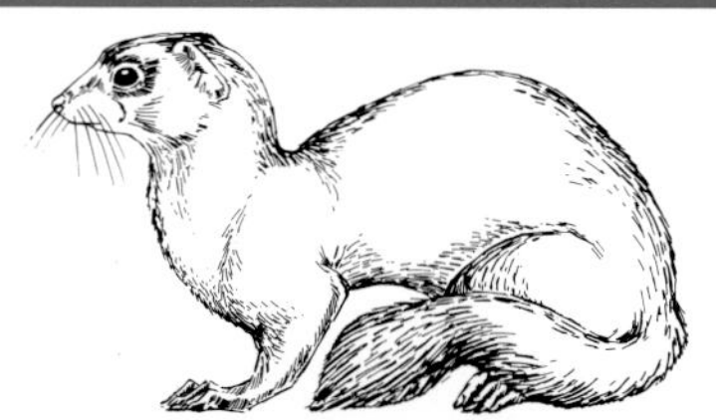

101

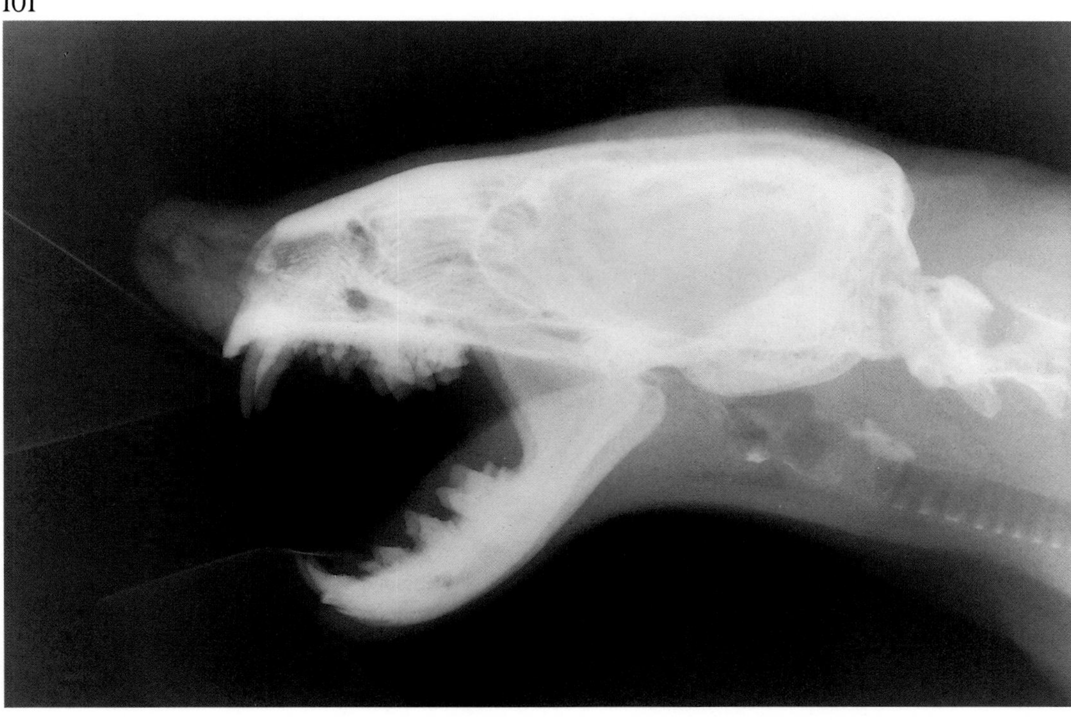

102

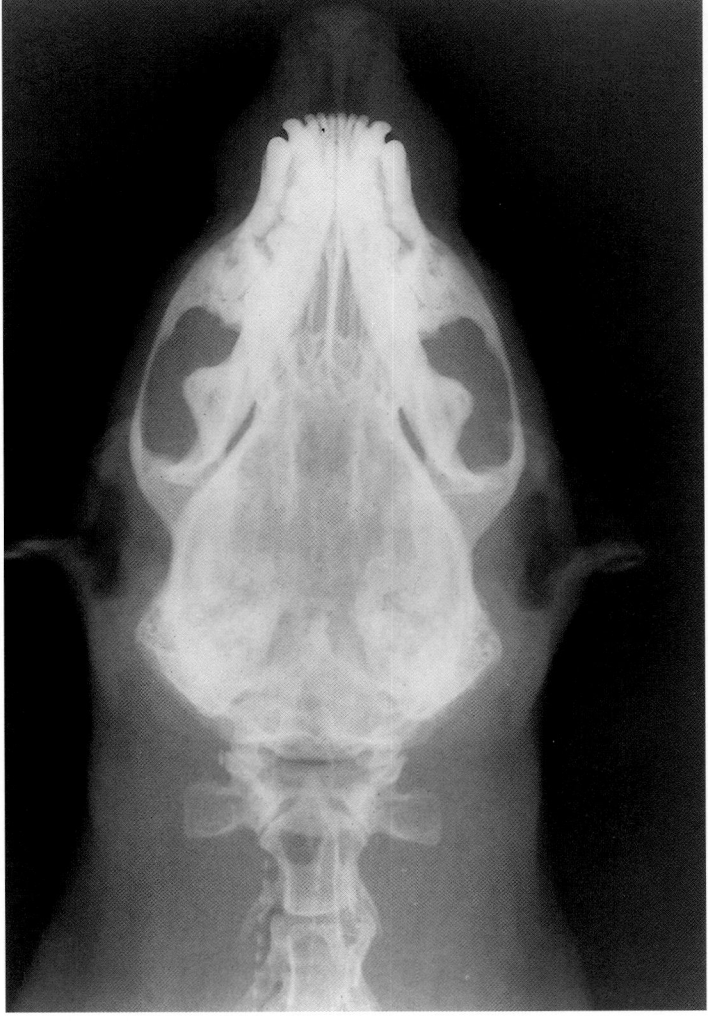

101/102 Skull: Normal Radiographic Appearance, lateral and dorsoventral.

Ferret *(Mustela putorius f. furo)*, female, adult.

The ferret has a short, compact skull, typical of carnivore, with prominent canines and a typical indentation behind the orbital cavity.

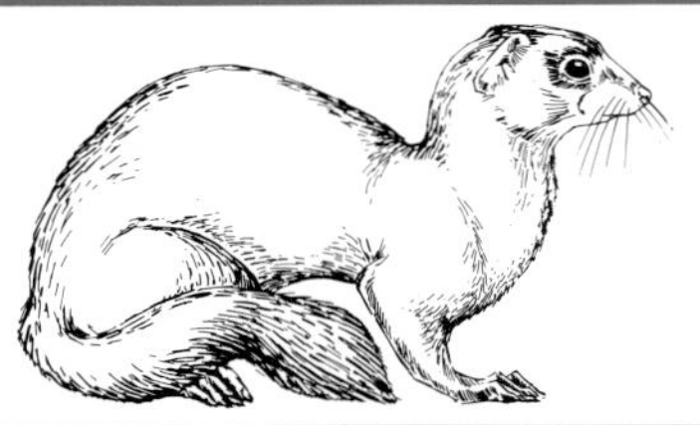

Small Mammals: Ferret

Radiographic Abnormalities

103

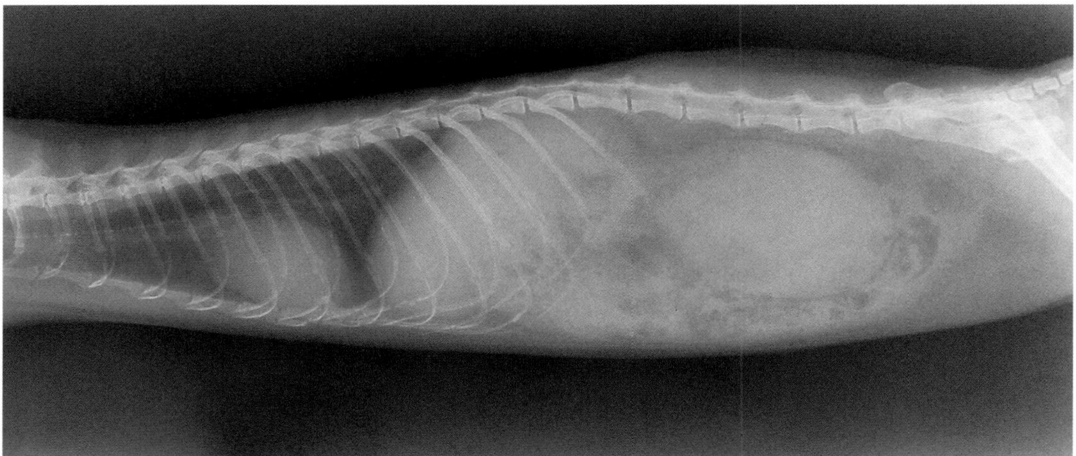

104

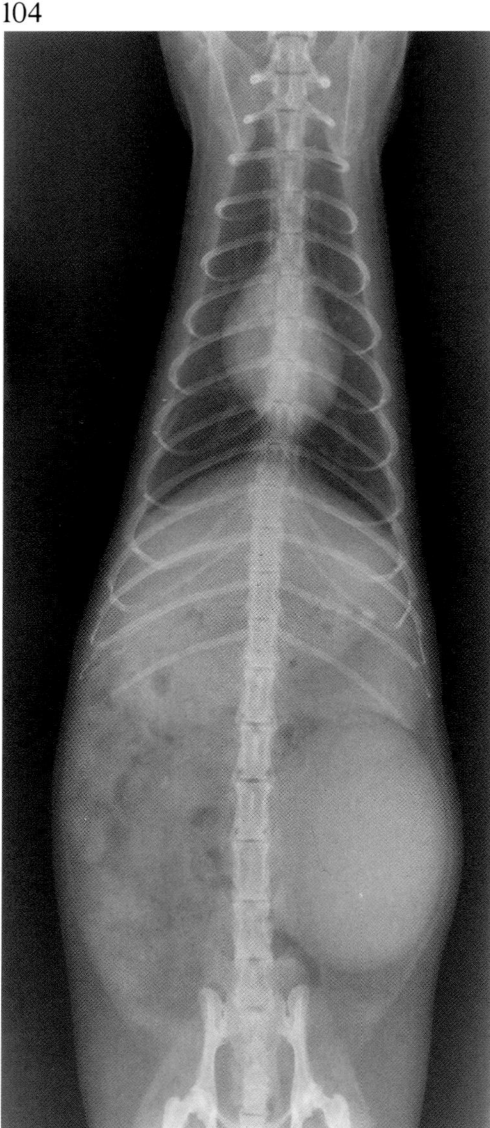

103/104 Perirenal Cyst.

Ferret *(Mustela putorius f. furo)*, female, adult.

A large soft tissue mass is visible on the level of the left kidney. This oval structure is well-defined in all directions.

The structure proved to be a perirenal cyst of the left kidney.

Note: On the ventrodorsal radiograph, the triangular shadow of the spleen is clearly visible between the stomach and the perirenal cyst.

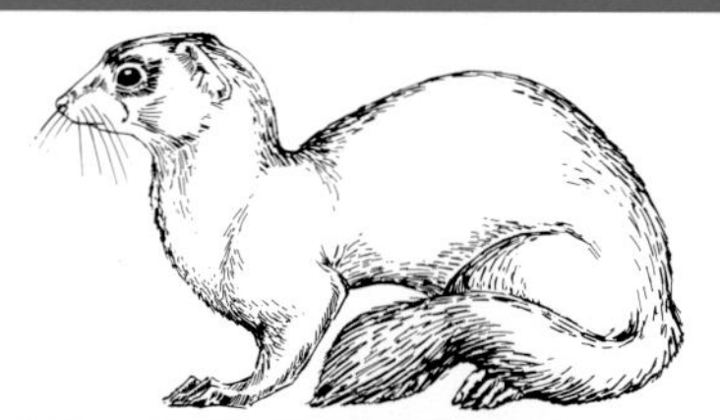

105

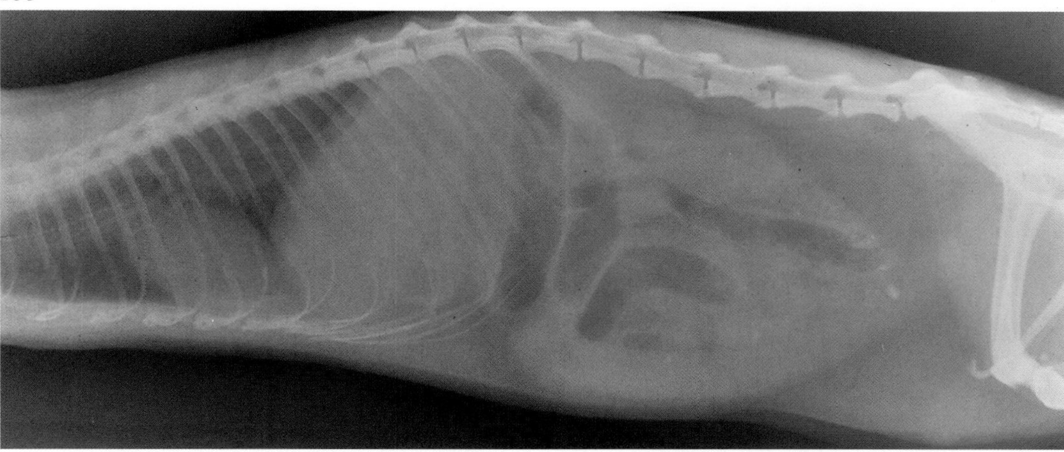

106

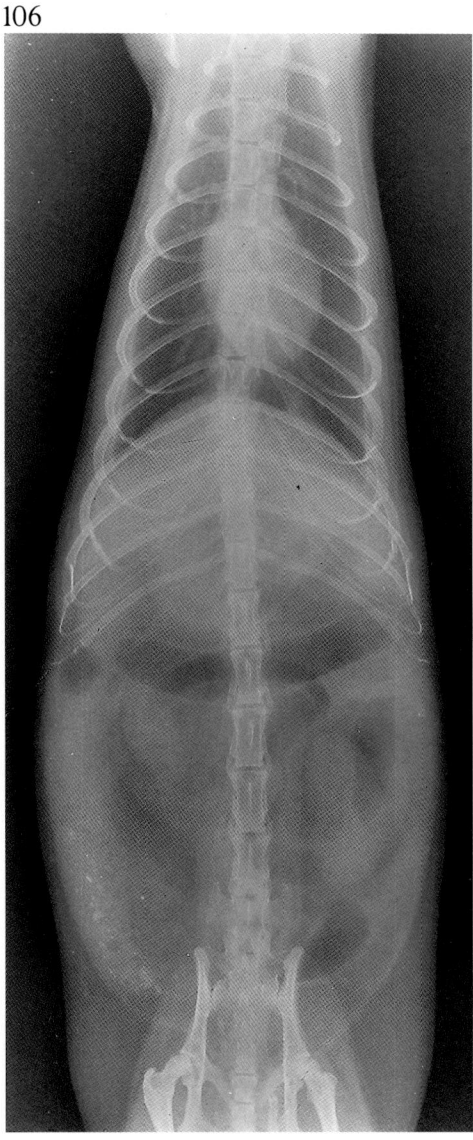

105/106 Ileus.

Ferret *(Mustela putorius f. furo)*, male, adult.

Various small intestinal loops in the mid-abdominal region are distended and gas-filled. There is also lack of definition in the mid-abdomen. These signs are indicative of localized peritonitis and ileus.

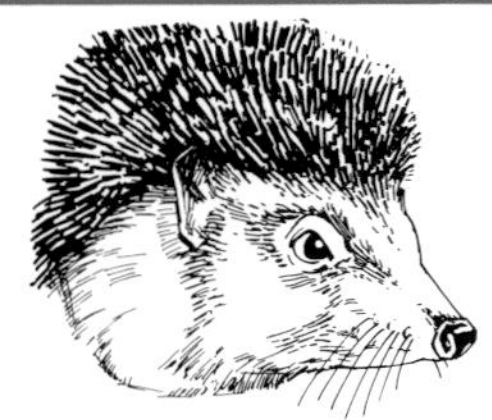

Small Mammals: Hedgehog

Radiographic Anatomy

107

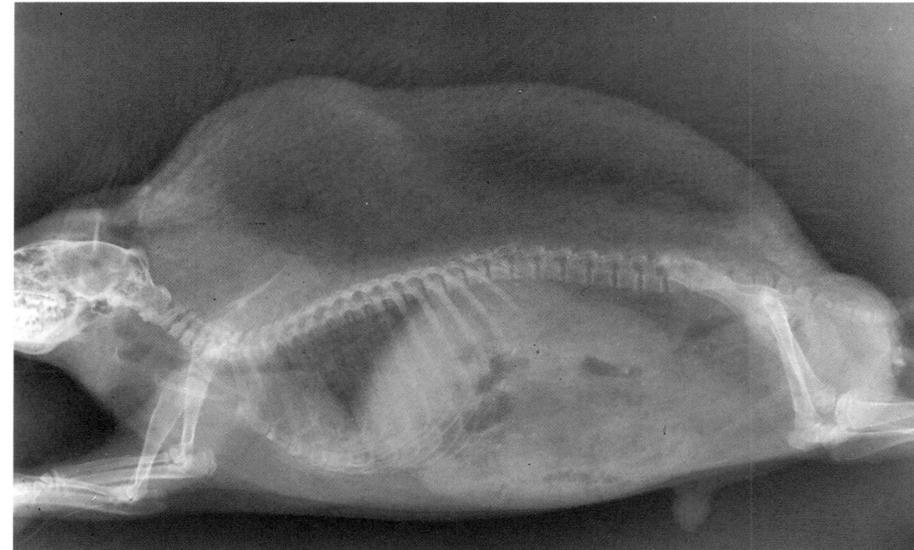

108

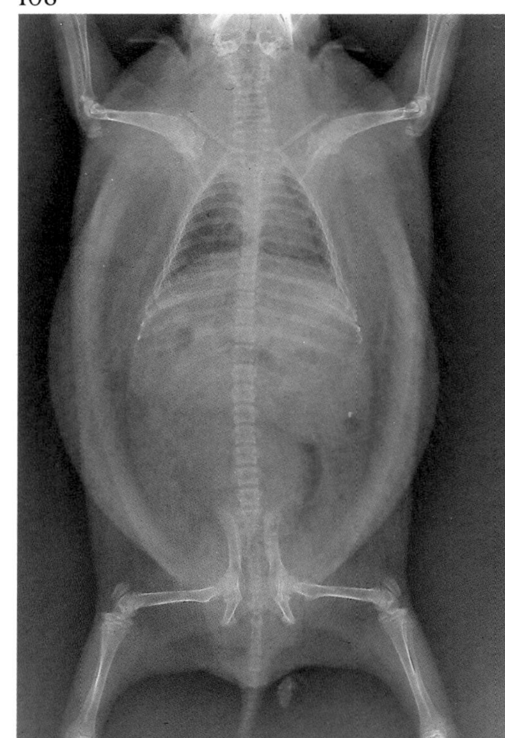

107 A

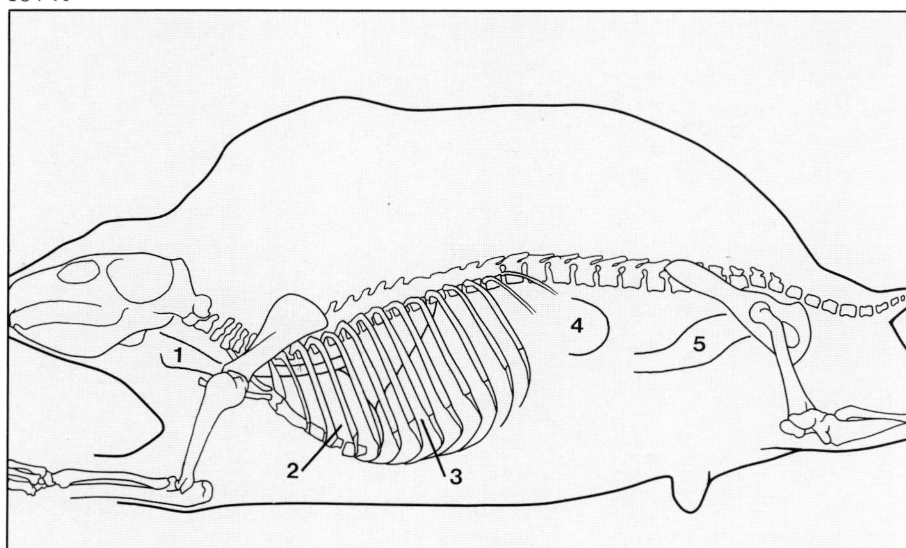

107/107A/108 Normal Radiographic Appearance, lateral and ventrodorsal.

Eurasian Hedgehog *(Erinaceus europaeus)*, male, 1 year.

The pericardial mediastinum encloses the thymus and the heart.

In the lateral projection, various organs such as the trachea (**1**), heart (**2**), liver (**3**), kidney (**4**), a few gas or feces-filled intestinal loops and the rectum (**5**) are visible.

In the ventrodorsal projection, differentiation between individual organs is more difficult due to superimposition of the muscle packets of the orbicular muscles, the cutis and the spines.

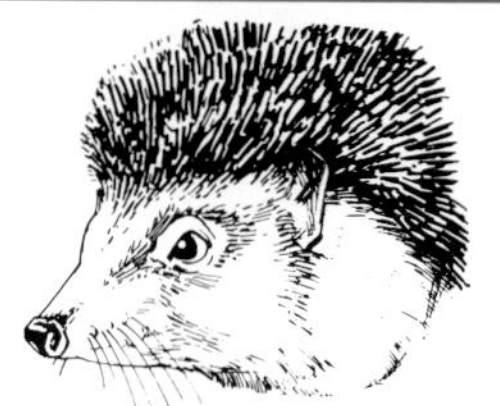

109

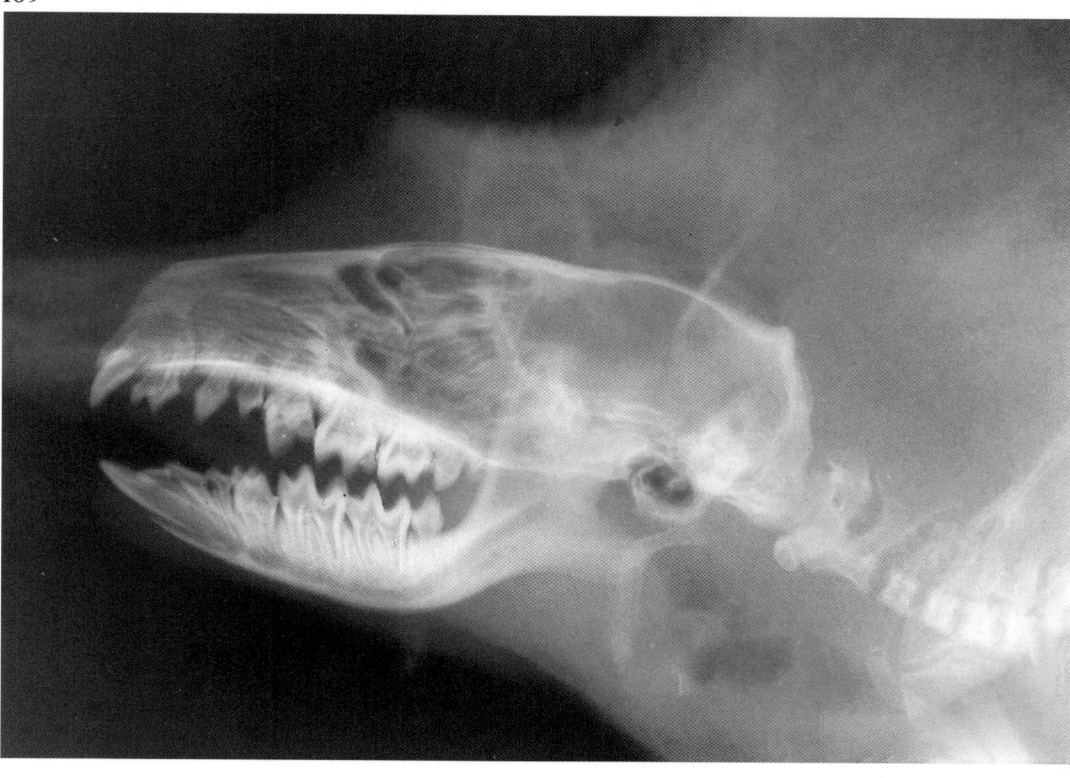

110

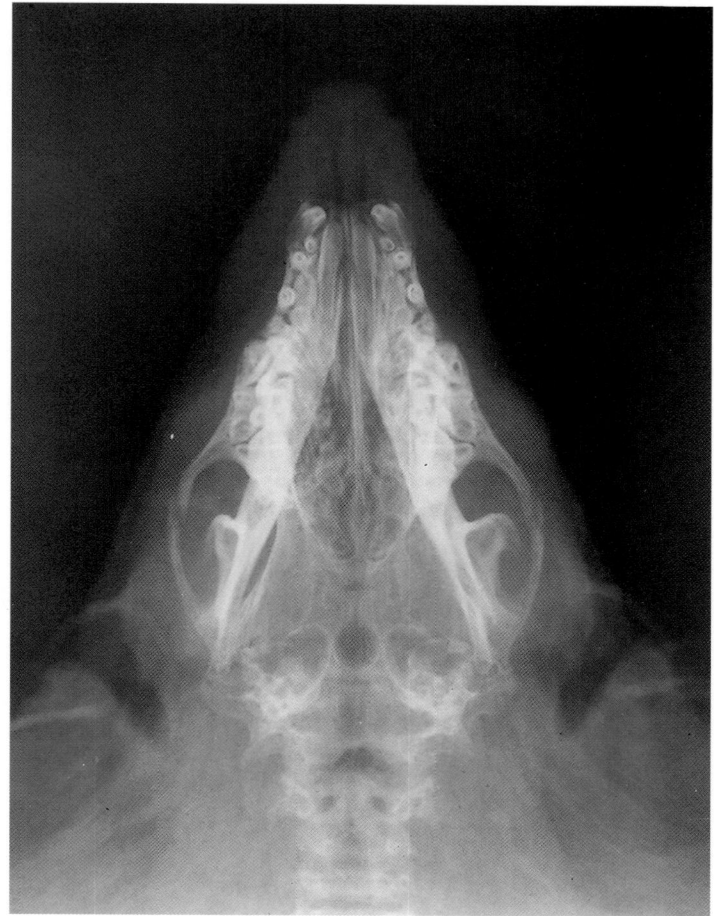

109/110 Skull: Normal Radiographic Appearance, lateral and dorsoventral.

Eurasian Hedgehog *(Erinaceus europaeus)*, adult.

The skull is typical of an insectivore: it is broad and powerful with pronounced cheek bones. This radiograph shows the teeth soon after the secondary dentition.

Note: The secondary dentition is complete within a year. In older animals, the teeth are worn down at a comparatively early age.

Contents

Birds

Radiographic Technique	76
Psittacines:	
Radiographic Anatomy	
Internal Organs	80
Contrast Radiography of the Alimentary Tract	82
Appendicular Skeleton	83
Skull	84
Radiographic Abnormalities	
Skull	86
Appendicular Skeleton	90
Lungs	94
Air Sacs	98
Heart and Vessels	102
Esophagus and Proventriculus	104
Ventriculus	106
Intestine	108
Cloaca	110
Liver	112
Spleen	114
Kidneys	116
Genital Organs	120
Miscellaneous	124
Contrast Radiography of the Alimentary Tract	126
Raptors:	
Radiographic Anatomy	
Internal Organs	138
Contrast Radiography of the Alimentary Tract	140
Axial Skeleton	142
Appendicular Skeleton	144
Skull	146
Radiographic Abnormalities	
Skull	147
Appendicular Skeleton	148
Miscellaneous	150
Woodcock/Raptors:	
Radiographic Abnormalities	
Miscellaneous	153
Hill-Mynah:	
Radiographic Anatomy	154
Radiographic Abnormalities	156
Pigeon:	
Radiographic Anatomy	
Internal Organs	158
Contrast Radiography of the Alimentary Tract	159
Radiographic Abnormalities	160
Fowl:	
Radiographic Anatomy	164
Radiographic Abnormalities	165
Waterfowl:	
Radiographic Anatomy	166
Radiographic Abnormalities	168
Long-legged Birds:	
Radiographic Anatomy	170
Radiographic Abnormalities	172

A

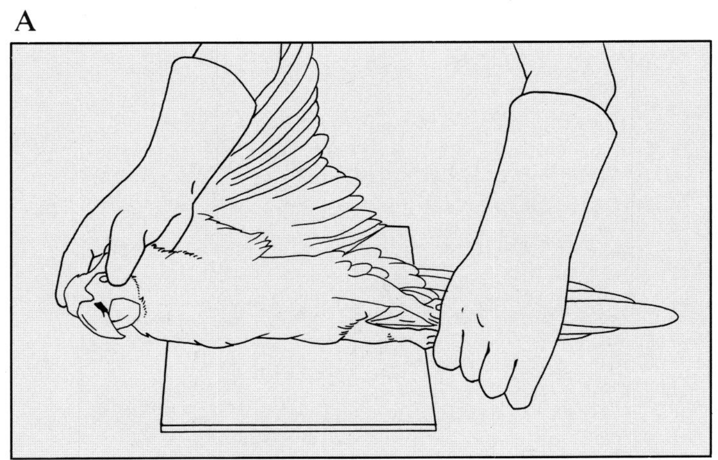

B

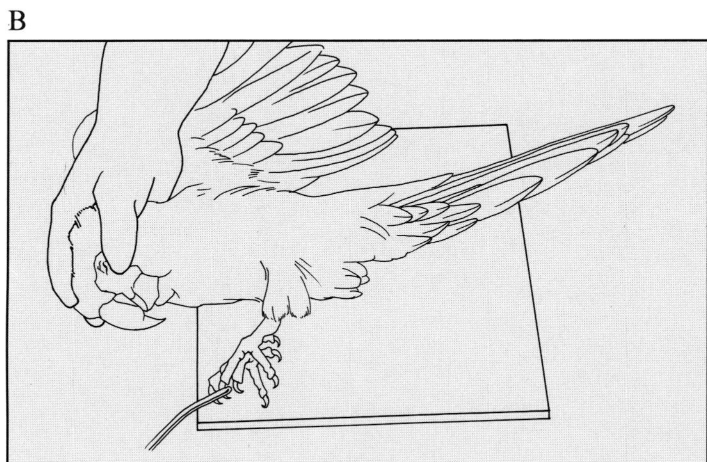

Introduction

Radiographic techniques in birds have given a new dimension to avian medicine. Most celomic organs are surrounded by air sacs providing excellent natural contrast. In small birds, where other diagnostics are limited, radiology can contribute important diagnostic information.

If the procedure is well organized and if the bird is handled competently, a radiographic investigation does not inflict any more stress upon the bird than general physical examination.

Preparation of the Avian Patient for Radiographic Examination

To prevent unwanted motion blurring of the radiograph or accidental induction of trauma to the restive patient, it is advisable to sedate the birds either by injecting diazepam or ketamine-HCl or by inhalation anesthesia with isoflurane, halothane or methoxyflurane. This is especially true for very active birds or for birds that will undergo a prolonged investigation. Chemically immobilized birds can be positioned directly on the cassette using radiolucent adhesive tape (FIG. **D** and **E**, see p. 78). If several views in the same projection are scheduled birds are fixated on a radiolucent plexiglass-plate. Birds with a filled proventriculus or ventriculus as well as birds that are scheduled for a contrast study should go without food for several hours before radiographic examination.

Note: Unstable, weak birds must be stabilized prior to the investigation.

Positioning

If the bird is held manually, one hand grasps the head from the back, holding the mandibular articulation between thumb and middle finger. The other hand takes the feet and carefully extends the legs fully.

For the lateral view (FIG. **A**), the bird is positioned on its right side to obtain radiographs that are consistent and comparable between individuals. Both wings are hyperextended over the back. The legs can be stretched caudally or cranially, depending on whether the cranial or caudal celomic cavity has to be evaluated. Suspected disorders of the cloaca and masses or eggs in this region can better be evaluated by pulling the legs cranioventrally (FIG. **B**). In this way, the organs of interest are not superimposed.

For the ventrodorsal view (FIG. **C**), the bird is positioned on its back with its wings slightly extended and held down by adhesive tape (FIG. **D** and **E**) or lead gloves.

By turning the body slightly away from the wing under investigation, an unobstructed view of the scapula can be obtained. Comparison of the abnormal wing with the opposite normal wing is very helpful for diagnosis. Sedated birds are positioned in the same manner as the ones that are held manually. They are restrained with adhesive tape.

C

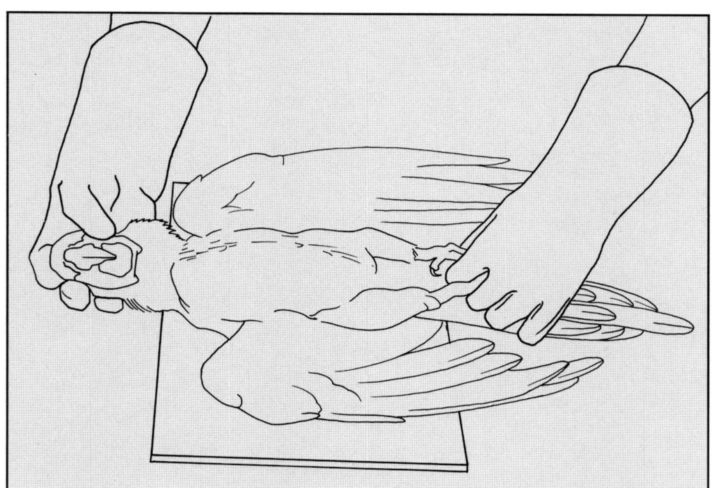

For radiographic examination of the limbs, the hind legs are stretched and pulled away from the body to avoid unwanted superimposition of the pelvic region.

A minimum of four views is needed for the radiographic evaluation of the avian skull: a lateral view, a ventrodorsal view, and one left and one right oblique view (FIG. **6A** till **8A**). For the lateral view, the beak is supported by a radiolucent sponge to keep the sagittal plane of the skull parallel to the X-ray cassette. The X-ray beam is centered at the caudal border of the orbit. For the ventrodorsal view, the neck is slightly hyperextended and the beak is taped to the cassette. This keeps the bony palate parallel to the cassette. Oblique ventrodorsal views are taken with the bird in dorsal recumbency: the head is rotated 15 degrees around its long axis to either side.

D

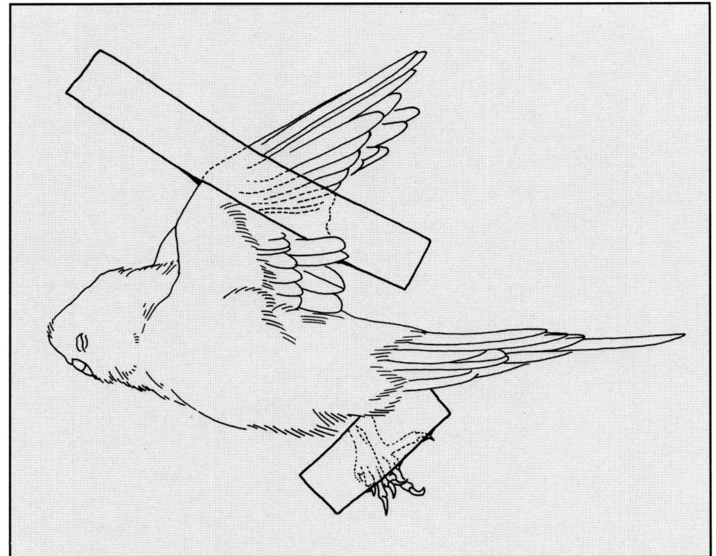

E

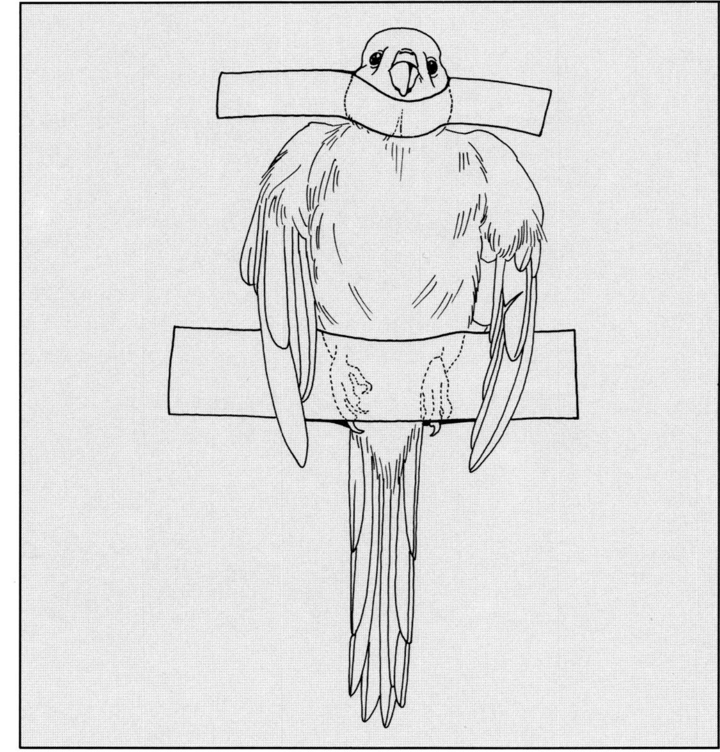

Radiographic Contrast Studies

As with mammals, positive-contrast studies such as gastrointestinal studies, angiography, urography and lymphography can be performed. The last three procedures have no great diagnostic significance and are not shown in this atlas. The crop can also be visualized by administration of air. Gastrointestinal studies with barium sulfate are very helpful diagnostic methods in birds and are easily performed. To fill the gastrointestinal tract, 25 ml/kg body weight of a barium sulfate suspension is instilled into the crop with a rigid stomach tube (FIG. **F**). The gastrointestinal contrast studies are also used to determine position and size of liver, urogenital organs, and to delineate suspected masses in the celomic cavity such as tumors. Radiographs are taken two and a half hours after the barium sulfate administration, when the entire gastrointestinal tract is filled with the contrast medium.

F

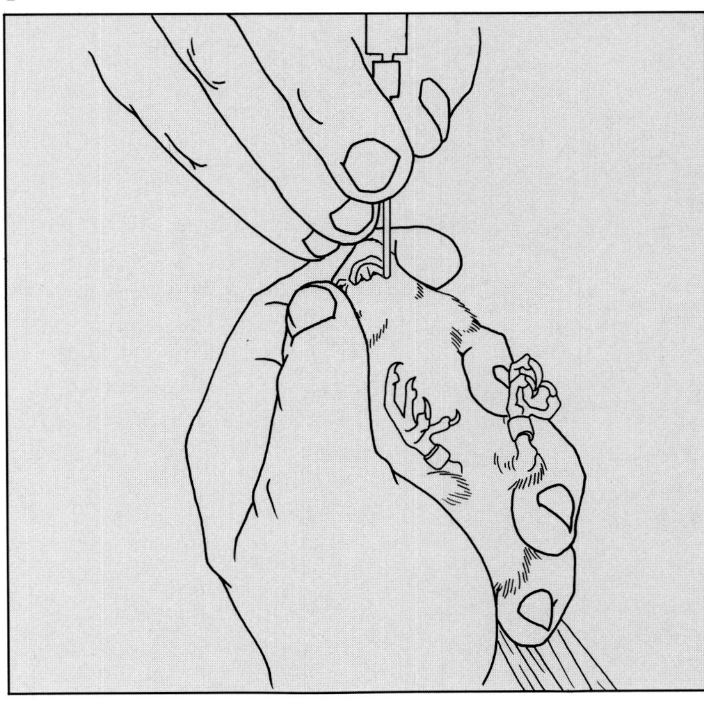

1

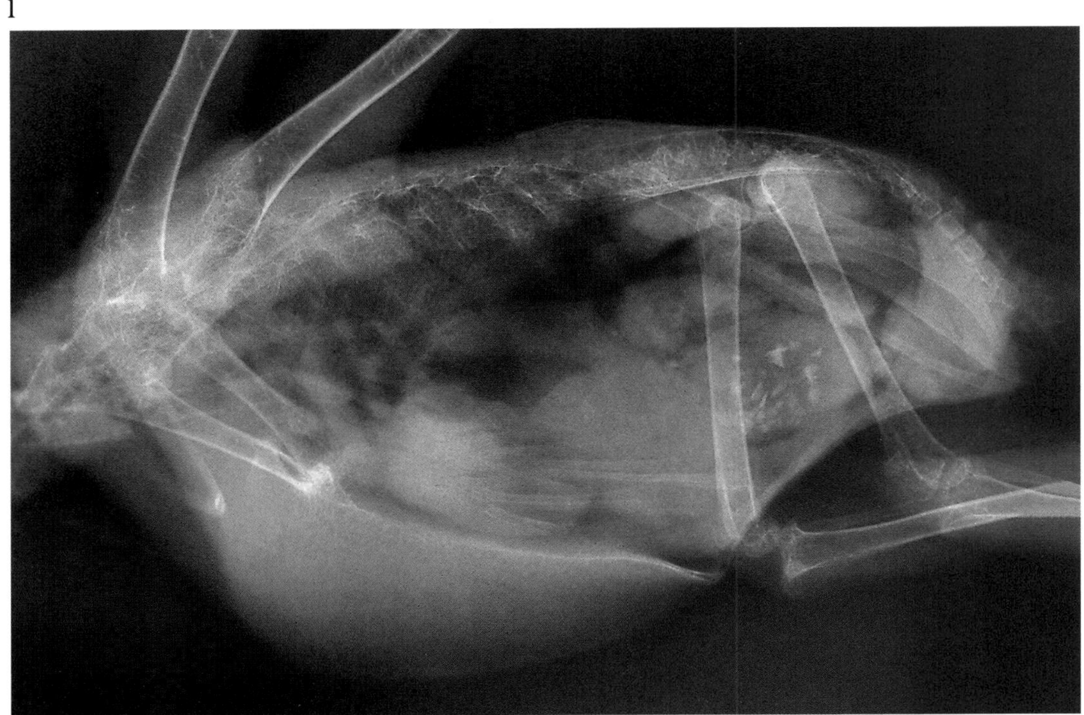

1 A

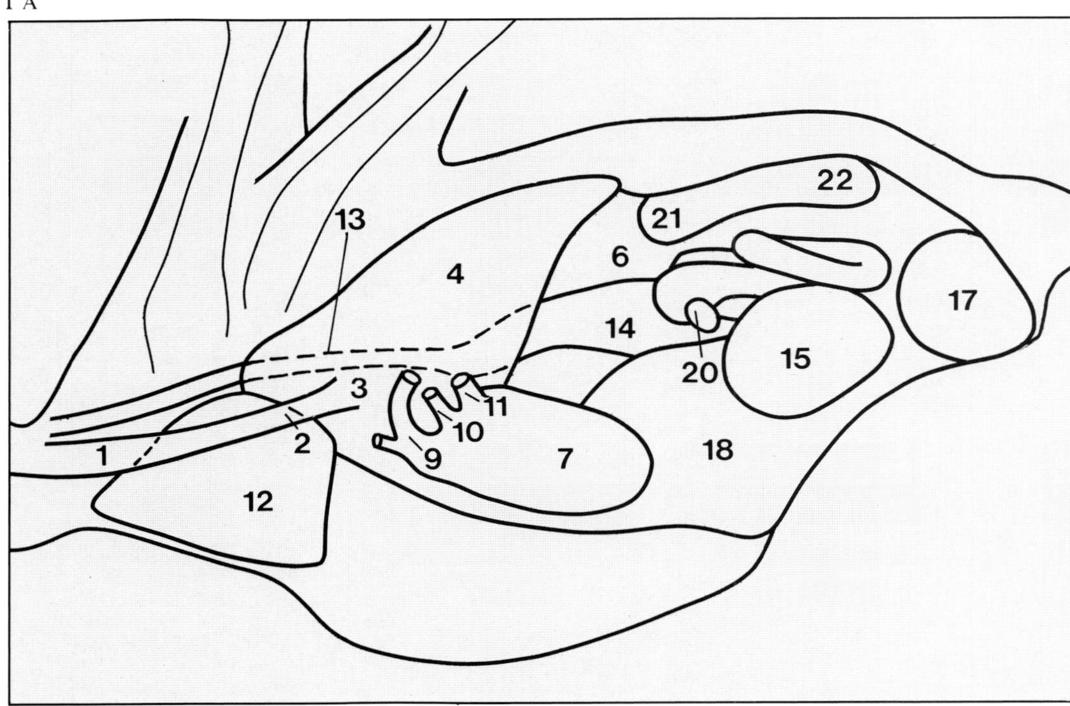

1/1A/2/2A Internal Organs: Normal Radiographic Appearance, lateral and ventrodorsal.

Lesser Sulfur-Crested Cockatoo *(Cacatua sulphurea),* adult.

Respiratory Organs

The trachea (**1**) follows the right side of the cervical spine, from the mandible to the syrinx, getting smaller at the celomic entrance (**2**). In the ventrodorsal projection, the syrinx, (**3**) located craniodorsal to the base of the heart, is superimposed by the sternum. On the lateral radiograph, it can easily be recognized in older birds by the calcified cartilage or in a singing or speaking bird by the large muscles around the syrinx. The lungs are attached to the thoracic wall and their volume remains unchanged during the respiratory cycle. The central parts of the lungs and the bronchi can best be examined on the lateral radiograph. The lungs (**4**) have a reticular pattern. Because of superimposition, the caudal limits of the lungs are difficult to evaluate. The radiolucencies of the clavicular air sacs (**5**) can be recognized in the axillary region. The borders of the different air sacs and the air sac walls between the two thoracic and abdominal air sacs on each side are usually not recognizable. Only in the lateral projection, the air sac walls can be seen as fine linear densities cranial to the kidney lobe. In the ventrodorsal projection, the air sacs (**6**) on both sides of the hourglass-shaped composite shadow of the heart, liver and gastrointestinal tract, can be easily compared and examined.

Heart and Vessels

On the ventrodorsal radiograph, the cardiac shadow (**7**) forms the cranial portion of the hourglass-shaped density located between the air sacs. It blends into the homogeneous soft tissue shadow of the bilobed liver and parts of the gastrointestinal tract. On the lateral radiograph, the heart can sometimes be evaluated without superimposition of the liver.

On the ventrodorsal radiograph, the right-sided aortic arch (**8**) is visible as a prominent round shadow. Sometimes, also the pulmonary arteries (**10**) can be seen. On the lateral radiograph, the ascending aorta (**9**) and aortic arch (**8**) are visible. Also, the pulmonic arteries (**10**) and caudal vena cava (**11**) can be recognized.

Birds: Psittacines

Radiographic Anatomy
Internal Organs

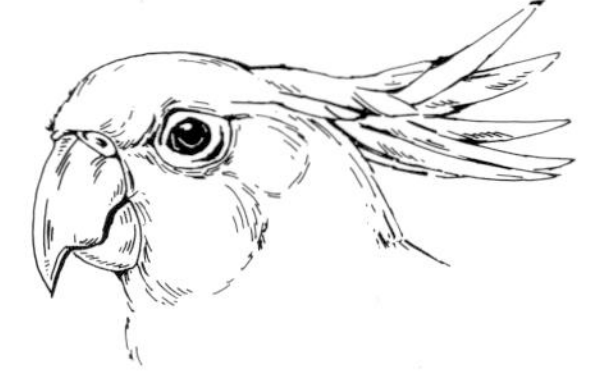

2

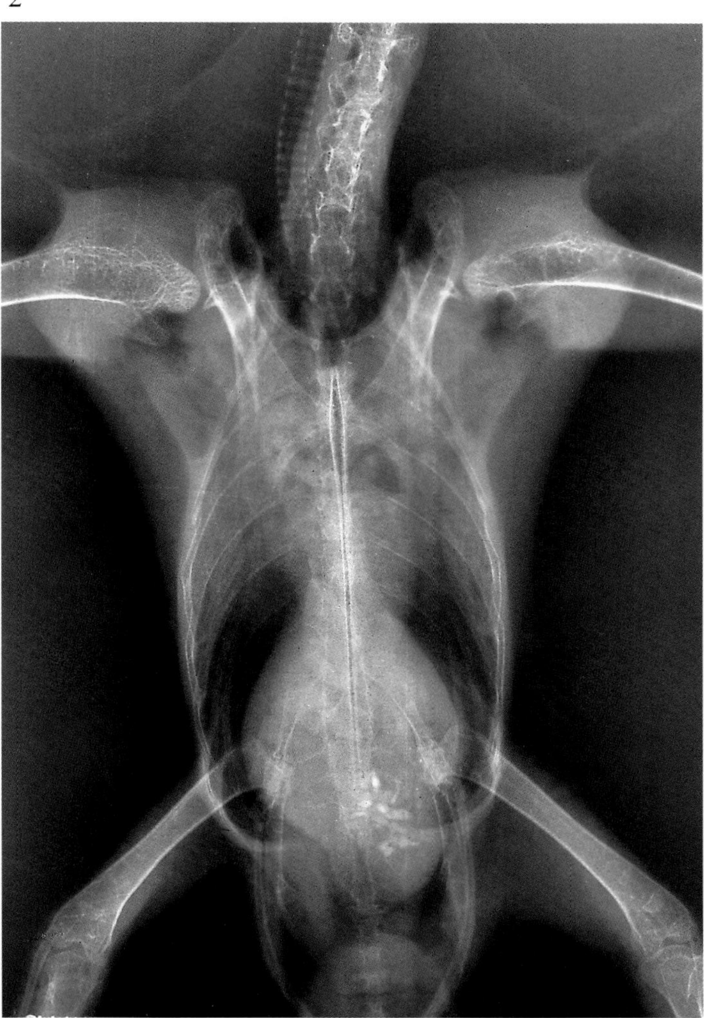

2A

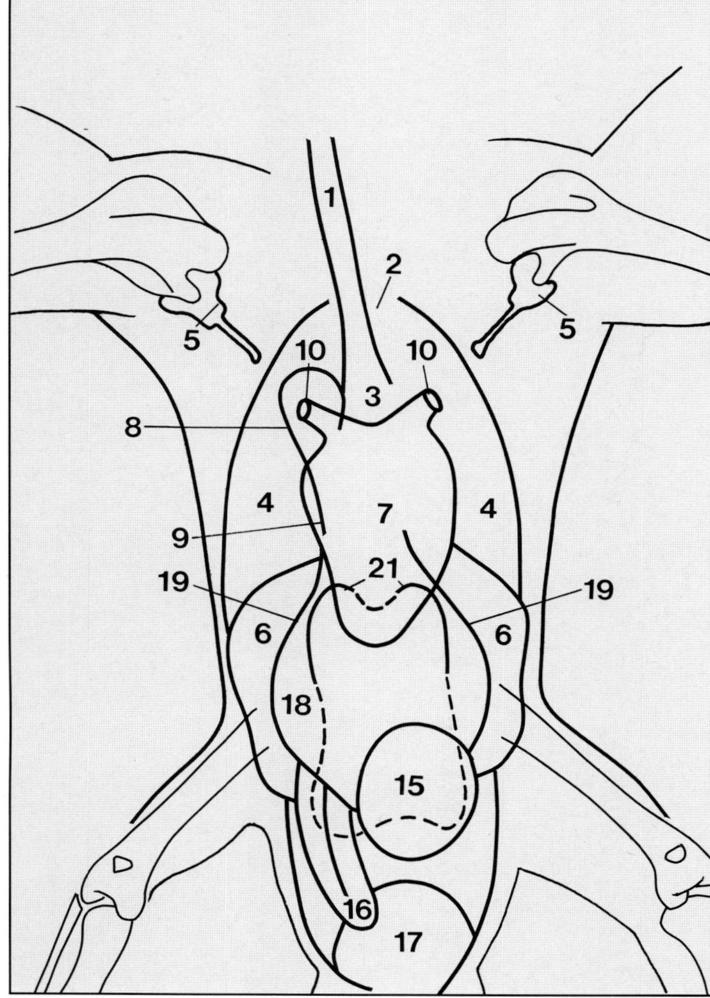

Gastrointestinal Tract

The crop (**12**) is lying for the better part to the right of the spine and can only be recognized by its contents (food, gas or contrast medium). On the lateral radiograph, both the esophagus (**13**) that crosses the lung shadow and the proventriculus (**14**) are recognizable as separate structures due to the negative contrast of the air sacs. On the ventrodorsal radiograph, esophagus and proventriculus are superimposed. The slightly oval ventriculus (**15**) can easily be spotted due to the presence of gravel. It is positioned on the left side. It is usually impossible to recognize individual segments of the intestinal tract. The duodenal loop (**16**), as an exception, is often seen on the ventrodorsal radiograph in the right celom. The intestines are displayed as a mass of mixed density and are superimposed by the liver and other organs. The cloaca (**17**) can be recognized as an oval shadow in the caudal celom.

Liver

On the lateral radiograph, the liver shadow (**18**) is fused with the cardiac and ventricular shadows. On the ventrodorsal radiograph, the craniolateral liver borders (**19**) are sharply outlined by the negative contrast of the air sacs. The caudal parts blend into the gastrointestinal viscera and cannot be recognized separately.

Spleen

On a good lateral radiograph, the spleen (**20**) is visible as a small spheric structure, located dorsal to the angle formed by liver and ventriculus.

Kidneys

On the ventrodorsal radiograph, the kidneys are superimposed by the gastrointestinal viscera. Only the two cranial lobes (**21**) can be recognized as superimposed semicircular densities. On the lateral radiograph, the cranial lobes (**21**) of the bean-shaped kidneys (**22**) extend into the radiolucent air sacs.

Genital Organs

Testes and ovary can be seen only in some species and then exclusively during the breeding season, when size reaches its maximum. They are located in the dorsal part of the celom between the lungs and kidneys, and are attached ventral to the cranial lobes of the kidneys. The oviduct is difficult to differentiate from the intestines.

3

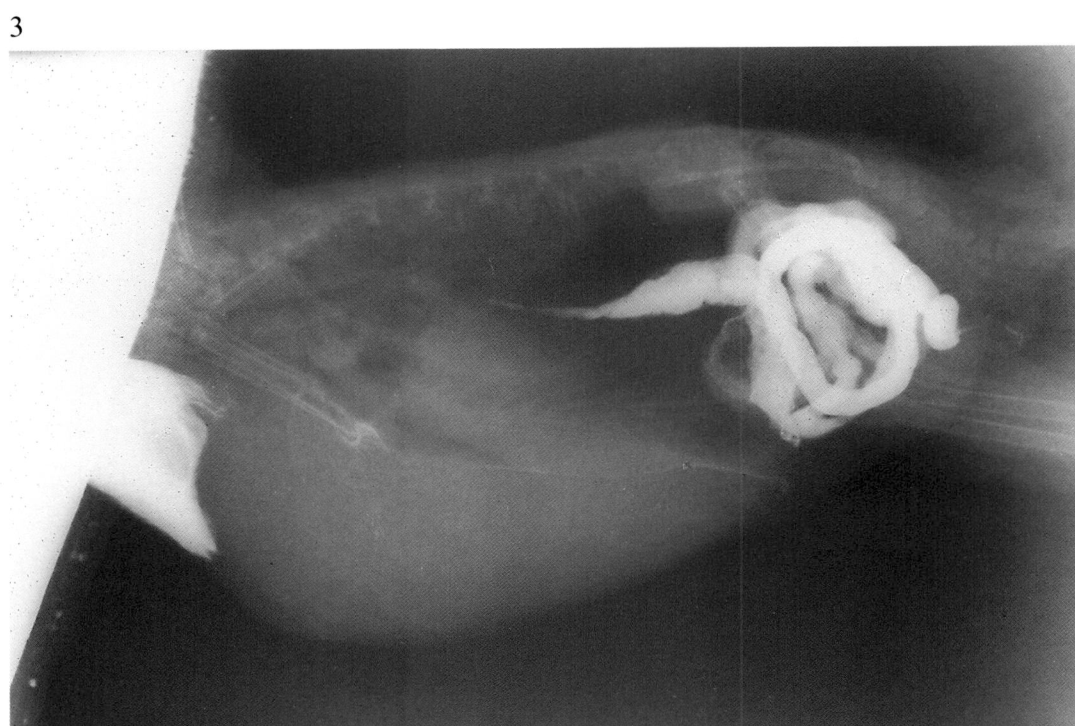

4

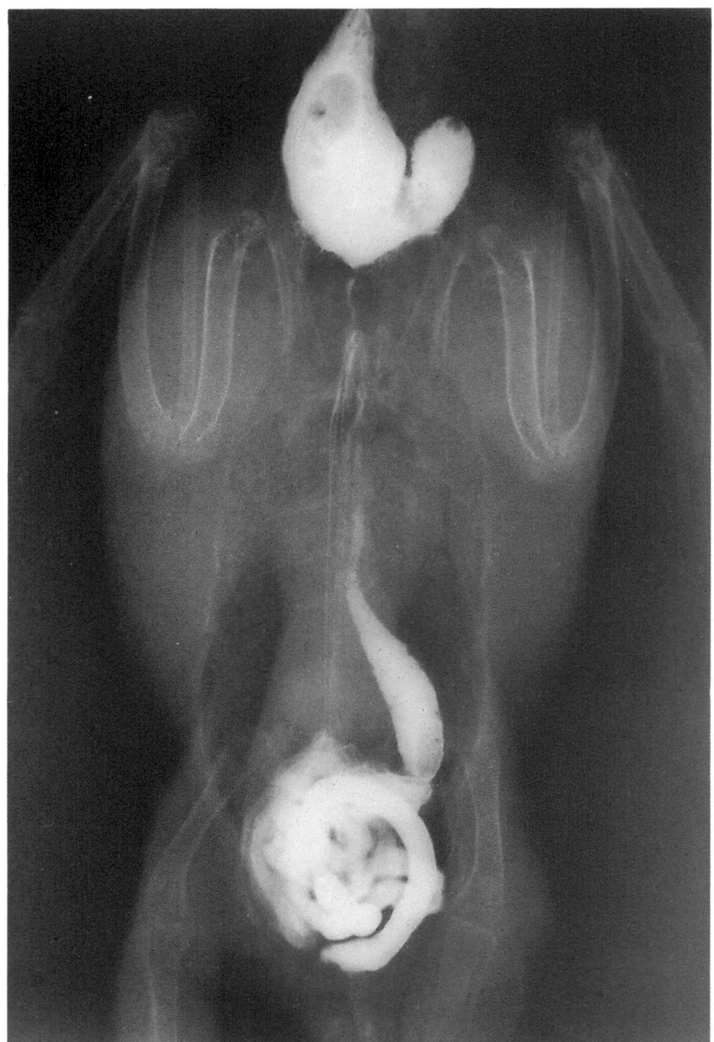

3/4 Normal Radiographic Appearance,
lateral and ventrodorsal: contrast study.

Budgerigar *(Melopsittacus undulatus)*, male, 3 years.

Radiographs were made 2$^1/_2$ h following administration of the barium sulfate contrast medium. The gastrointestinal tract can be evaluated to its full extent.

Note: In the budgerigar, the visceral organs occupy a larger part of the celom than in large psittacines. This reduces the size of the air sacs especially on the lateral radiograph.

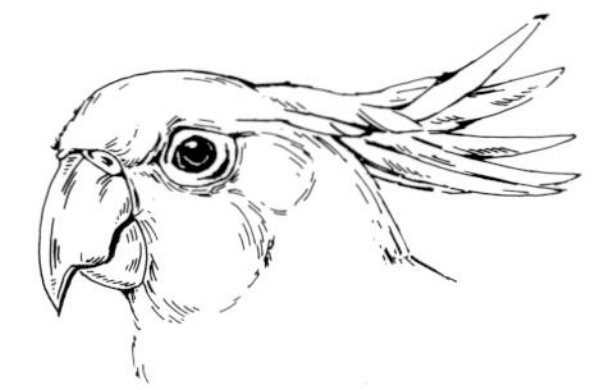

5-1

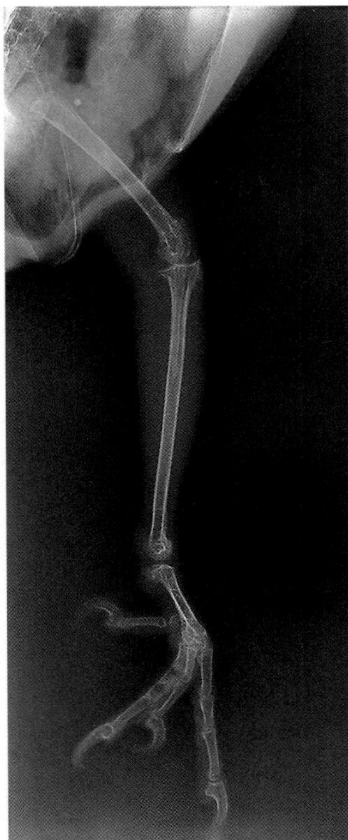

5-1 A

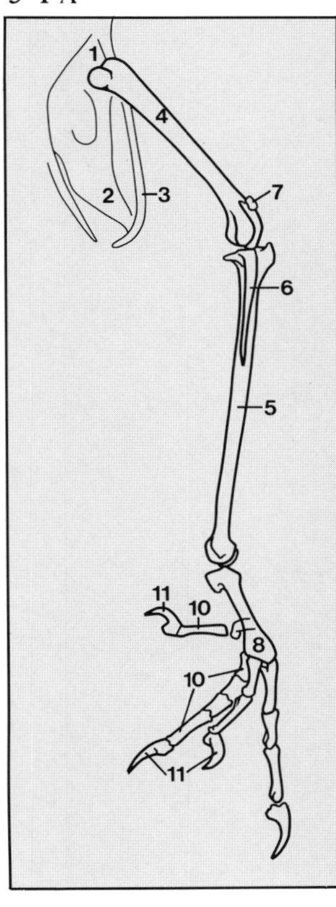

5-2

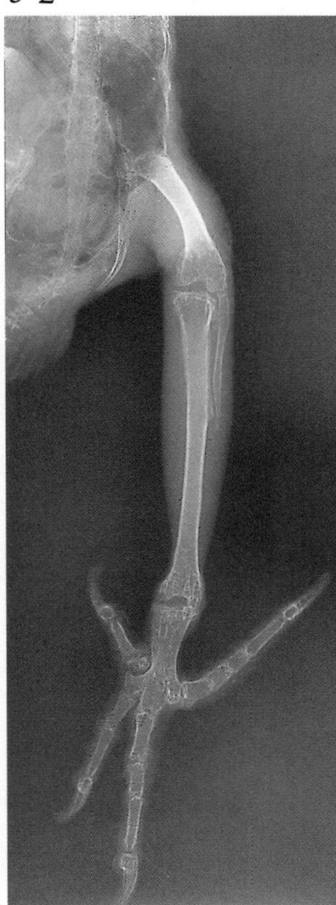

5-2 A

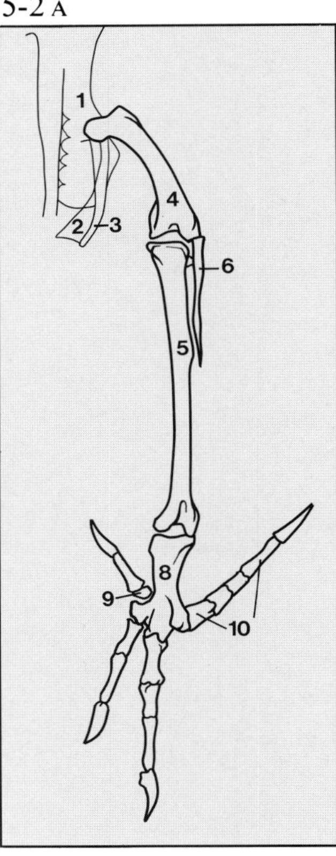

5-1/5-1A/5-2/5-2A Left Leg:
Normal Radiographic Appearance,
mediolateral and dorsoplantar.

Greater Sulfur-Crested Cockatoo *(Cacatua galerita)*, adult.

In psittacines, the acetabulum is formed by the ilium (**1**), the ischium (**2**) and the pubis (**3**). The ischium is difficult to see because of its fine structure.

The stifle joint is formed by the femur (**4**), the tibiotarsus (**5**), the fibula (**6**) and the patella (**7**). Usually, the fibula is united with the tibiotarsus.

The large tarsometatarsus (**8**), including the metatarsals II to IV, articulates with the phalanges (**10, 11**) of the corresponding digits. The small bone proximal to digit I represents metatarsal I (**9**).

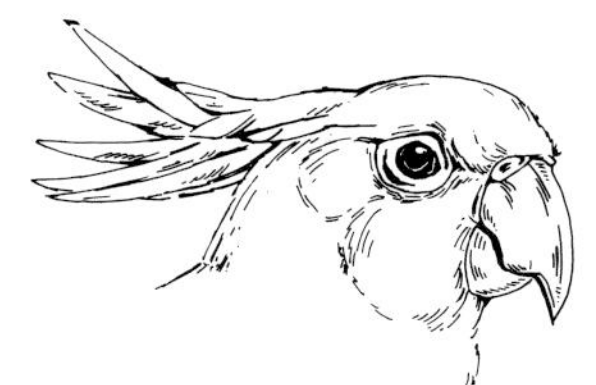

6

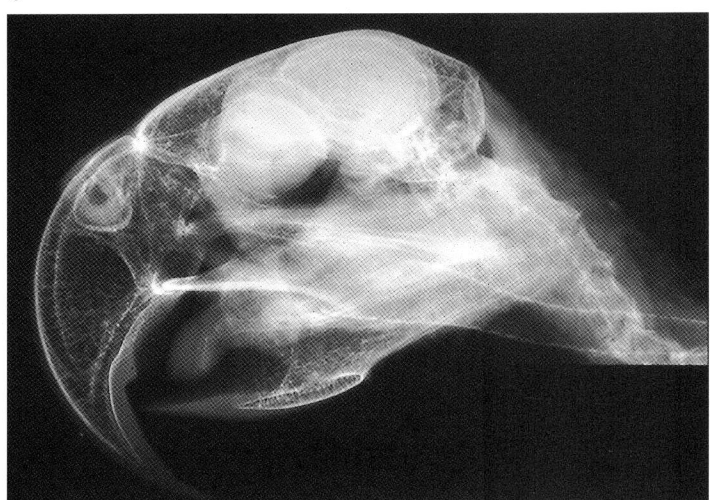

6 A

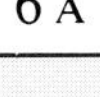

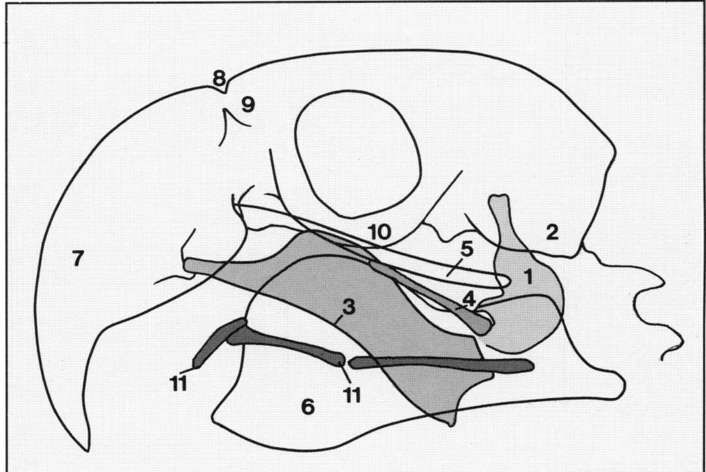

7

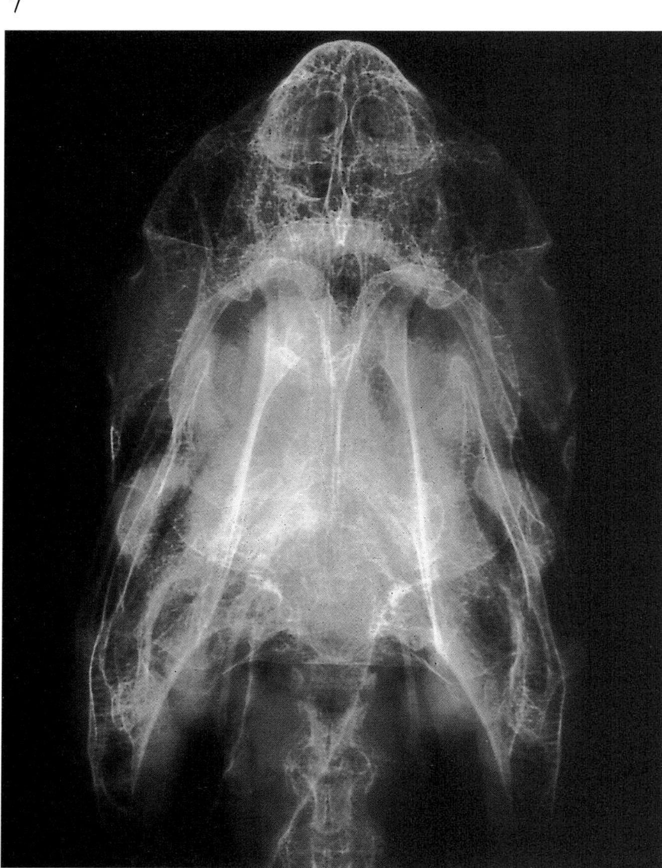

7 A

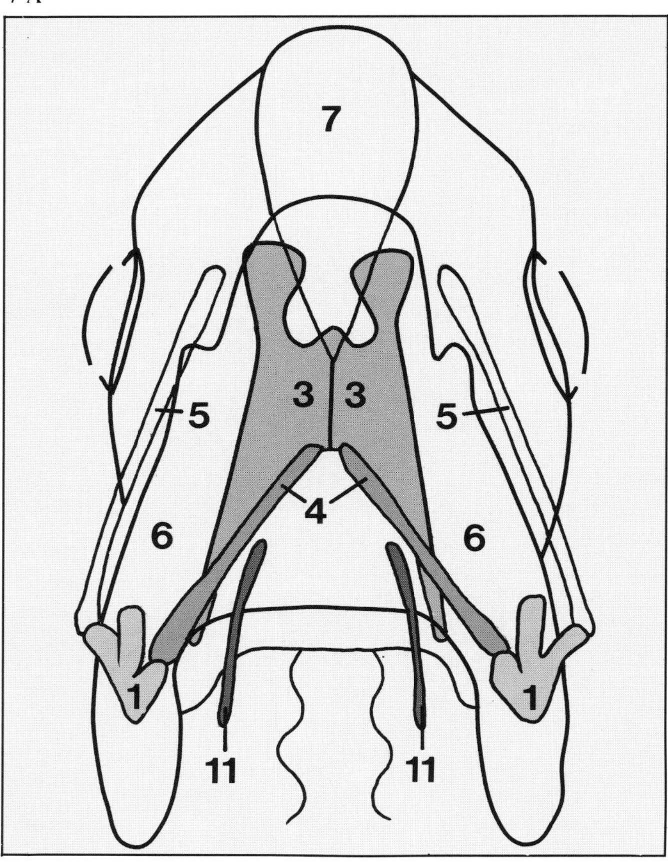

6/6A/7/7A/8/8A Skull: Normal Radiographic Appearance, lateral, ventrodorsal and left oblique.

Blue and Yellow Macaw *(Ara ararauna).*

The avian skull is a dynamic structure. The quadrate bone (**1**) has a dorsal otic process which articulates with the squamous part of the temporal bone (**2**). The quadrate bone also articulates with the palatine (**3**) and pterygoid (**4**) bones, with the zygomatic arch (**5**), and also suspends the mandible (**6**). The quadrate bone is best evaluated in the lateral and the oblique projections.

The upper jaw is primarily formed by the premaxilla (**7**). The nasal bones form the dorsal and lateral portion of the osseous nasal cavity. The nasofrontal hinge (**8**) is a synovial articulation between the upper beak and the frontal bone (**9**). In psittacines, the palate is an incomplete shelf made of two broad plates. The palatine bones articulate rostrally with the premaxilla and caudally with the pterygoid bones.

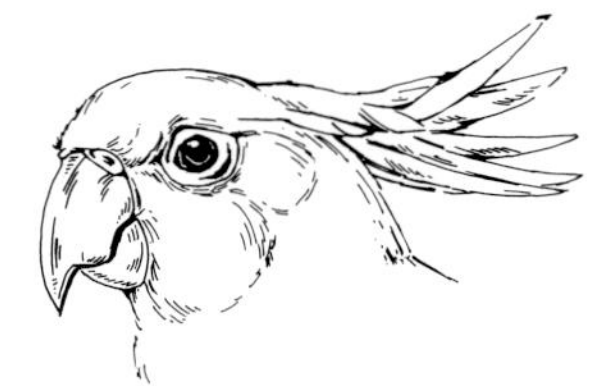

8

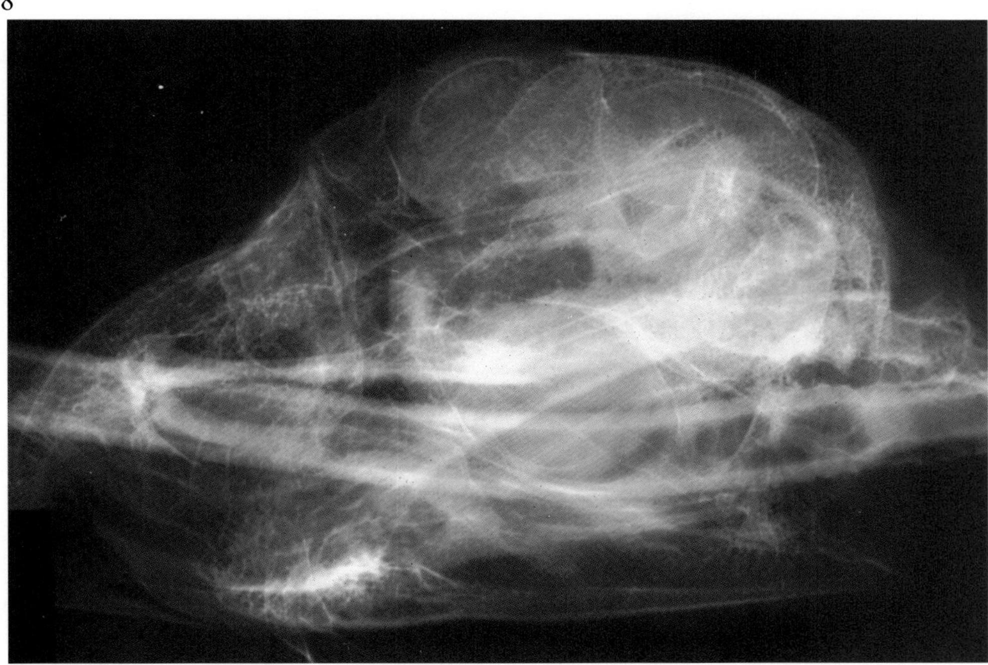

8 A

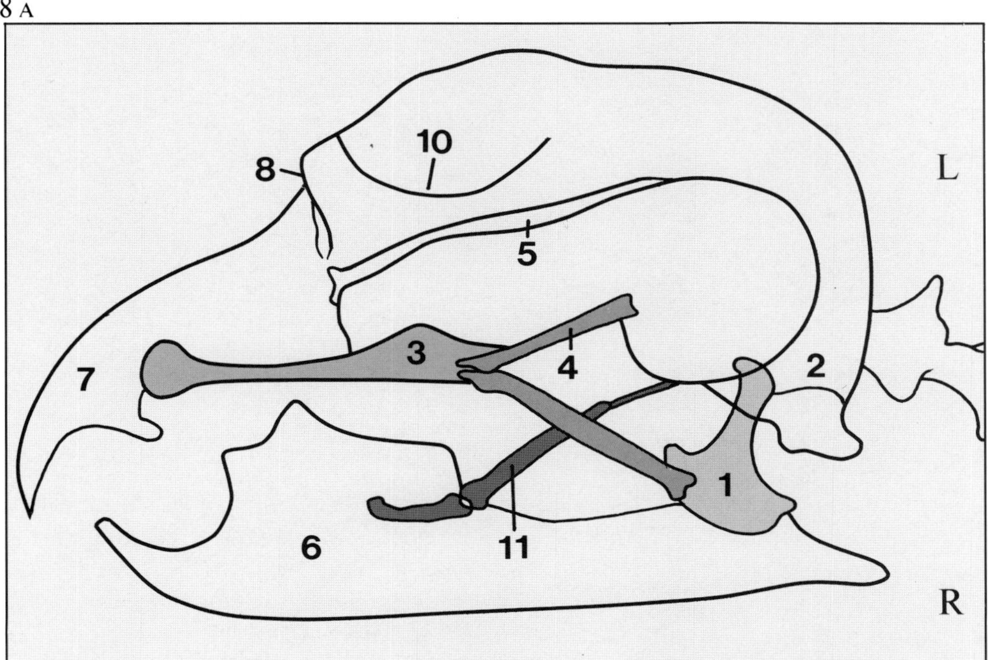

The suborbital arch (**10**) forms the ventral portion of the orbit. Scleral ossicles are composed of 10-18 overlapping bony plates that form a ring within the sclera (not shown here). Paranasal sinuses are difficult to identify radiographically unless they become distended when pathology is present. The shape of the hyoid bones (**11**) varies among species and often extends to the tip of the tongue. Avian tracheal rings are ossified and complete.

9

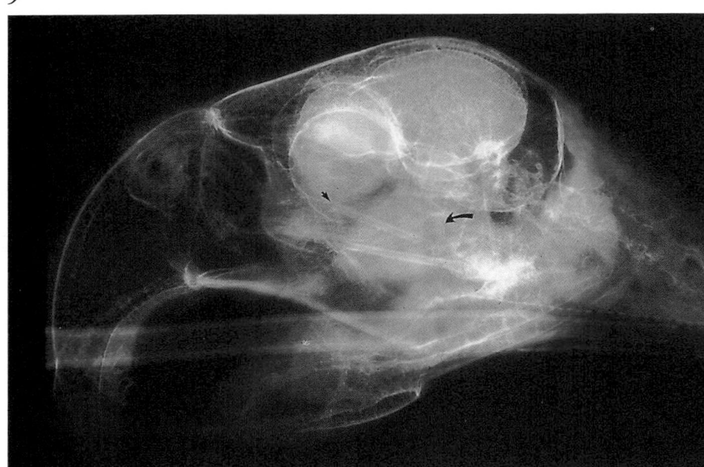

11

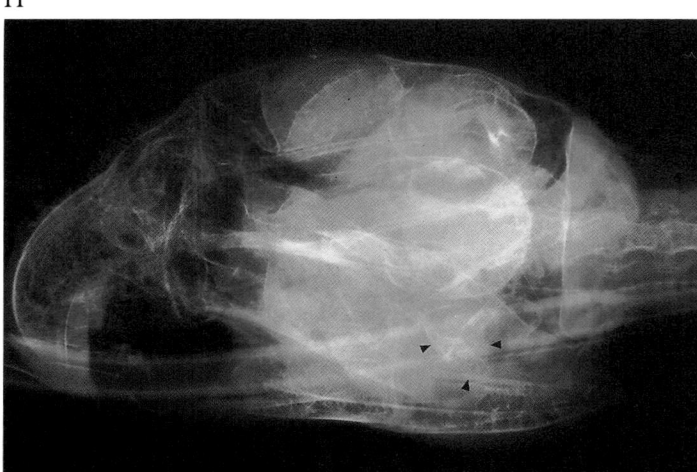

12

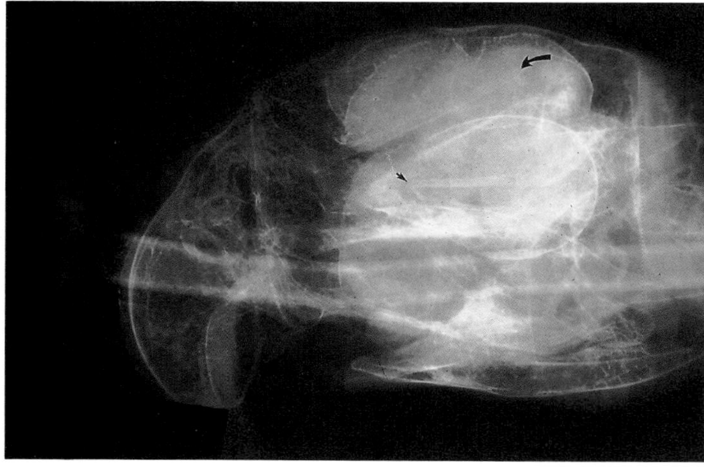

10

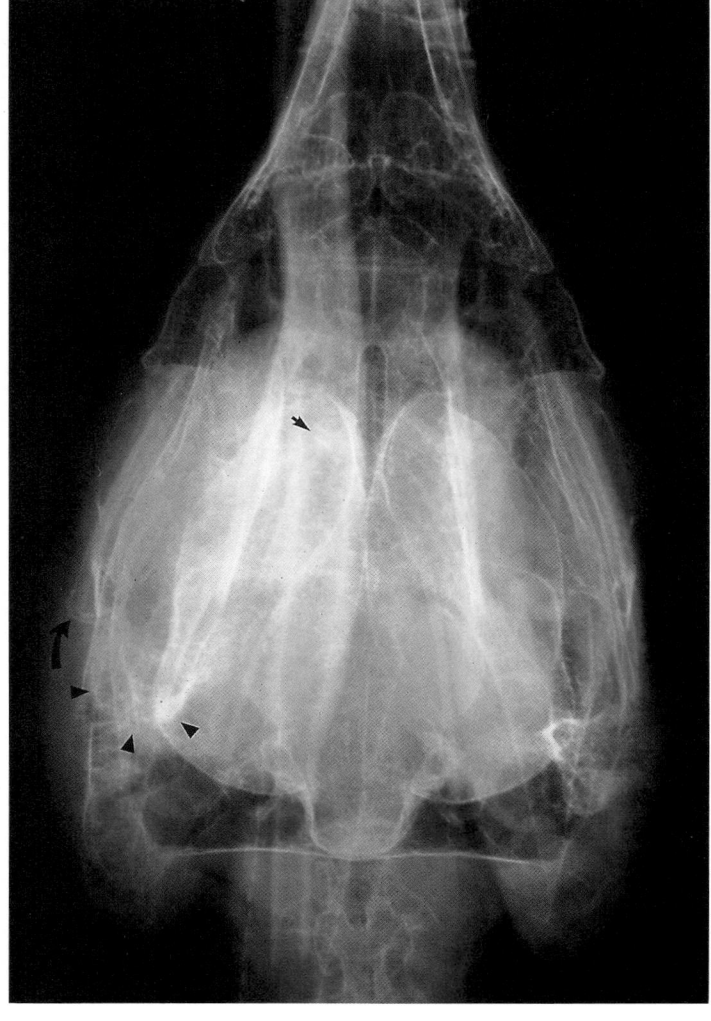

9/10/11/12 Multiple Fractures.

Blue and Yellow Macaw *(Ara ararauna)*, 2 years.

Due to its location the folding fracture of the caudal right zygomatic arch (curved arrow) can best be seen on the lateral (FIG. **9**), ventrodorsal (FIG. **10**) or left oblique (FIG. **11**) view. A fracture of the rostral right pterygoid bone (straight arrow) is also visible on the same radiographs. The right quadrate bone is displaced cranially (arrowheads) due to a compound fracture (FIG. **12**). The displacement is best visualized by comparing the left (FIG. **11**) and right (FIG. **12**) oblique views. The right quadrate bone is less distinct and positioned more rostrally.

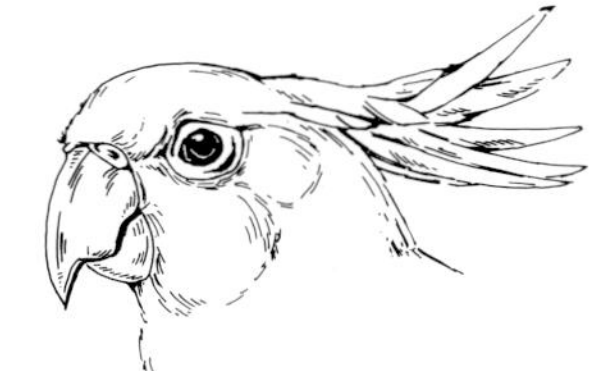

13

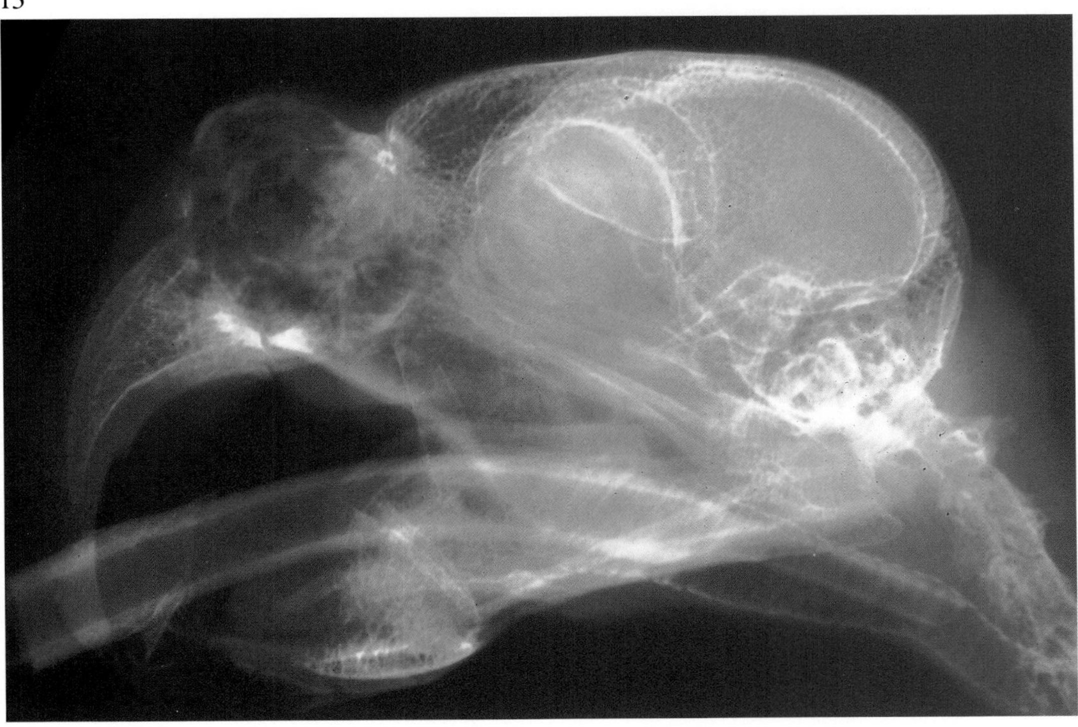

14

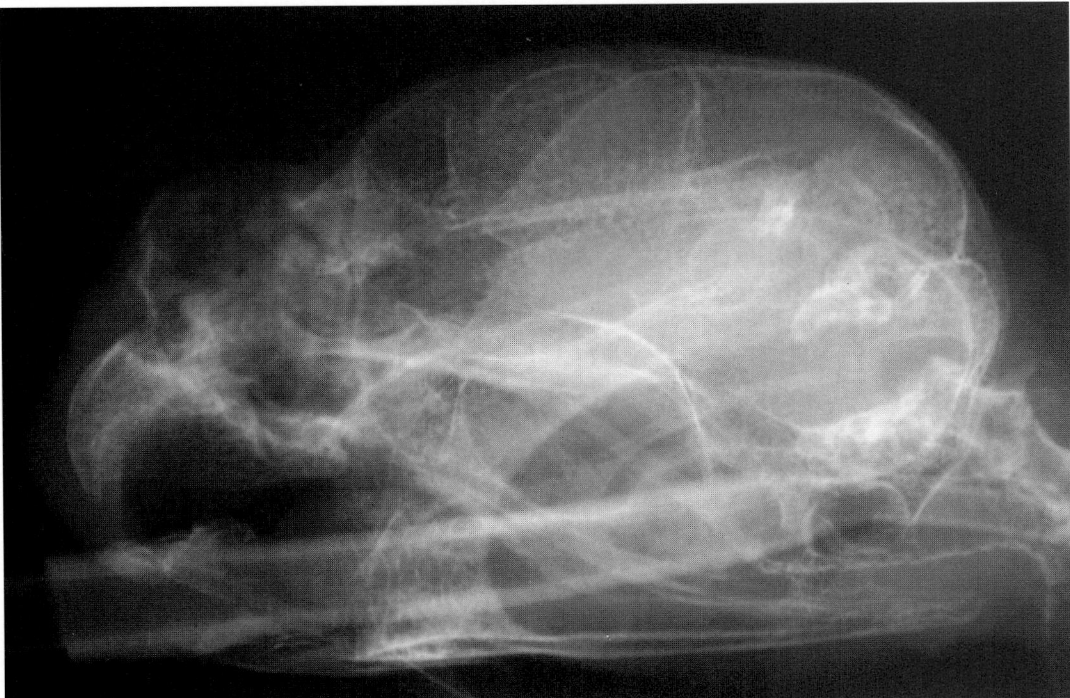

13/14 Infectious Rhinitis and Osteomyelitis.

African Grey Parrot *(Psittacus e. erithacus)*, 28 years.

A lesion with expansive, productive and destructive features involves the nares, nasal bones, operculum, nasal concha, portions of the premaxilla and maxilla. The rostral diverticulum of the infraorbital sinus and proximal articulating areas of the left zygomatic arch and palatine bone are destroyed. There is soft tissue swelling of the rostral choanal field.

From the lesion, a necrotic granuloma was removed by curretage.

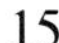

15

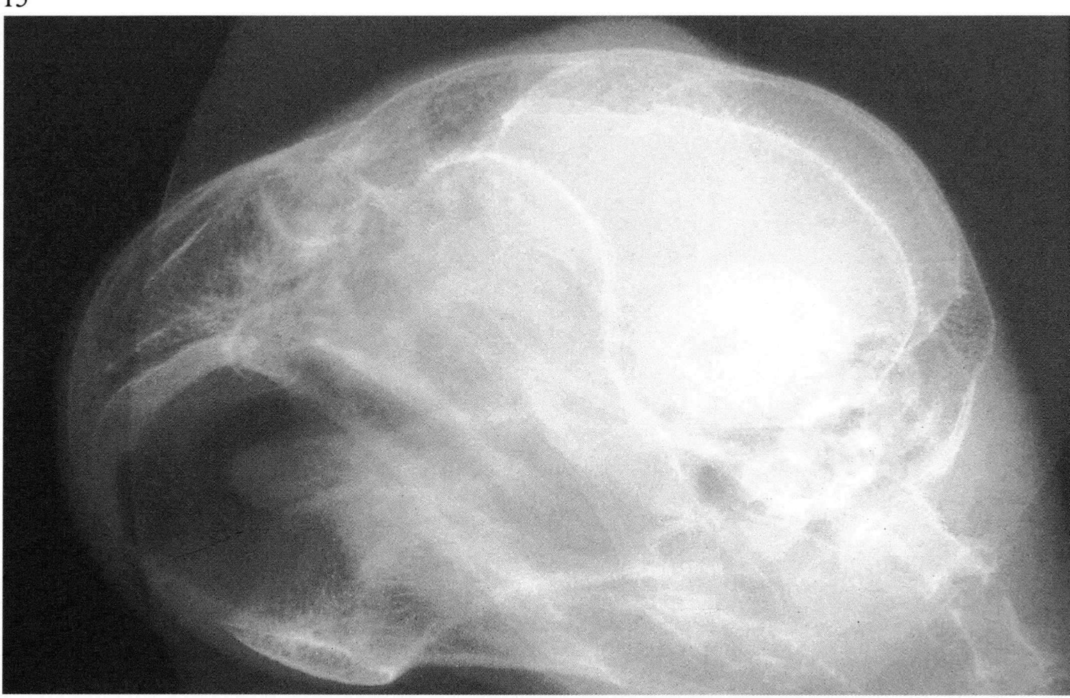

16

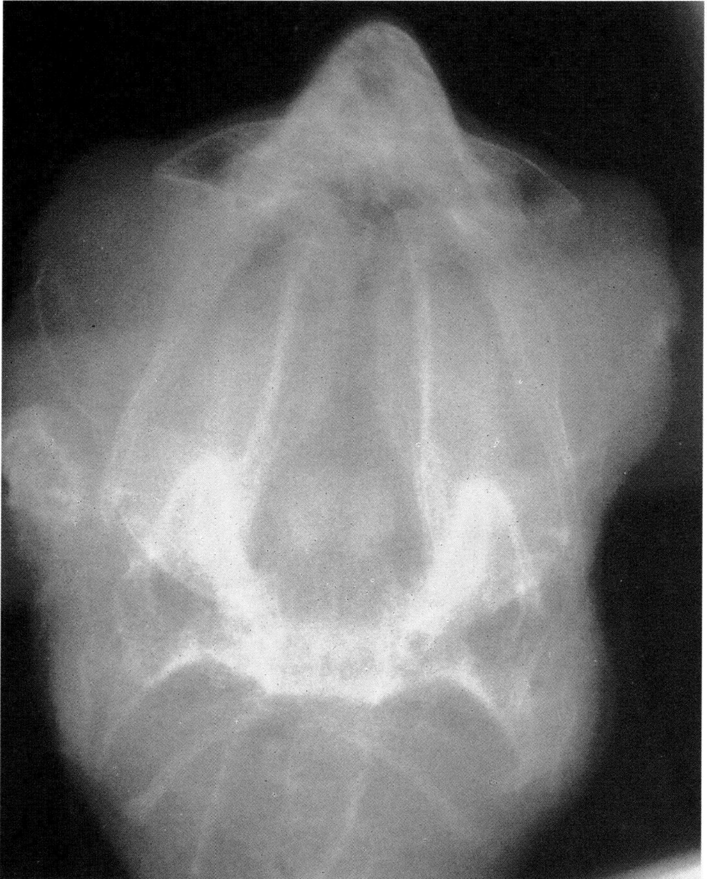

15/16 Soft Tissue Infection.

African Grey Parrot *(Psittacus e. erithacus)*, 5 years.

Soft tissue swelling is prominent rostral and dorsal to the left and right orbit in the region of the preorbital diverticulum of the infraorbital sinus. The infraorbital diverticula medial to each globe are enlarged, which accounts for the caudolateral displacement of the scleral rings. Focal mineralization is present in the soft tissue of the infraorbital sinus. The underlying bony structures appear uninvolved.

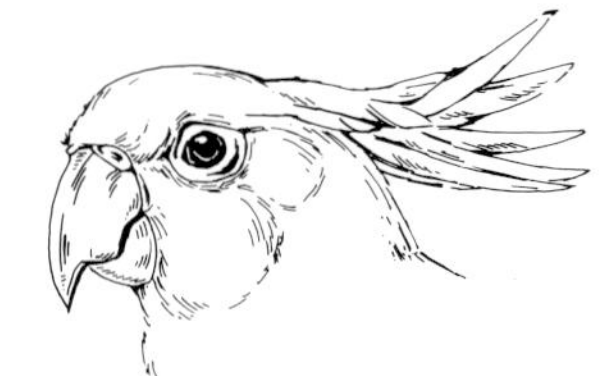

17

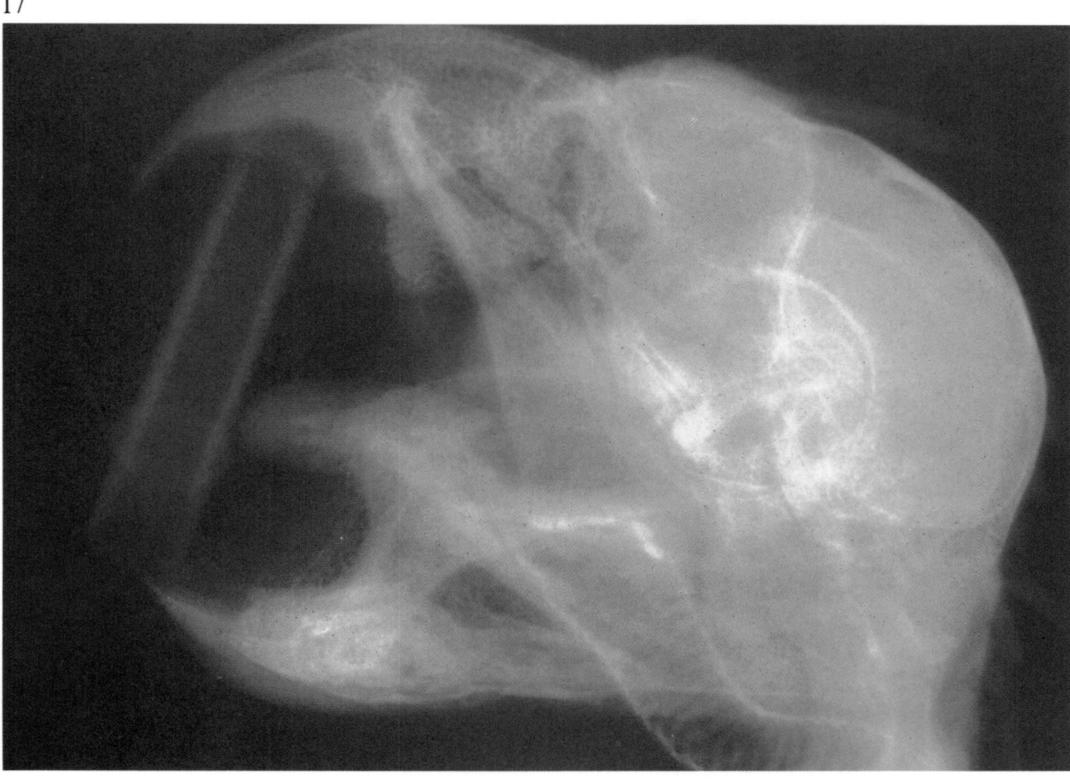

18

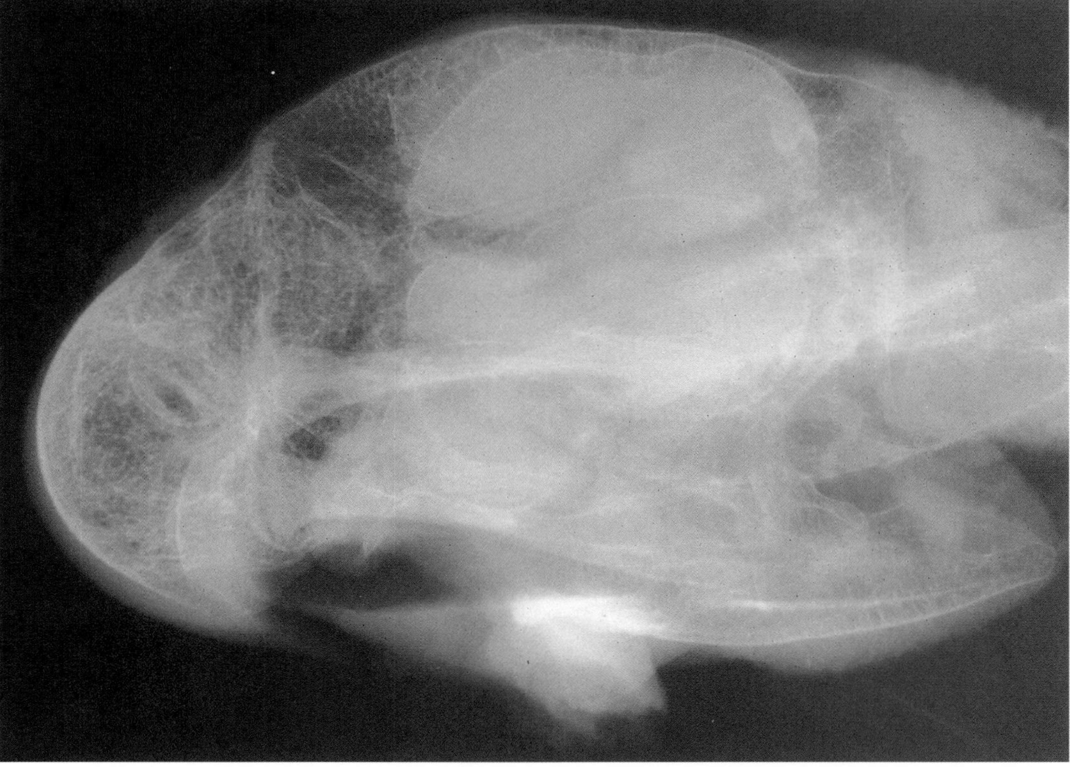

17 Osteomyelitis.

Cockatiel *(Nymphicus hollandicus)*, 2 years.

A bony lesion containing productive and destructive changes involves the base of the mandible and extends along the right ventral ramus. Several small fragments of sequestered bone are also present.

18 Squamous Cell Carcinoma.

Scarlet Macaw *(Ara macao)*, adult.

An irregular soft tissue mass extends along the left lower beak. The mandibular bone has an irregular outline with areas of lysis and sclerosis. Periosteal involvement is not visible. The histological examination showed a squamous cell carcinoma.

19

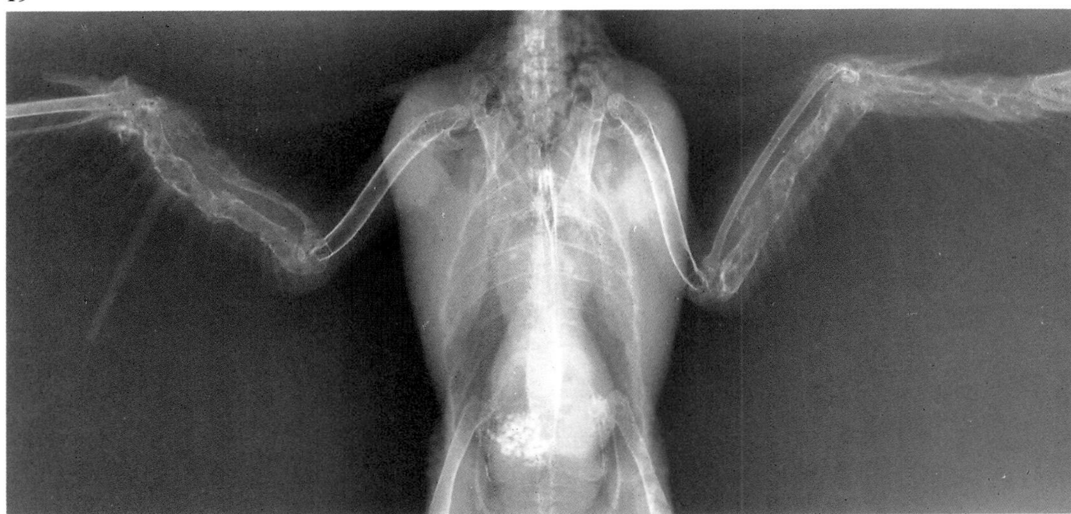

20

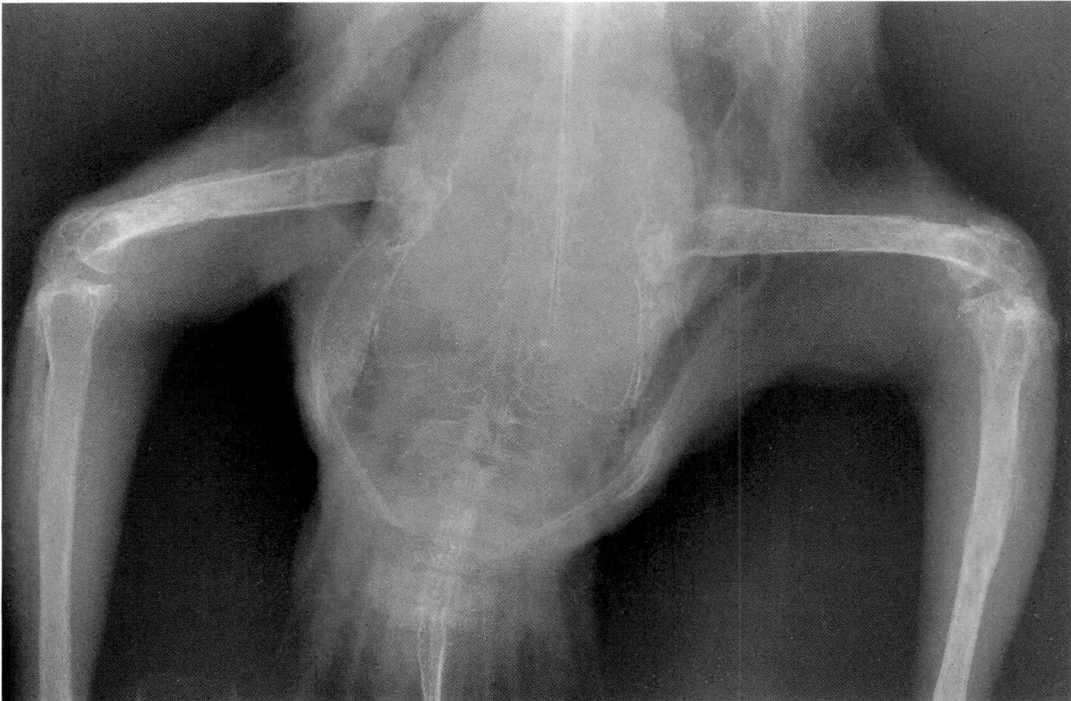

19 Metabolic Bone Disease.

Cockatiel *(Nymphicus hollandicus)*, adult.

The radius, ulna, and distal bones of the wings are strongly deformed by extensive lytic and sclerotic bony changes. The left femur is also affected. The findings are consistent with metabolic bone disease such as osteomalacia.

It is striking that the partially pneumatized humerus is little or not affected.

20 Metabolic Bone Disease.

Yellow-collared Macaw *(Ara auricollis)*, adult.

The skeleton has a generalized diminished density. There are no signs of malformation. The cortices of both femurs have a rough outline due to consolidated periosteal new bone formation.

Postmortem diagnosis was nutritional secondary hyperparathyroidism.

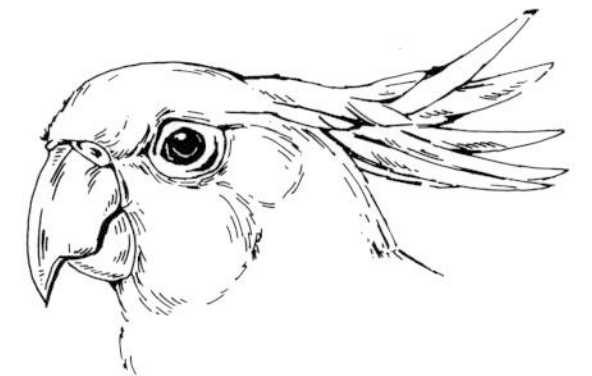

21

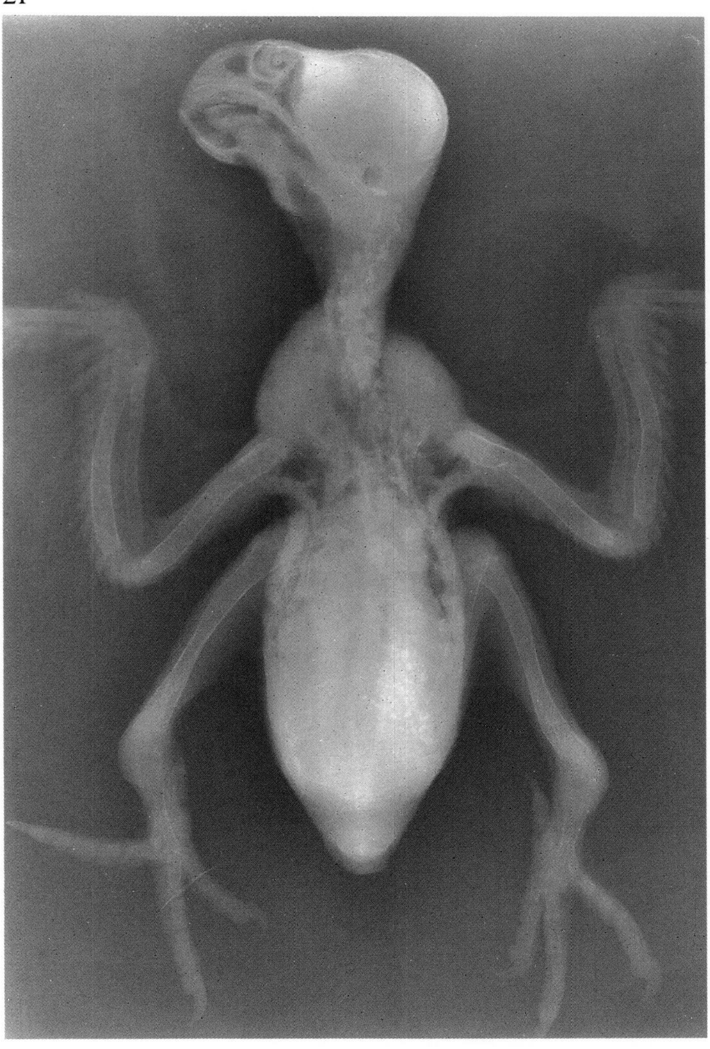

22

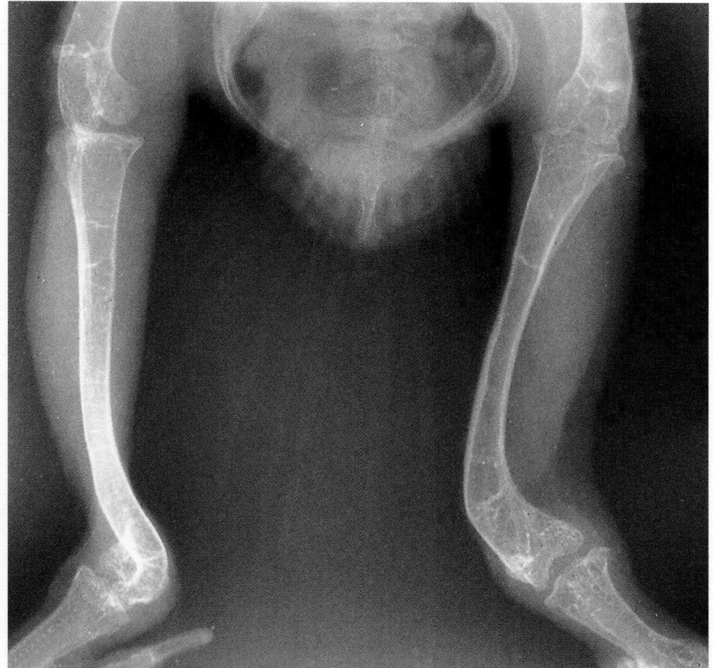

21/22 Metabolic Bone Disease.

Grey Parrot *(Psittacus e. erithacus).*

FIG. **21** shows the parrot at the age of two months. The overall density of the skeleton is decreased. The cortical outlines of the long bones are barely visible. Most of the long bones are abnormally bent. In the proximal left humerus, a folding fracture is present. FIG. **22** shows part of the skeleton of the same parrot at the age of one year after correction of the feeding regimen. The cortices of the femurs and tibiotarsi are of normal density. However, malformation of the bones persists.

23

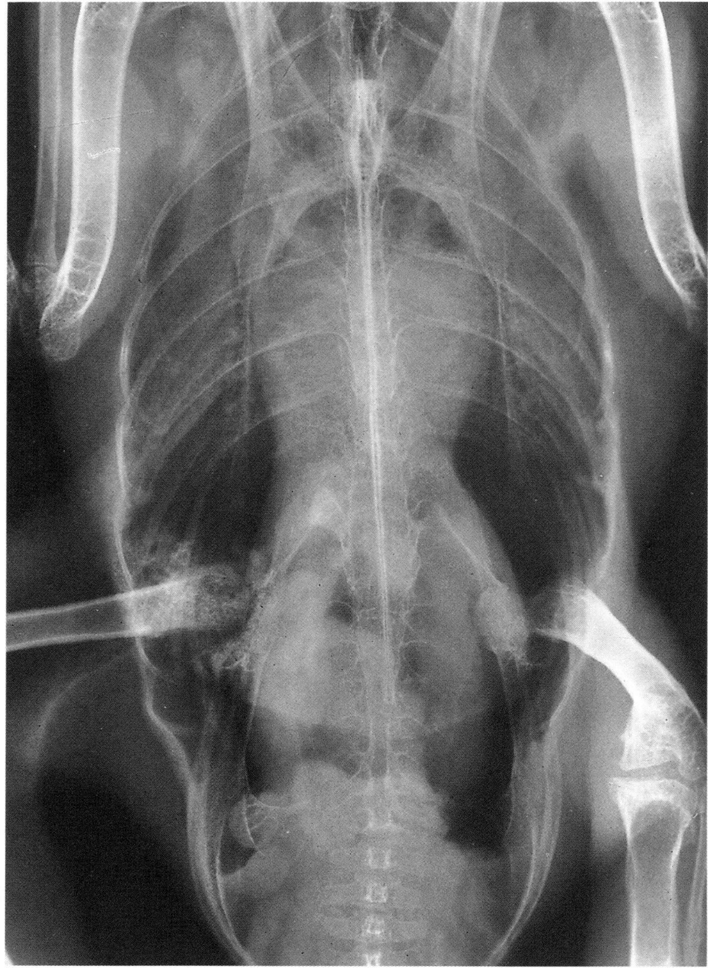

24

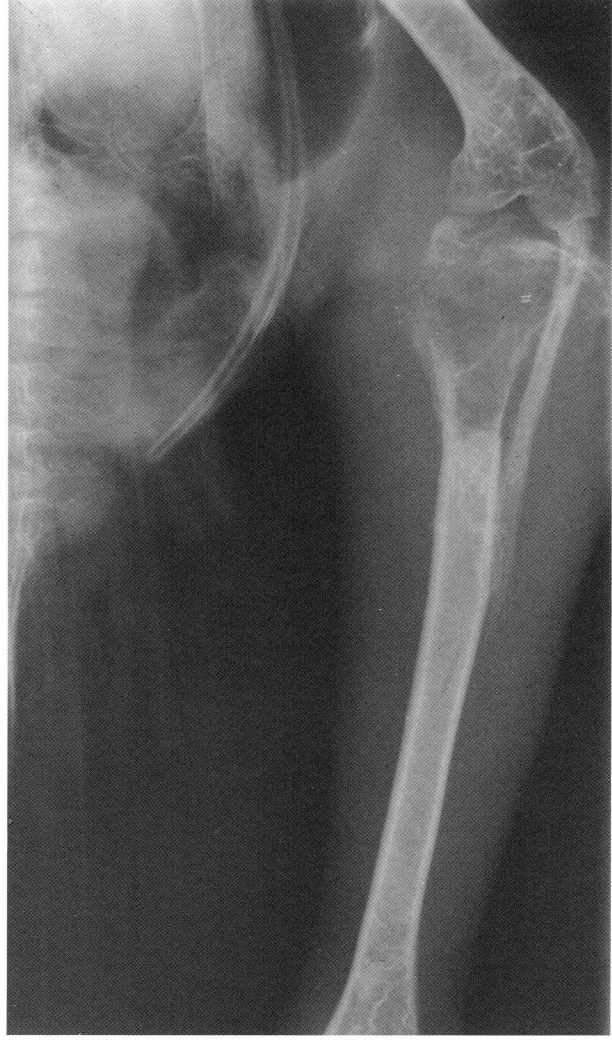

23 Coxarthrosis.

Blue-fronted Amazon *(Amazona aestiva).*

Extensive bone destruction in the proximal right femur and acetabulum is visible. Focal calcifications are present in the soft tissues around the joint.

Note: The histological examination showed necrotic areas with local calcifications, but no inflammatory changes.

24 Osteosarcoma.

Hyacinth-Macaw *(Anodorhynchus hyazinthinus)*, 8 years.

The radiograph reveals an area of osteolysis in the proximal left tibiotarsus. Periosteal new bone formation is present on the medial side. In the mid-diaphyseal region, several radiolucencies are recognizable. Periosteal new bone formation can also be seen distal to the area where the fibula is fused with the tibiotarsus. An osteosarcoma was diagnosed.

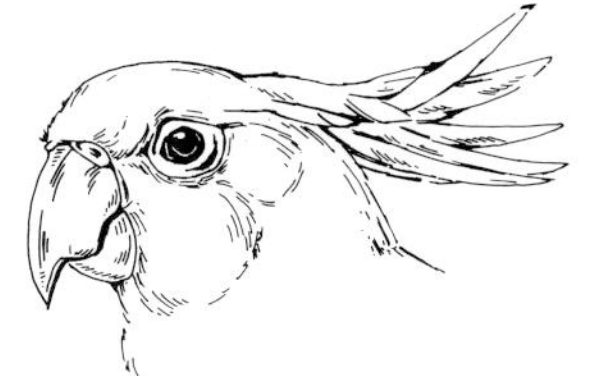

25

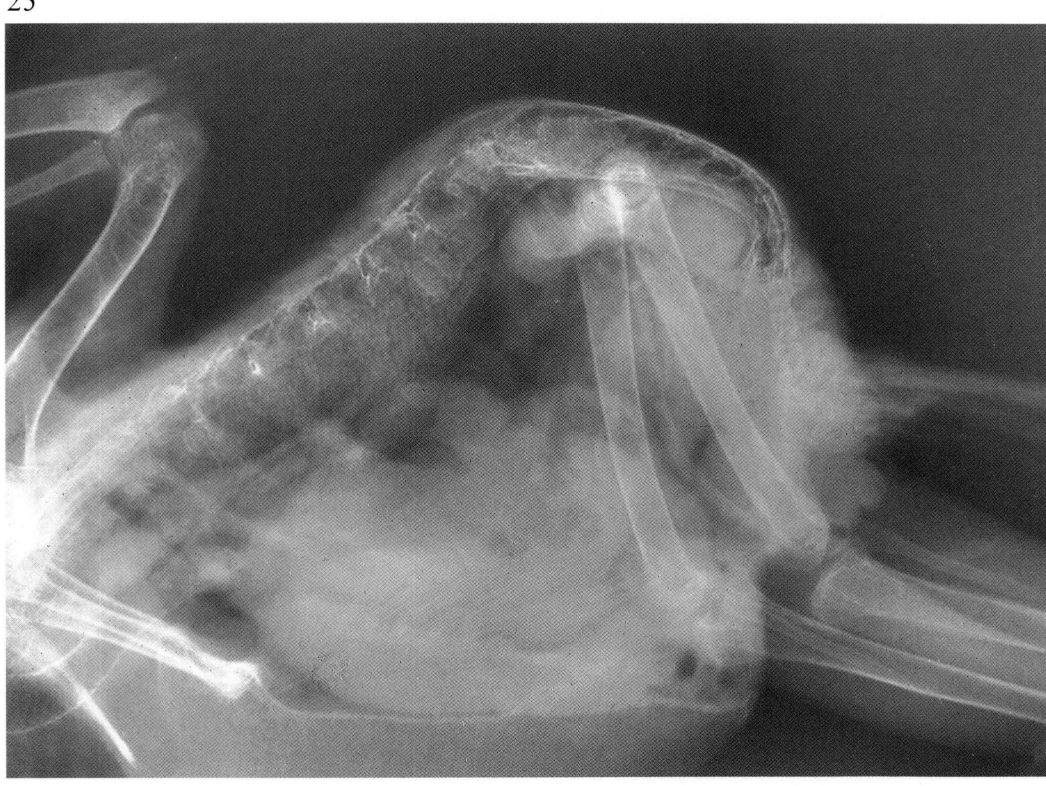

26

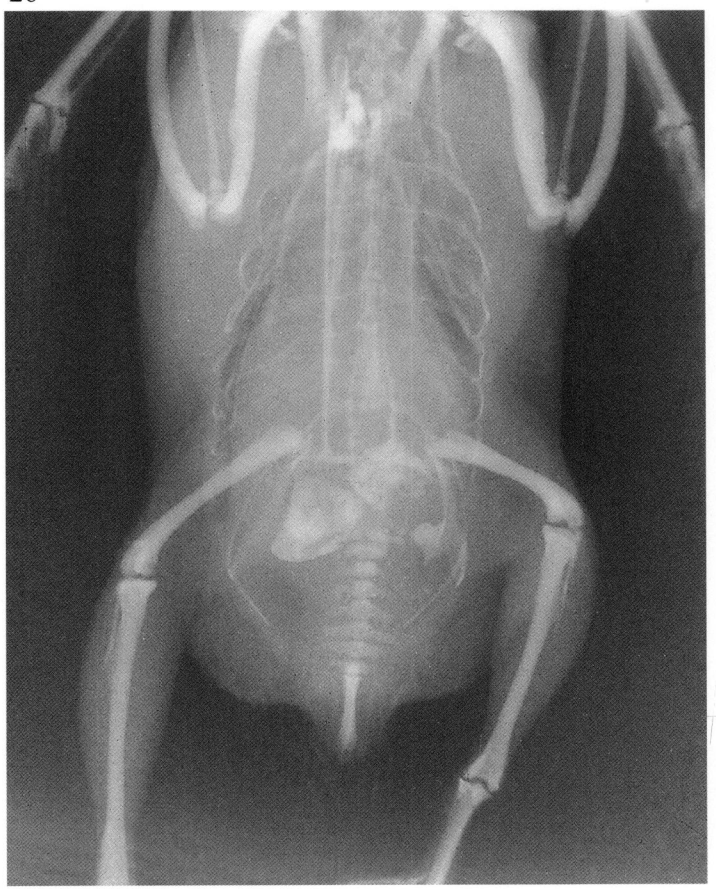

25 Kyphosis.

Blue-fronted Amazon *(Amazona aestiva)*, 12 years.

Distortion of the cranial and caudal parts of the synsacrum has resulted in severe deformation.

26 Osteosclerosis.

Budgerigar *(Melopsittacus undulatus)*.

All the long bones, the sternum, and the synsacrum show an increased bone density involving the medullary cavity. Some periosteal new bone formation is also present. The new bone formation of the synsacrum expands into the right celomic cavity. The caudal part of the celomic cavity has an increased density and the cardio-hepatic "hourglass"-shape has disappeared. A cystic degeneration of the ovary caused the bony abnormalities.

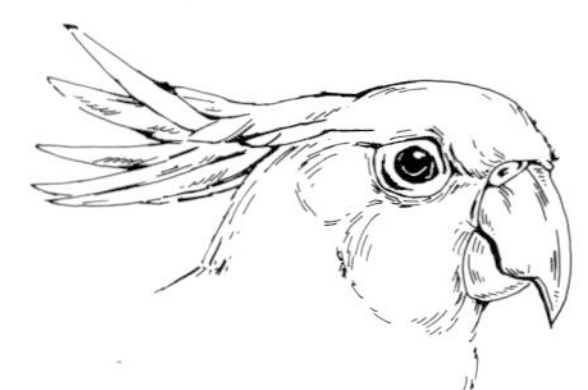

27

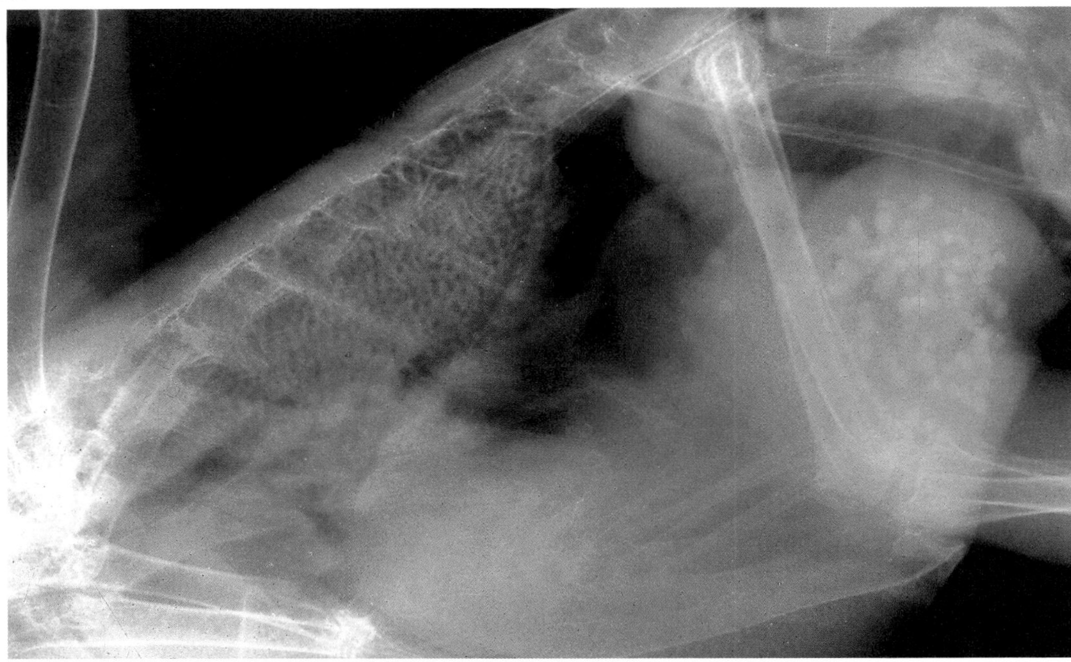

28

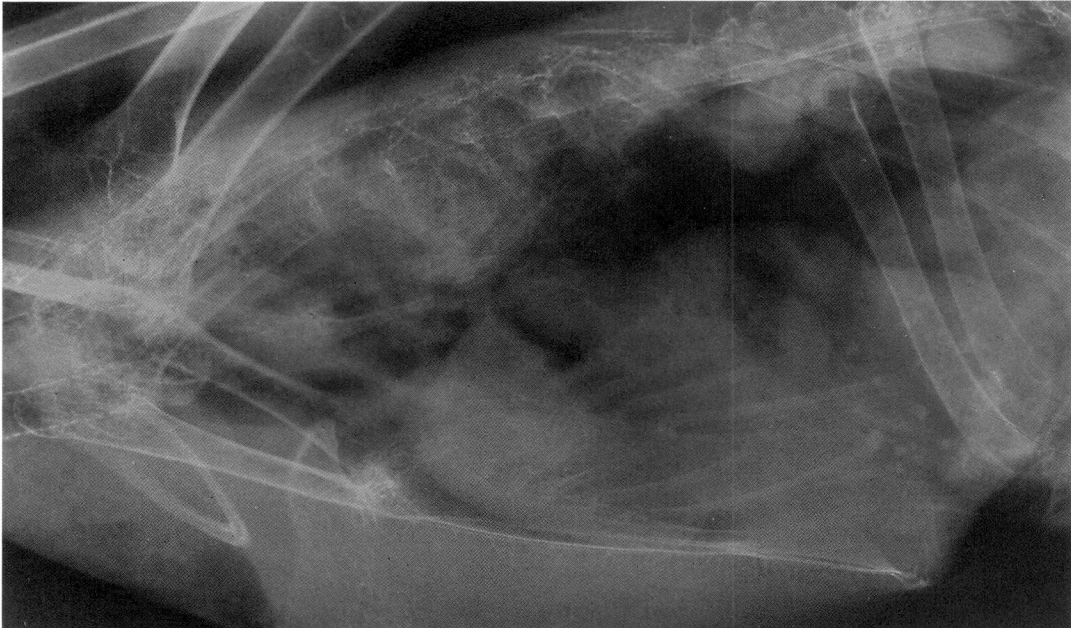

27 Pulmonary Congestion.

Blue-fronted Amazon *(Amazona aestiva)*, male, 15 years.

The reticular pattern of the lungs is accentuated. The caudal lung borders are outlined by fine linear shadows. Increased densities are also present in the central parts of the lungs and at the base of the heart.

Note: Pulmonary congestion is often seen in cases of cardiomyopathy and severe arteriosclerosis.

28 Pneumonia.

Blue-fronted Amazon *(Amazona aestiva)*, 3 years.

A large homogeneous radiodensity extends from the tracheal bifurcation to the periphery of the dorsocaudal parts of the lung. This was due to aspergillosis pneumonia.

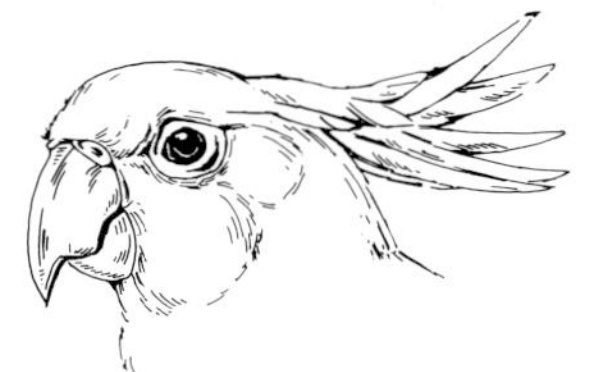

29

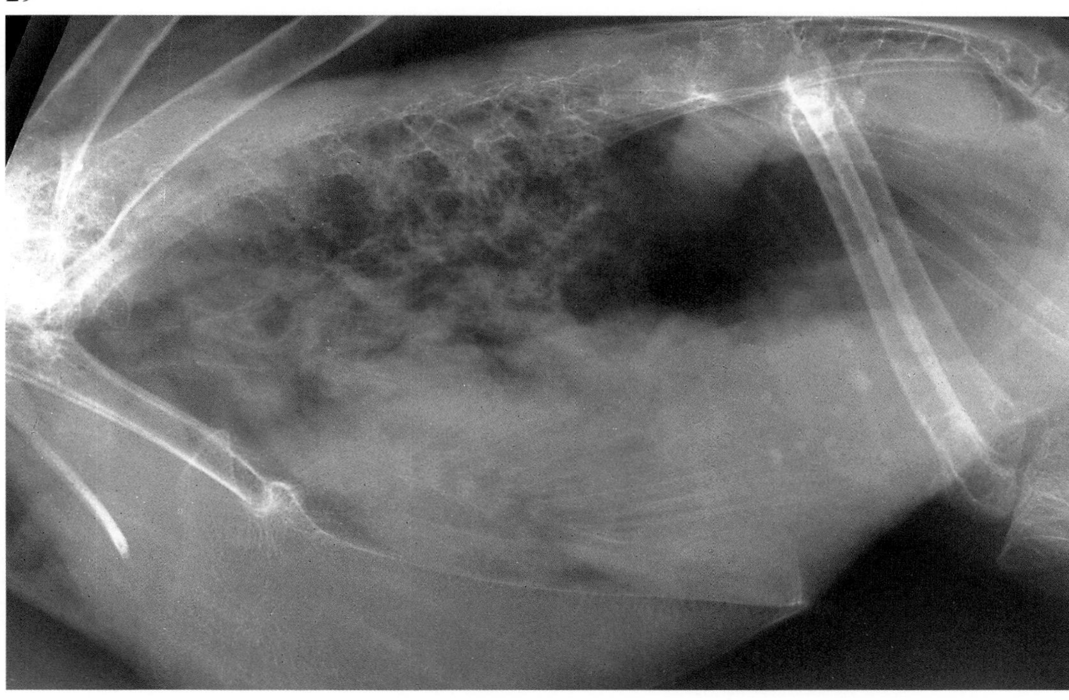

30

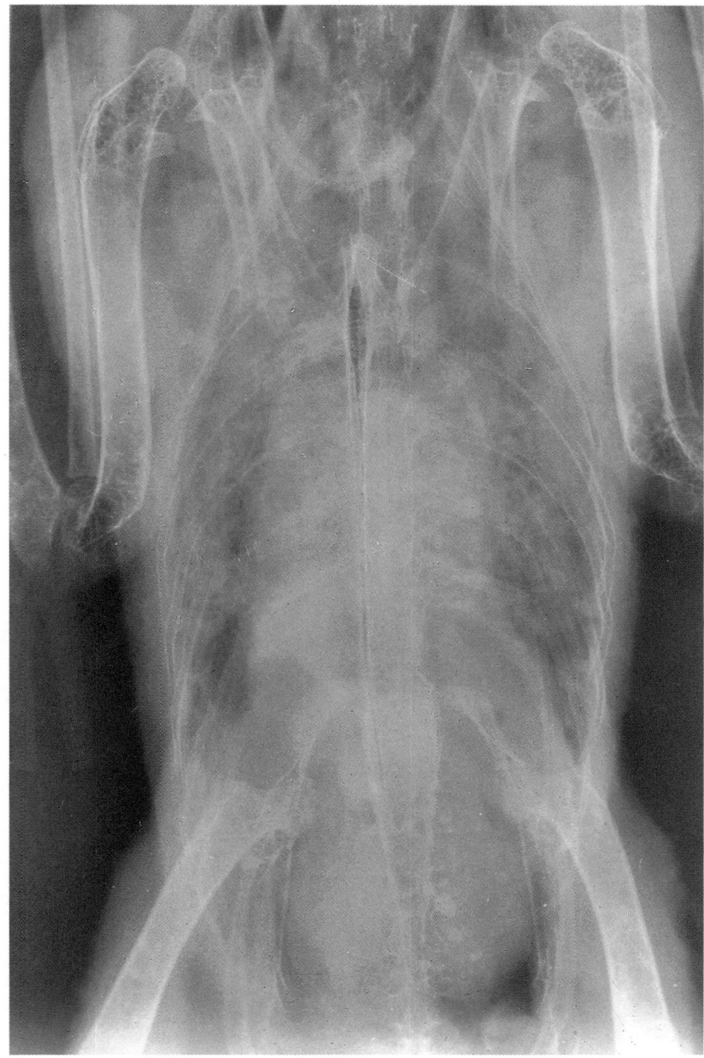

29/30 Pneumonia.

Yellow-crowned Amazon *(Amazona ochrocephala).*

Irregular confluent densities are distributed throughout the lungs and extend into the air sacs. On the ventrodorsal radiograph, the cardiac outline and the hourglass-shaped heart and gastrointestinal tract are poorely demarcated by the surrounding lungs and air sacs. On the lateral radiograph, the heart is visualized poorly because of opacities in the region of the main bronchi.

Note: This amazon is not positioned ideally (sternum and spine are not superimposed), but the density of the right and left lung and air sacs can be compared nonetheless.

31

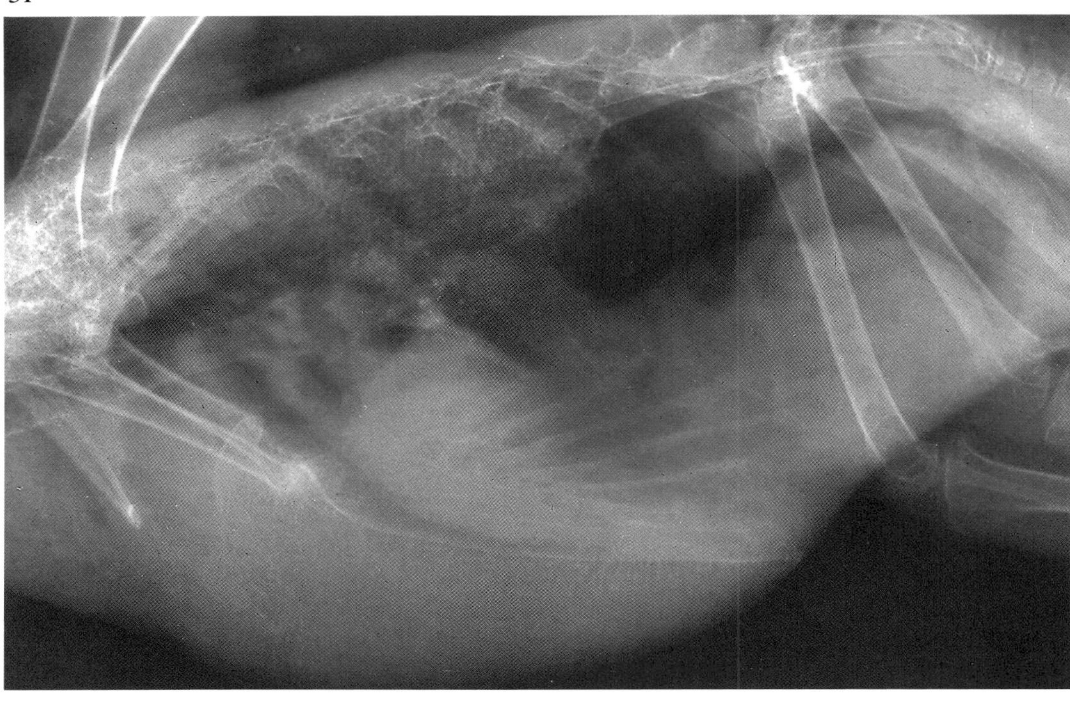

32

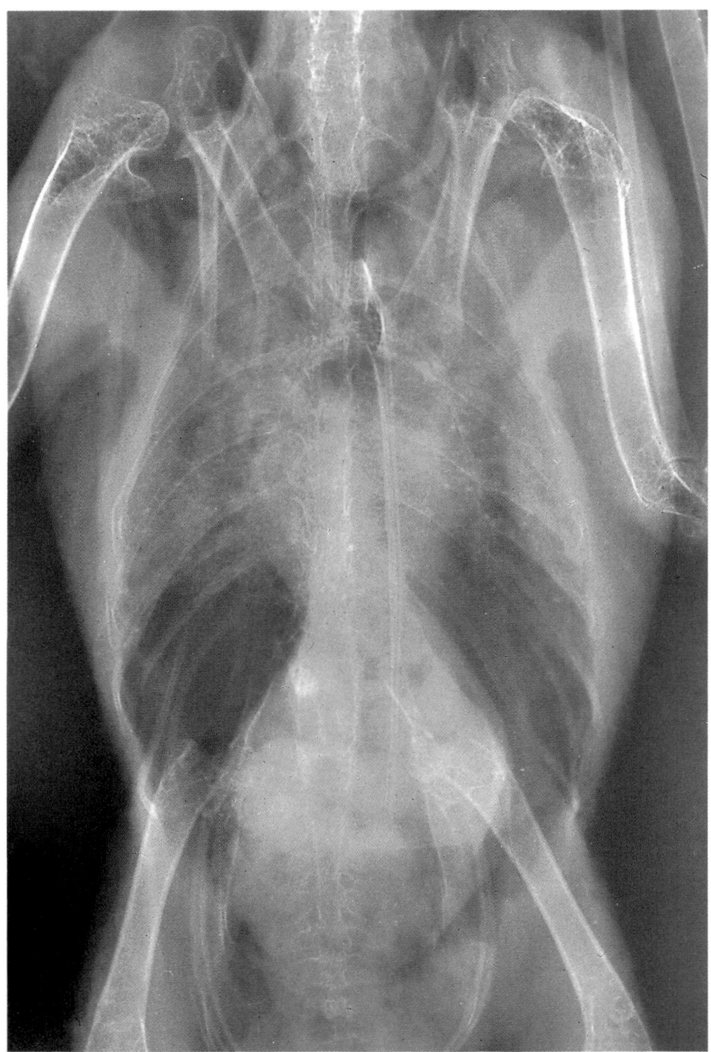

31/32 Pneumonia.

Orange-winged Amazon *(Amazona amazonica)*, 15 years.

Focal calcifications can be recognized in both projections. On the lateral radiograph, they are concentrated in the hilar region and on the ventrodorsal radiograph they are more evenly distributed throughout the lungs. These calcifications represent granulomas that are the result of chronic bacterial pneumonia.

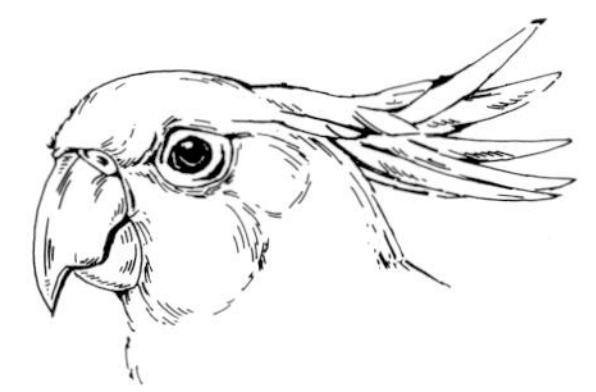

33

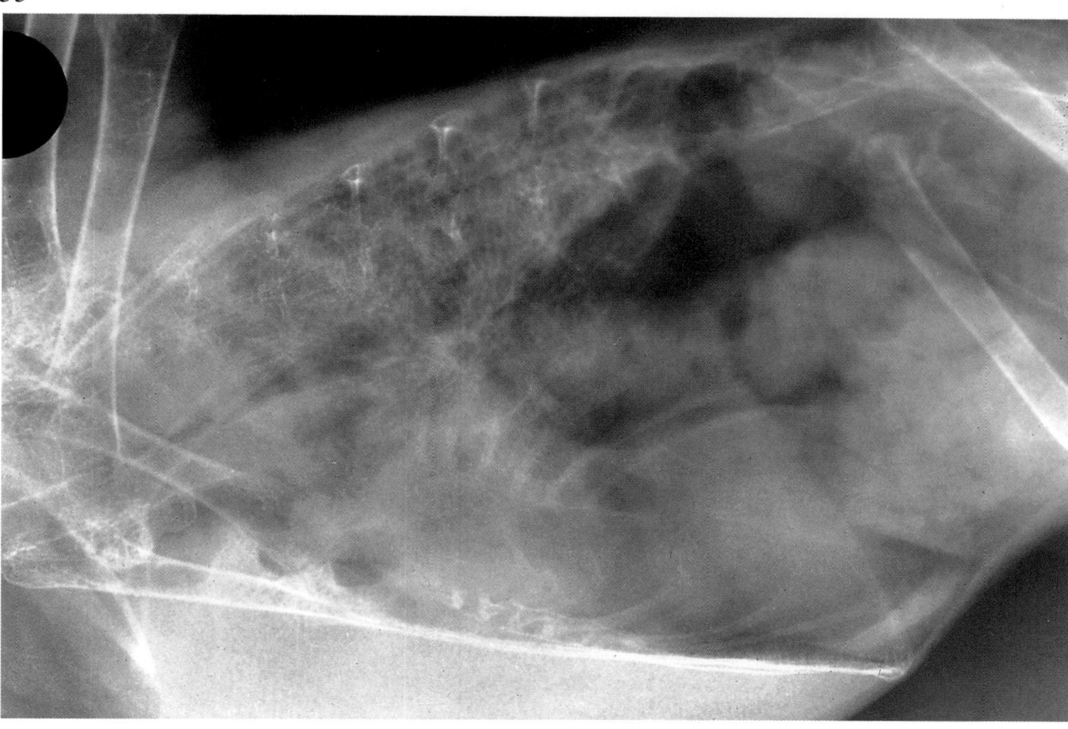

34

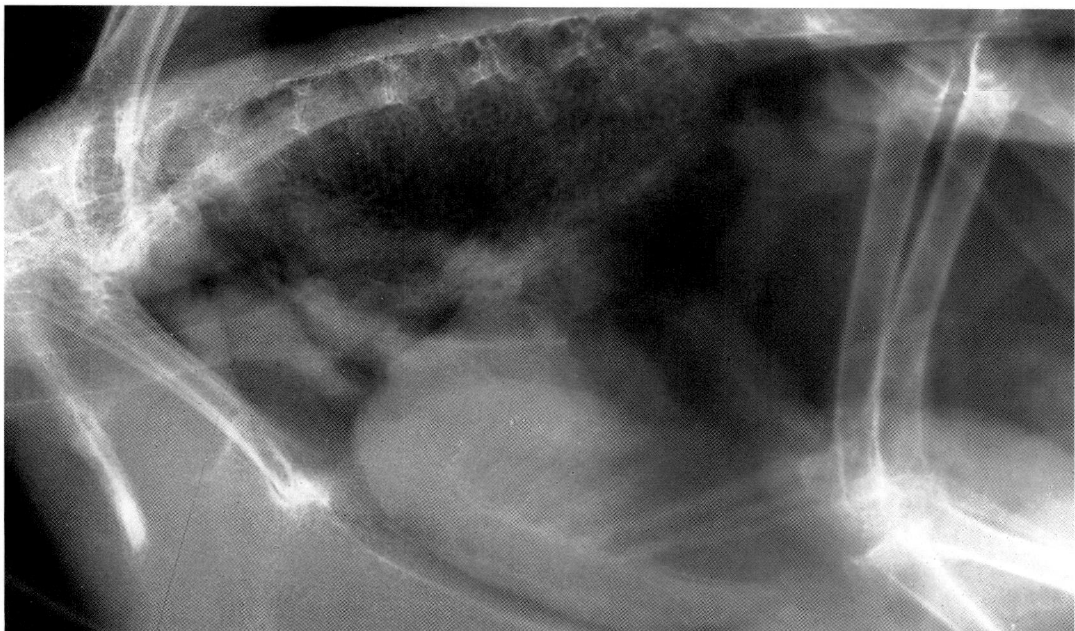

33 Bronchopneumonia.

Yellow-crowned Amazon *(Amazona o. ochrocephala),* 5 years.
In the hilar region, the walls of the main bronchi are thickened, presenting a "doughnut" sign. The density of the lungparenchyma is increased and the caudal lung-border is visible.

Note: Together with the clinical findings a pulmonary aspergillosis infection was diagnosed.

34 Bronchial Occlusion.

Grey parrot *(Psittacus e. erithacus).*

In contrast to FIG. **33** pulmonary details are clearly visible. The cardiac shadow is clearly defined. In the region of the tracheal bifurcation a distinct soft tissue shadow extends cranially and caudally. The main bronchi were occluded by mycotic hyphi.

35

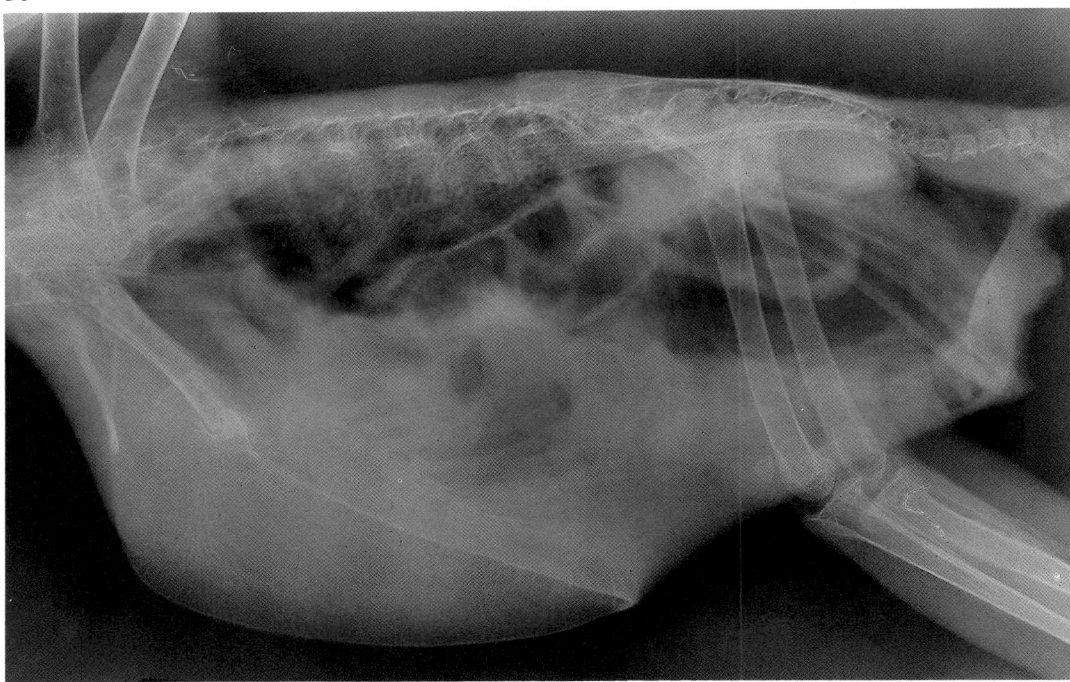

36

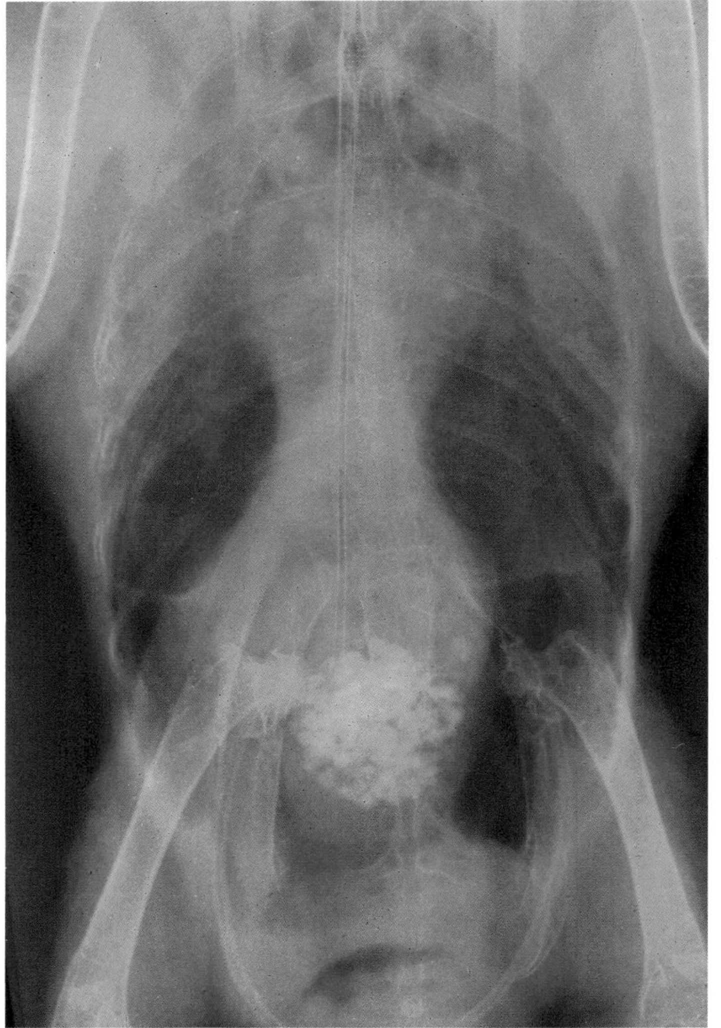

35 Air Sacculitis.

Blue-headed Parrot *(Pionus menstruus)*.

The increased soft tissue density of the lungs prevents visualization of the heart. The caudal borders of the lungs are opacified. In the hilar region, the main bronchi cannot be seen. In the enlarged air sacs of the caudal celomic cavity, linear densities are present, especially around the cranial lobe of the kidney. These findings suggest that the air sac walls are covered by fungal hyphi. The abdominal air sacs are enlarged due to "air trapping" caused by obstruction to the lumen of main bronchi.

36 Air Sacculitis.

Blue-fronted Amazon *(Amazona aestiva)*.

A distinct linear density is traversing the radiolucent air sacs bilaterally. This density is an end-on reflection of the thickened wall between cranial and caudal thoracic air sacs.

Note: The air sac walls are normally not recognizable. They can only be seen if they are thickened by inflammatory changes.

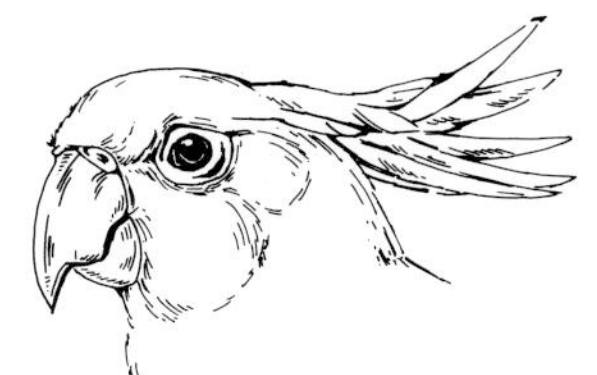

37 Air Sacculitis.

Grey Parrot *(Psittacus e. erithacus).*

Comparison of the symmetrical left and right air sacs reveals a generalized increased density of the left air sacs. This asymmetric density pattern is often found in mycotic air sacculitis.

37

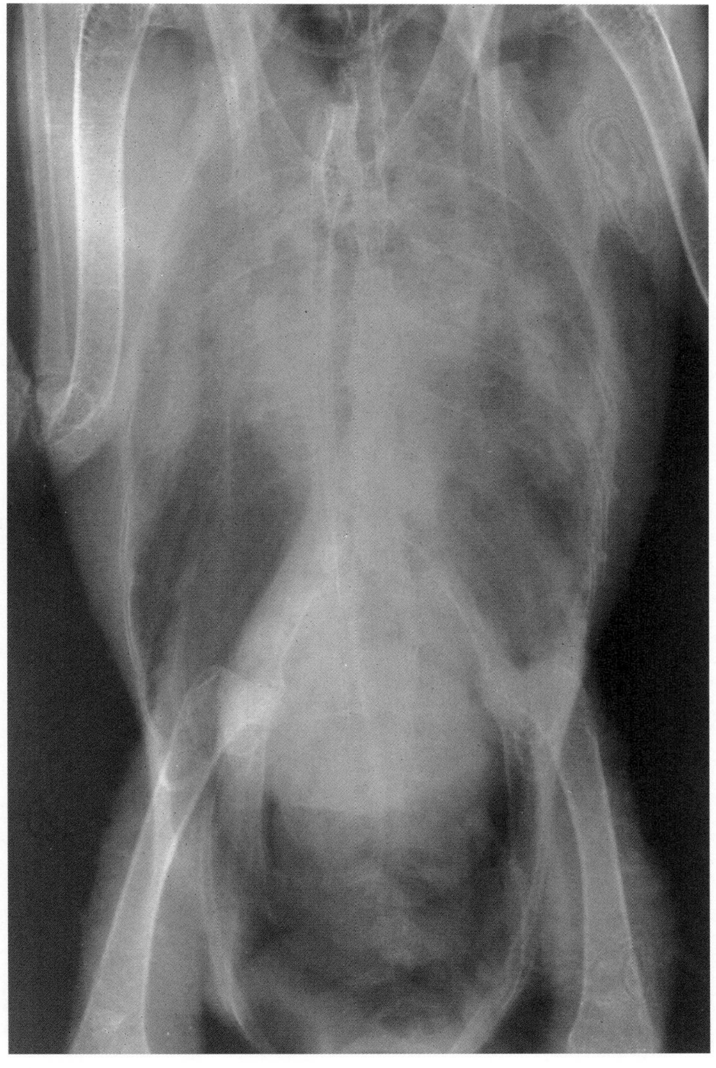

38

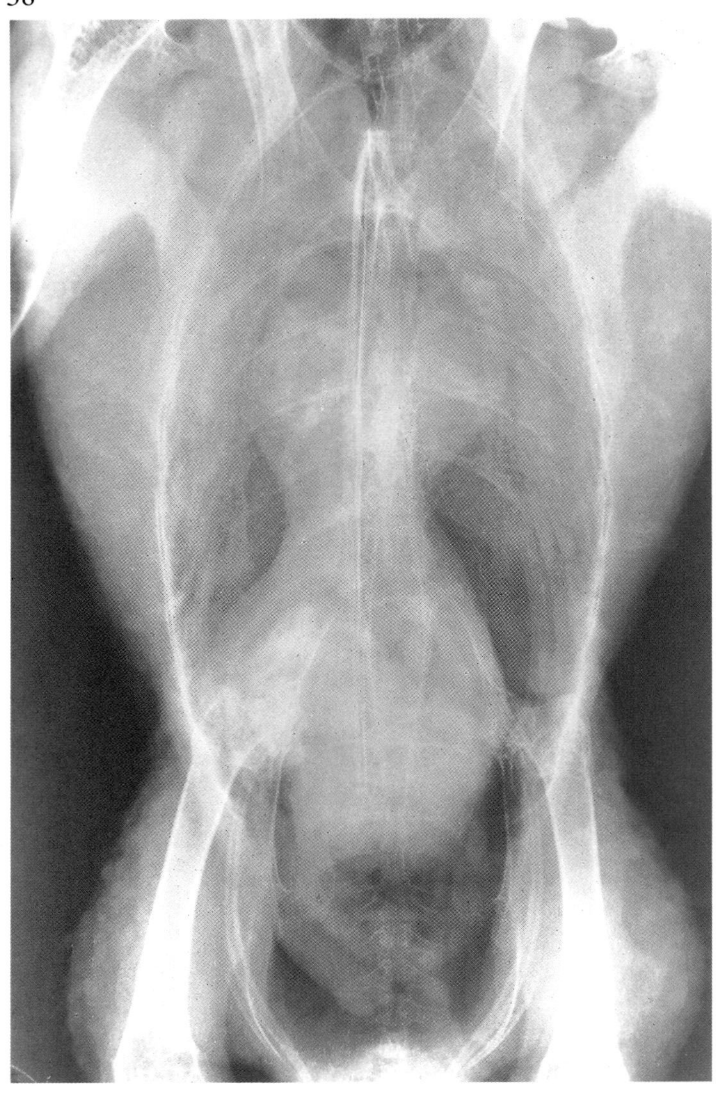

39

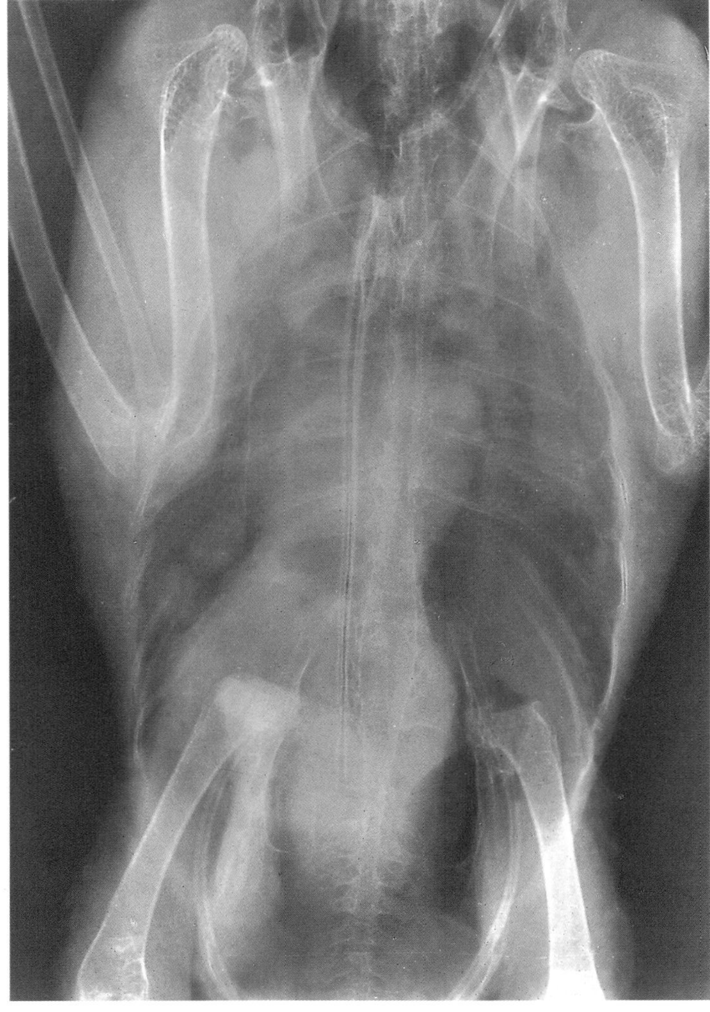

38 Air Sacculitis.

Grey Parrot *(Psittacus e. erithacus).*

The right caudal thoracic air sac, which is superimposed by the right femur and hip joint, contains a localized soft tissue density. The asymmetry in this region is significant. Also, a small focal shadow is present in the right cranial thoracic air sac. The air sacs of the left side are normal.

39 Air Sacculitis.

Grey Parrot *(Psittacus e. erithacus).*

Despite poor positioning, a distinct soft tissue density can be seen in the right caudal thoracic air sac that is superimposed by the head of the right femur. In the right cranial thoracic air sac, two well-defined round opacities are visible. Biopsy identified these masses as aspergillomas. The lungs are normal.

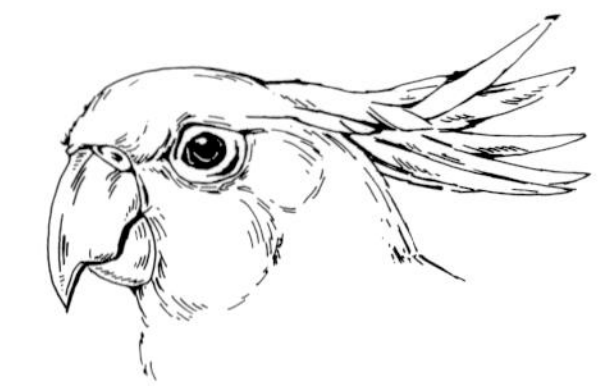

40

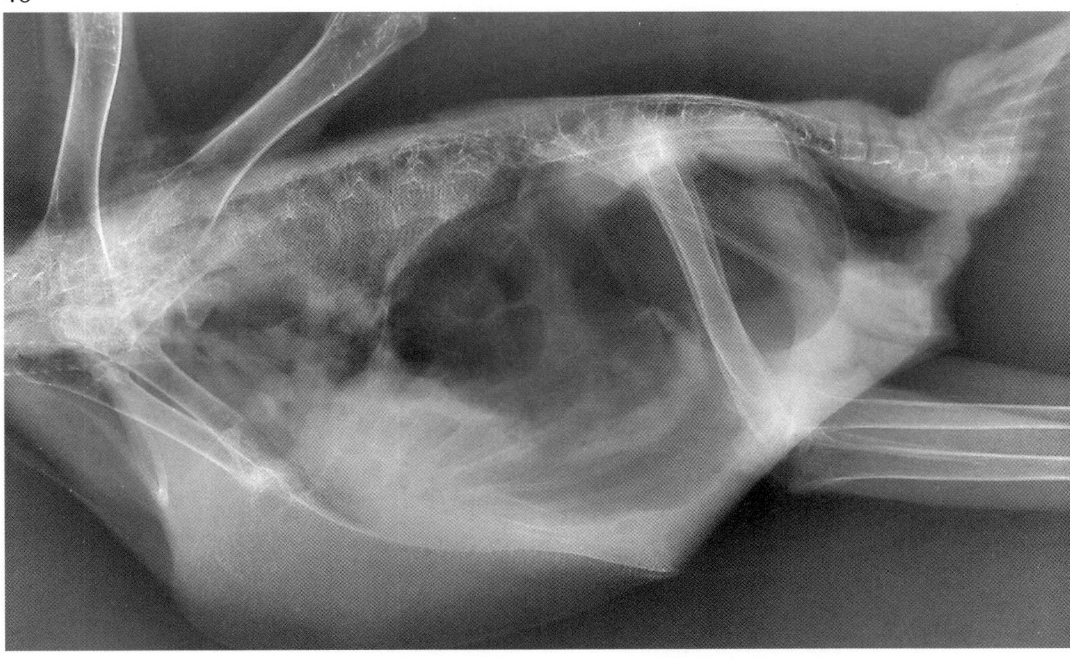

41

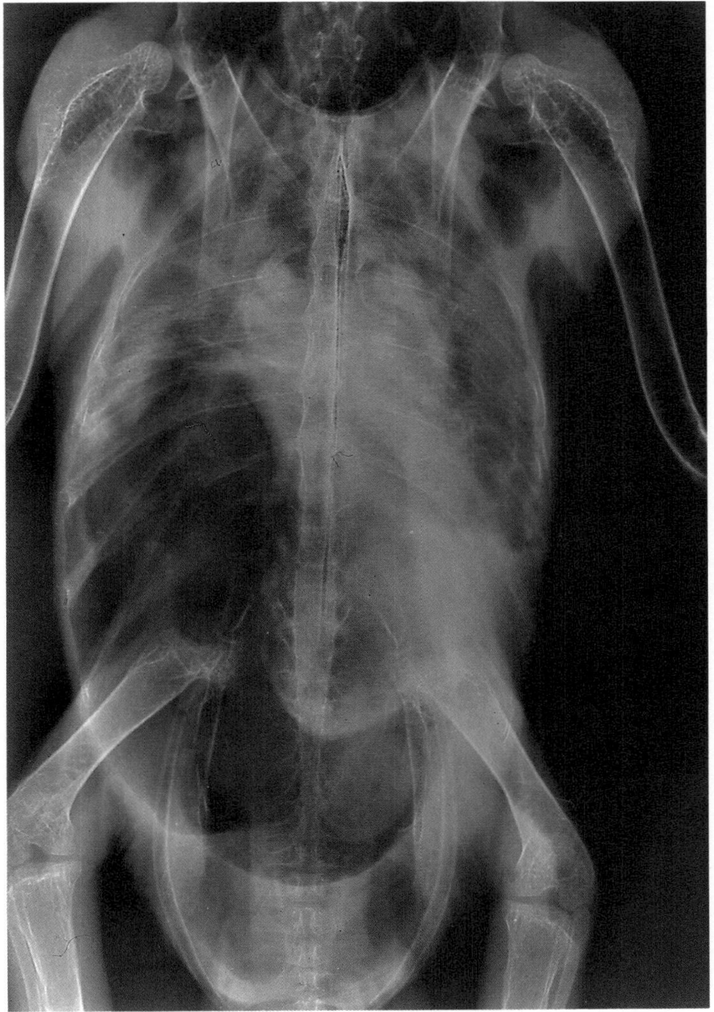

40/41 Air Sac Overexpansion.

Blue and Yellow Macaw *(Ara a. ararauna).*

Although the macaw is correctly positioned, on the ventrodorsal radiograph a significant asymmetry of the air sacs can be seen. The left air sacs are collapsed due to bronchial obstruction. The right air sacs are overexpanded, as a consequence of 'air trapping'. On the lateral radiograph, the overexpansion is significant. In the hilar region, the bronchi show minor opacities and the pulmonary density is increased.

Note: Birds with overexpansion of the caudal air sacs usually present with respiratory distress. Mucosal proliferations in the syrinx or the main bronchi, producing a valve effect, are often small and not recognizable on radiographs. "Air trapping" in the caudal air sacs is therefore an excellent diagnostic sign of changes in the central parts of the lungs.

42

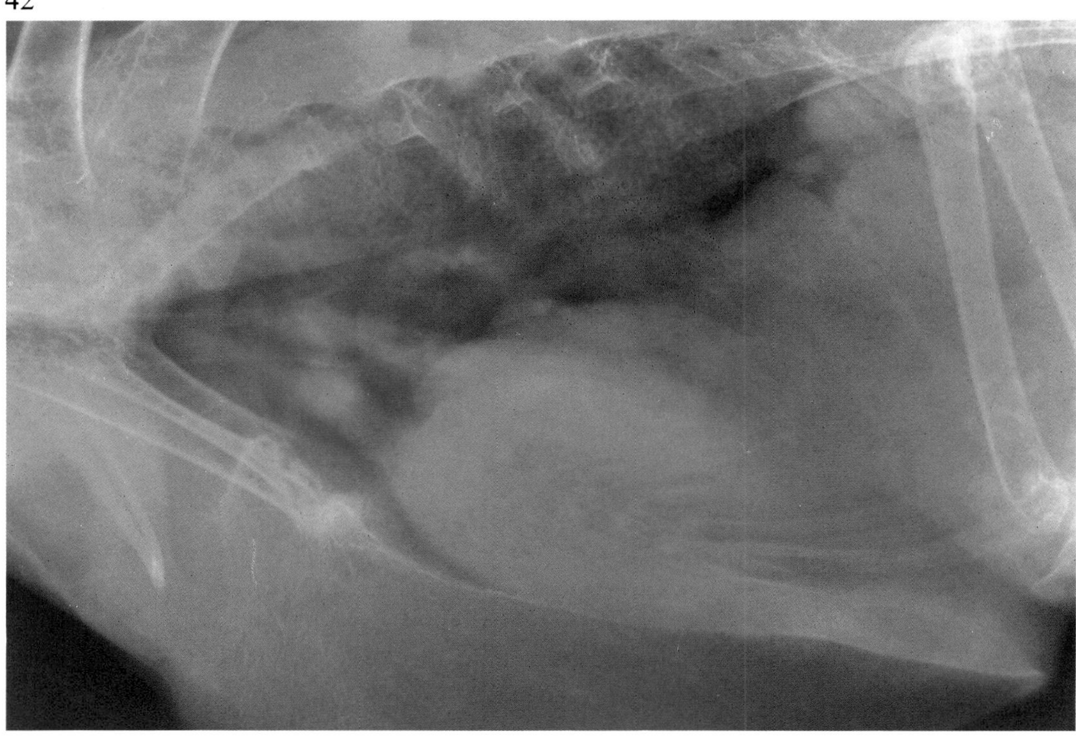

43

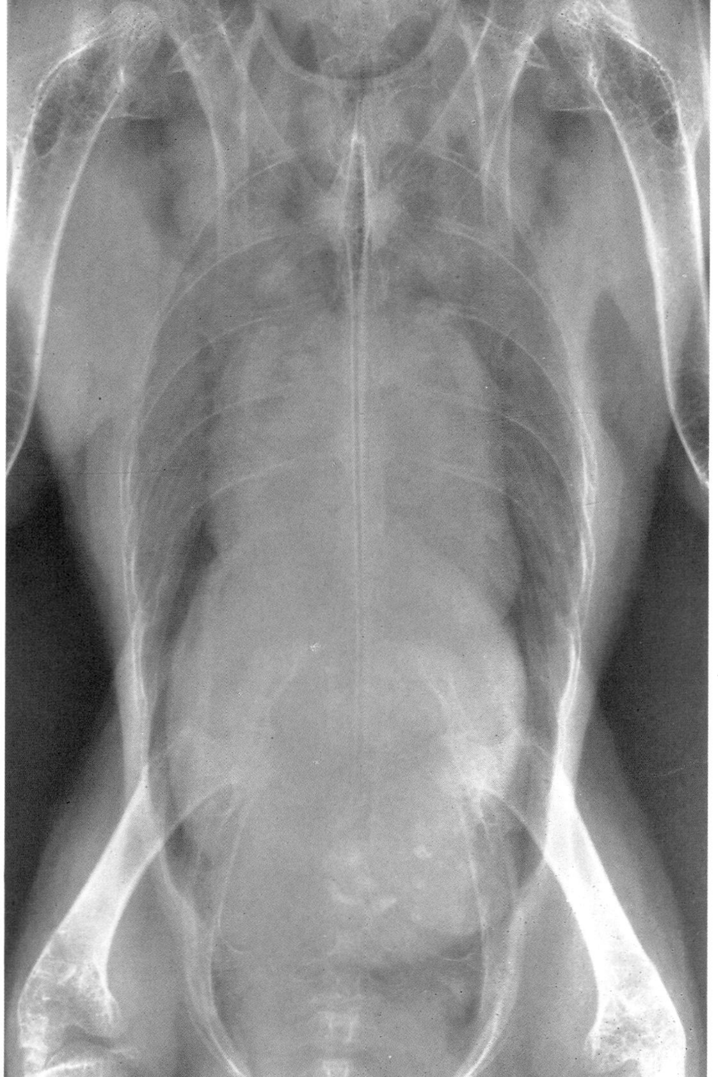

44

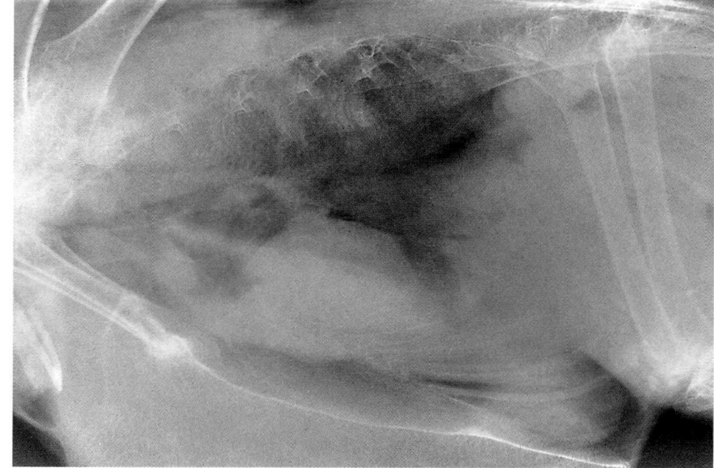

42/43/44 Hydropericardium.

Blue and Yellow Macaw *(Ara a. ararauna)*.

The cardiac shadow is enlarged and appears very dense. It also has an abnormal shape and expands over the midline to the left side (FIGS. **42, 43**).

The pericardium was punctured and 20 ml of fluid was aspirated. After this procedure, the cardiac shadow regained normal size (FIG. **44**). However, the heart has not yet returned to the normal position.

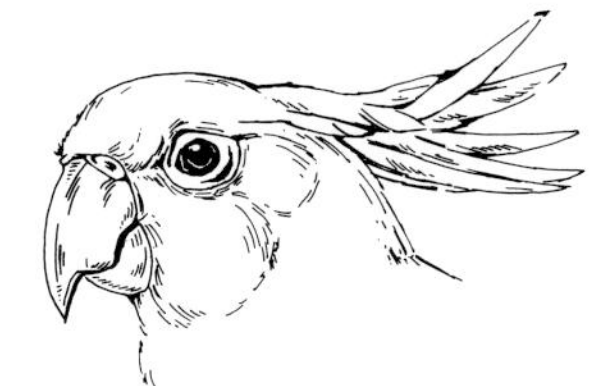

45

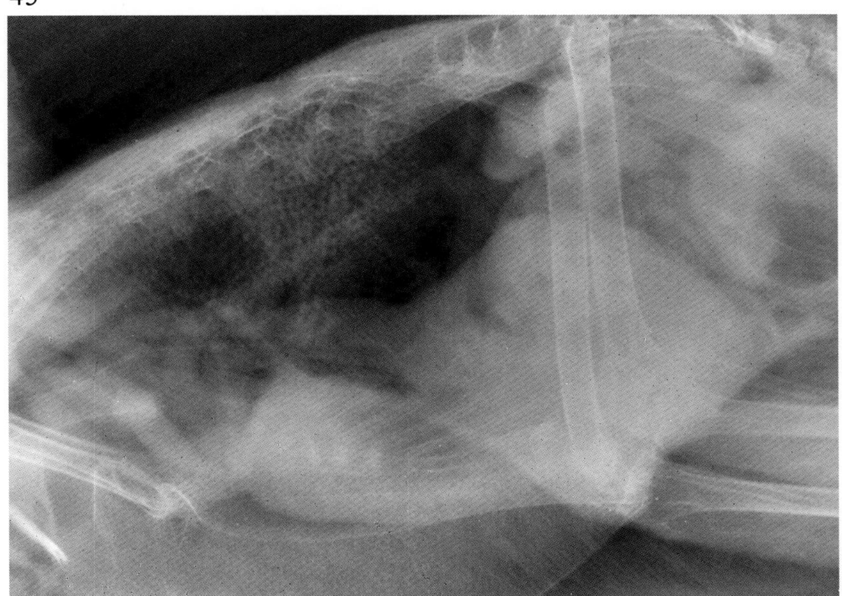

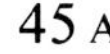

45 A

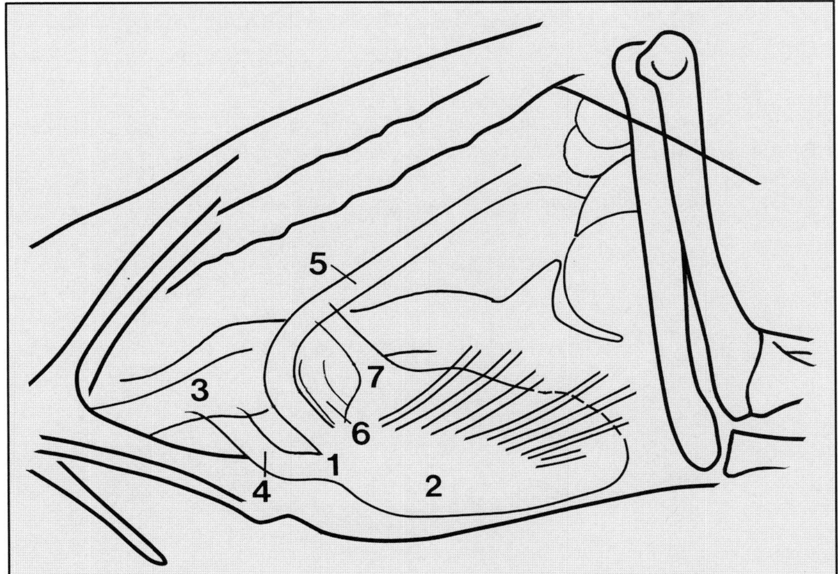

45/45A Arteriosclerosis.

Grey Parrot *(Psittacus e. erithacus).*

The radiopacity of the large arteries and veins is abnormally increased. As a result they can be seen easily. The aorta (**1**) leaving the heart (**2**) divides shortly before it reaches the trachea (**3**) into the brachiocephalic artery (**4**) and descending aorta (**5**). The pulmonary arteries (**6**) can also be recognized as very dense vessels. Further caudally, the vena cava (**7**) is visible.

This radiograph shows the typical signs of arteriosclerosis.

46

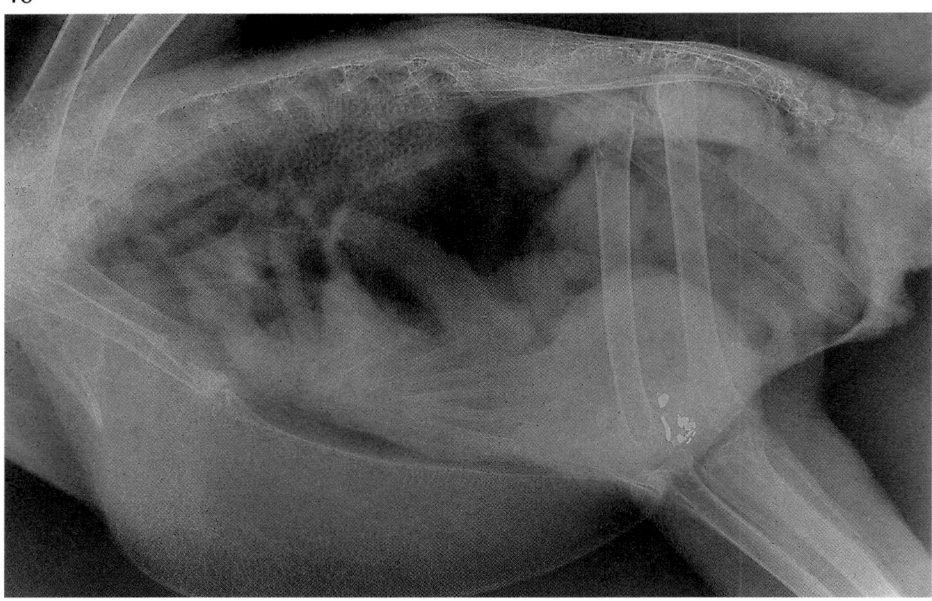

47

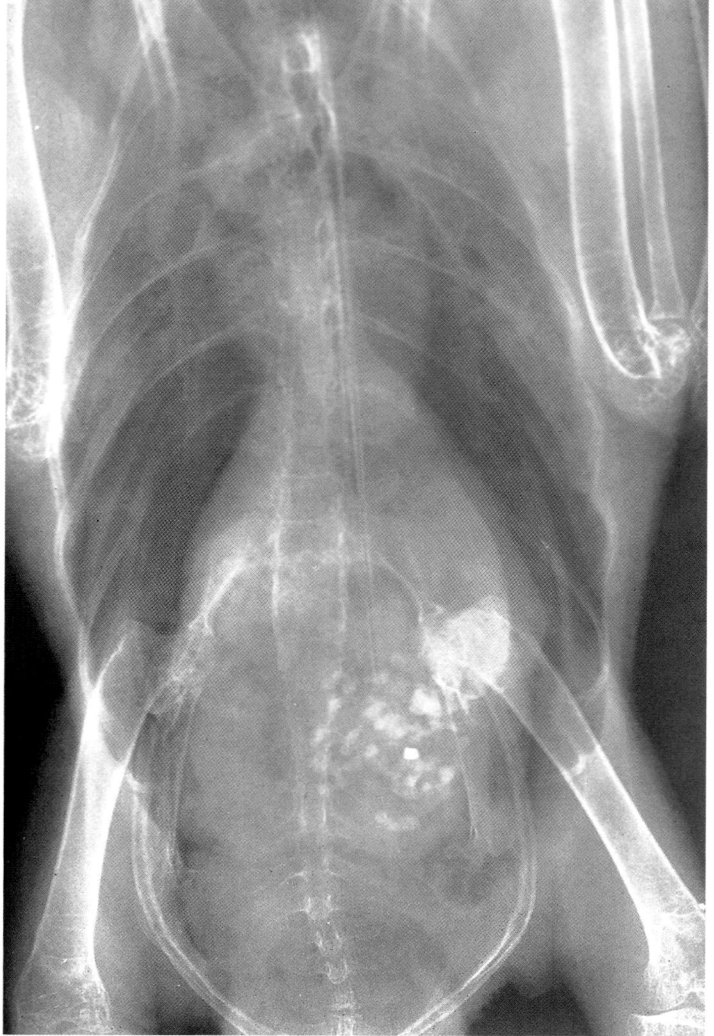

46 Wall Thickening of Esophagus and Proventriculus / Hypovitaminosis A.

Grey Parrot *(Psittacus e. erithacus).*

Esophagus and proventriculus cast very dense shadows. This type of high radiodensity is often found with hypovitaminosis A, when the mucous membranes have become metaplastic resulting in increased wall thickening.

47 Dilatation of Proventriculus.

Grey Parrot *(Psittacus e. erithacus).*

On this ventrodorsal radiograph, the proventriculus is visible. Its left border extends beyond the liver shadow. The visibility of the proventriculus lateral to the liver border indicates slight enlargement of the proventriculus.

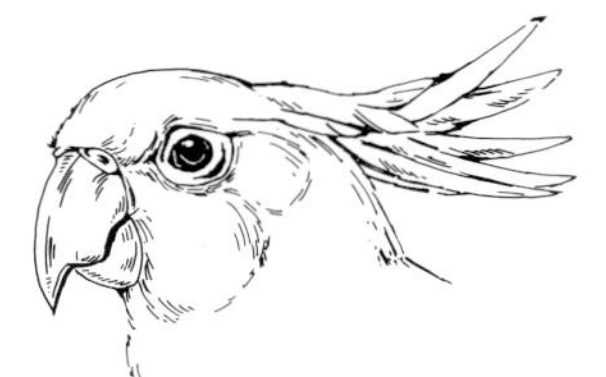

48

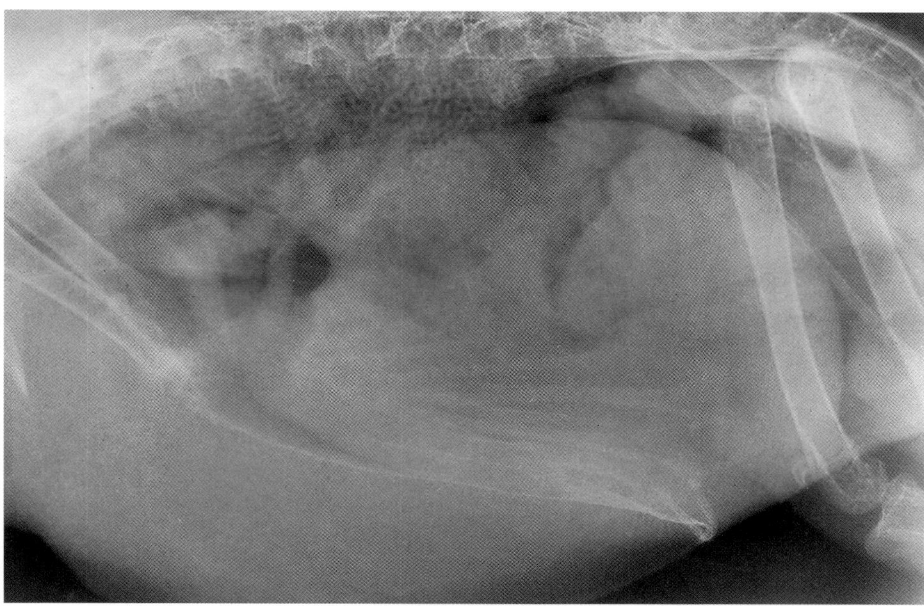

49

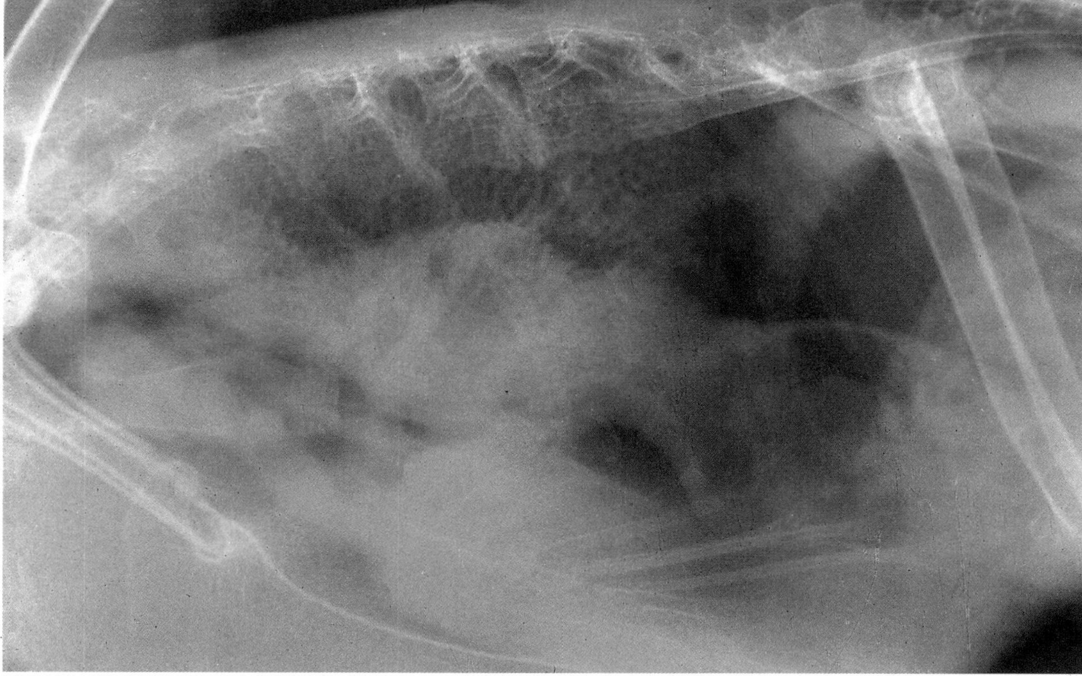

48 Dilatation of Proventriculus.

Grey Parrot *(Psittacus e. erithacus).*

Caudal to the syrinx the esophagus expands and joins a severely dilatated proventriculus that is delineated by the lungs dorsally. The proventriculus contains a large amount of food.

Note: In psittacines, severe enlargement of the proventriculus is found in cases of Candida-infections or "Macaw wasting disease", a viral infection.

49 Esophageal Neoplasm.

Blue-fronted Amazon *(Amazona aestiva)*, 12 years.

Dorsal to the heart a well-defined soft tissue density is present that seems to be part of the esophagus. Caudal to this mass, the esophagus passes into the dilated air-filled proventriculus. The proventricular wall is distinctly outlined. Histologically, the mass proved to be a poorly differentiated carcinoma, probably a squamous cell carcinoma.

50

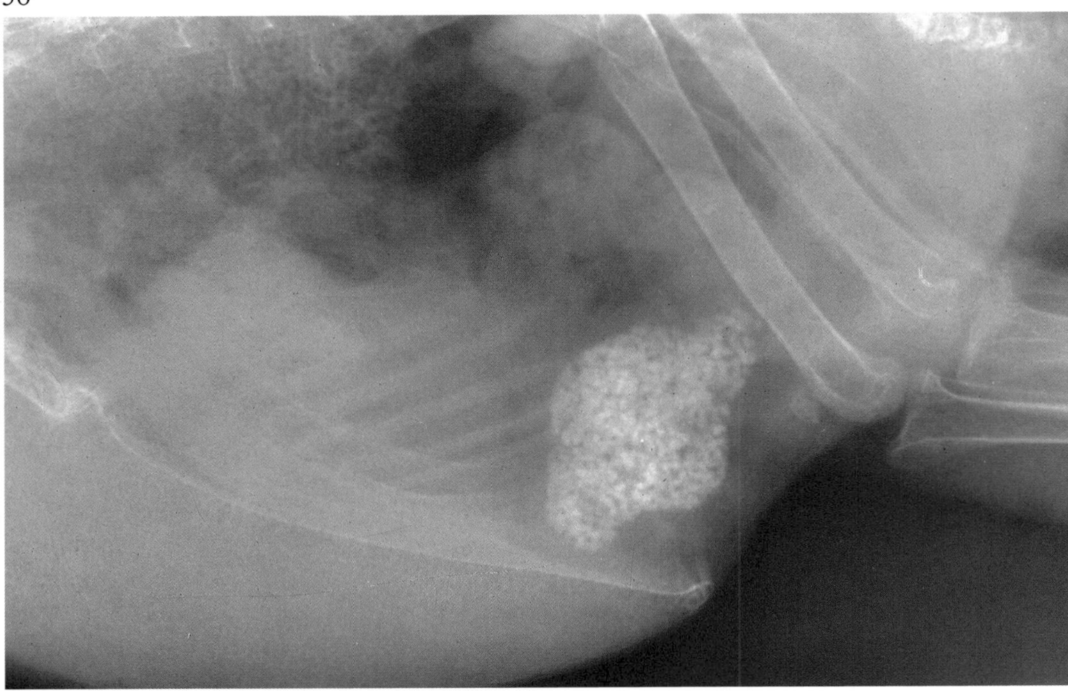

51

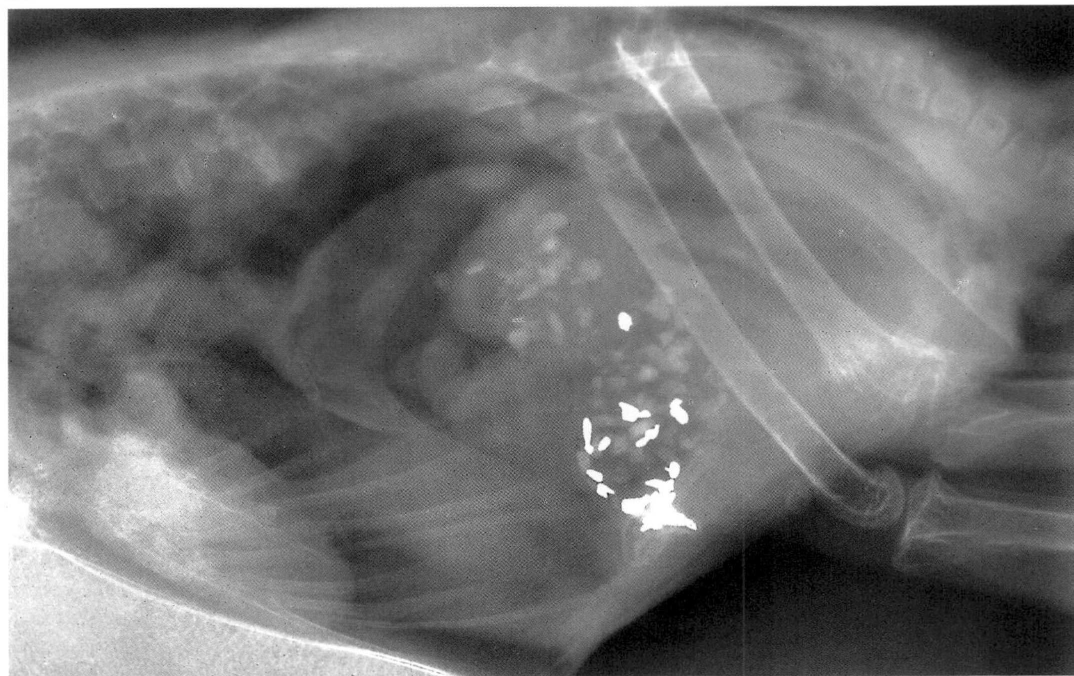

50 Gravel in the Ventriculus.

Blue-fronted Amazon *(Amazona aestiva).*

Some gravel in the ventriculus is a normal finding in seed-eating birds. In this bird, however, the ventriculus is filled with an excessive amount of gravel delineating the shape of the ventricular cavity.

Note: An excessive accumulation of gravel in the ventriculus is not physiologic. In cases of intestinal inflammation, some birds eat large amounts of gravel. Therefore, excessive accumulation of gravel may be interpreted as a sign of inflammatory bowel disease.

51 Lead Poisoning.

Larger Sulfur-Crested Cockatoo *(Cacatua galerita).*

In addition to gravel stones several highly radiopaque particles are visible in the ventriculus.

Note: This radiographic finding in combination with an appropriate history and clinical findings suggests a diagnosis of lead poisoning.

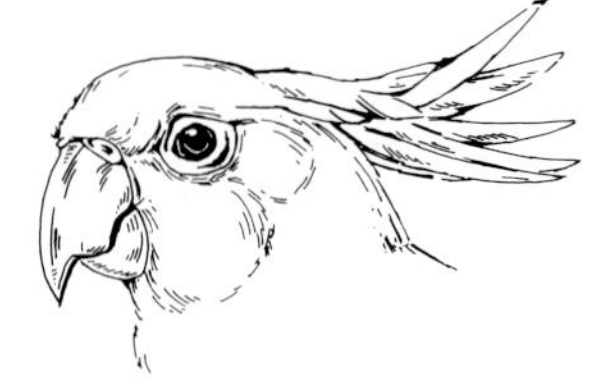

52

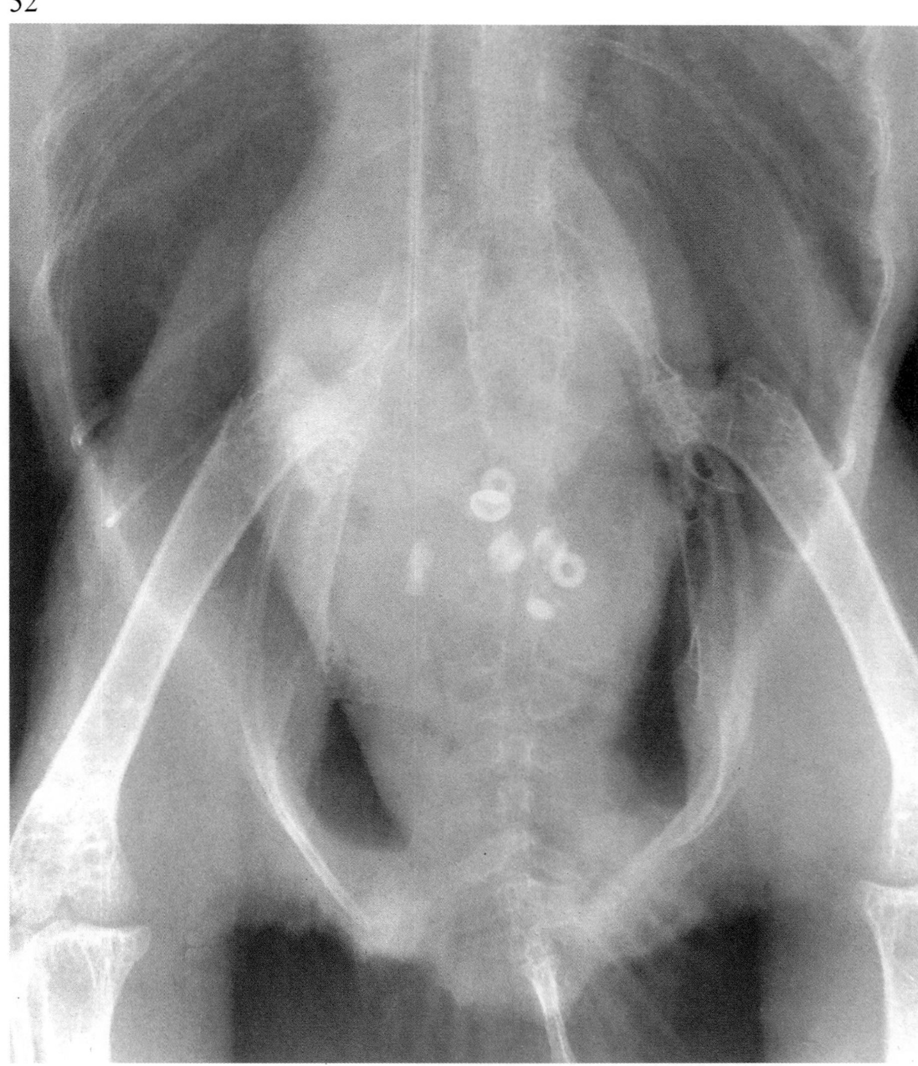

52 Foreign Body in the Ventriculus.

Yellow-crowned Amazon *(Amazona ochrocephala oratrix).*

Dense particles representing plastic beads are visible in the ventriculus. The ventriculus has an unusual caudal position. The proventriculus extends beyond the liver shadow indicating dilatation. The plastic beads were an incidental finding.

53

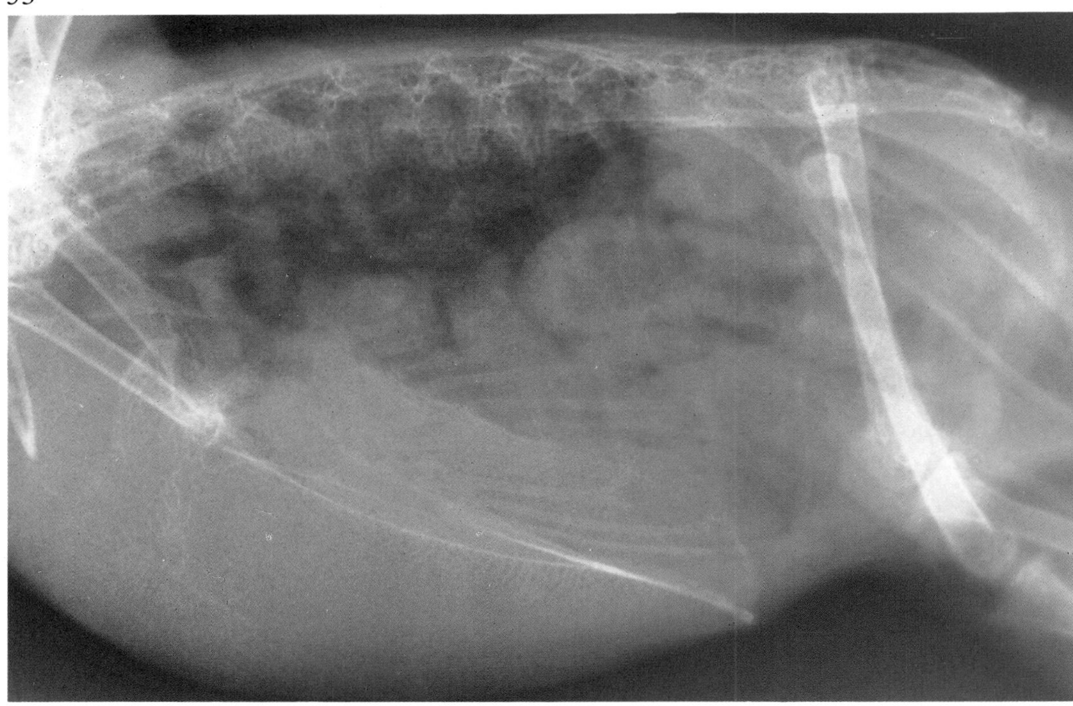

54

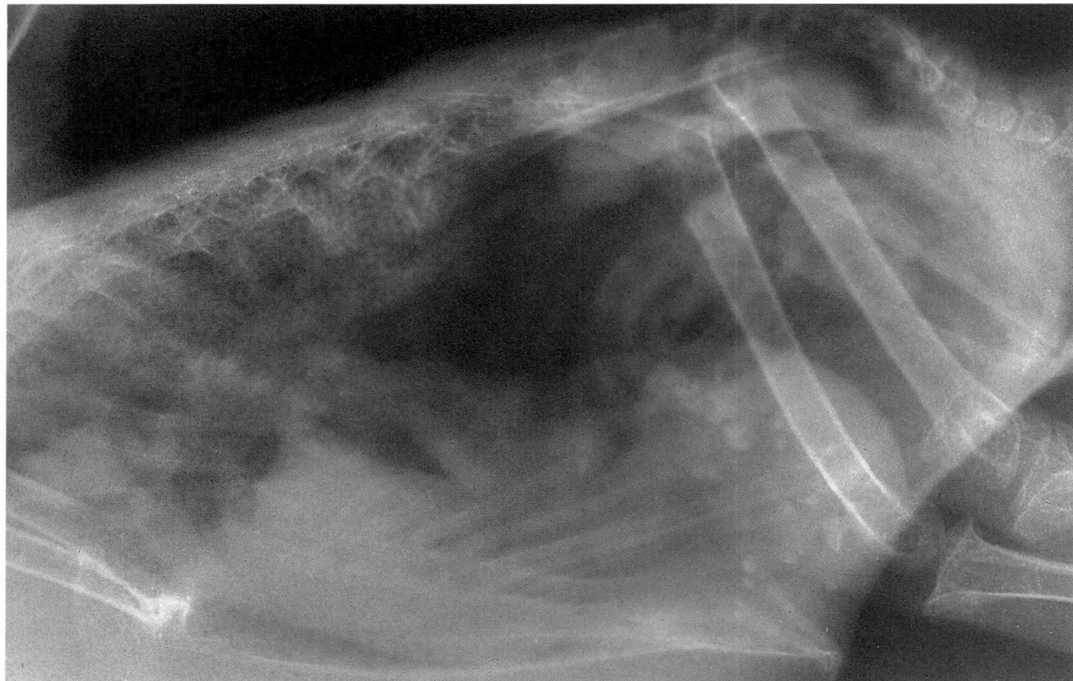

53 Intestinal Parasitosis.

White-fronted Amazon *(Amazona a. albifrons).*

A distended, gas-filled small intestinal loop extends caudally in the centre of the celom. The intestinal tract occupies more space than usual.

Note: Radiodense, slightly distended intestinal loops are important signs of parasitic infestations.

54 Enteritis, lateral.

Grey Parrot *(Psittacus e. erithacus).*

Air-filled intestinal loops are recognized as radiolucent tubelike structures. Increased amounts of air in the intestines of psittacines are usually a sign of pathology. In this case an E. coli infection was present.

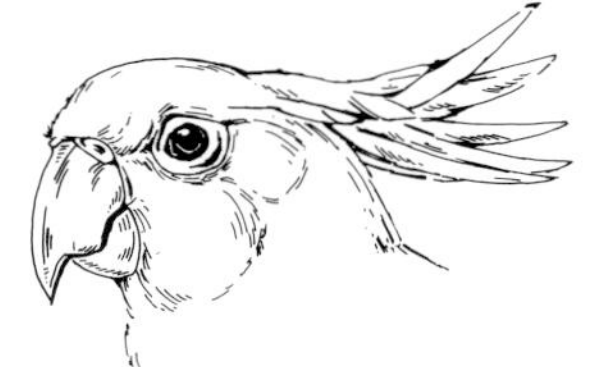

55

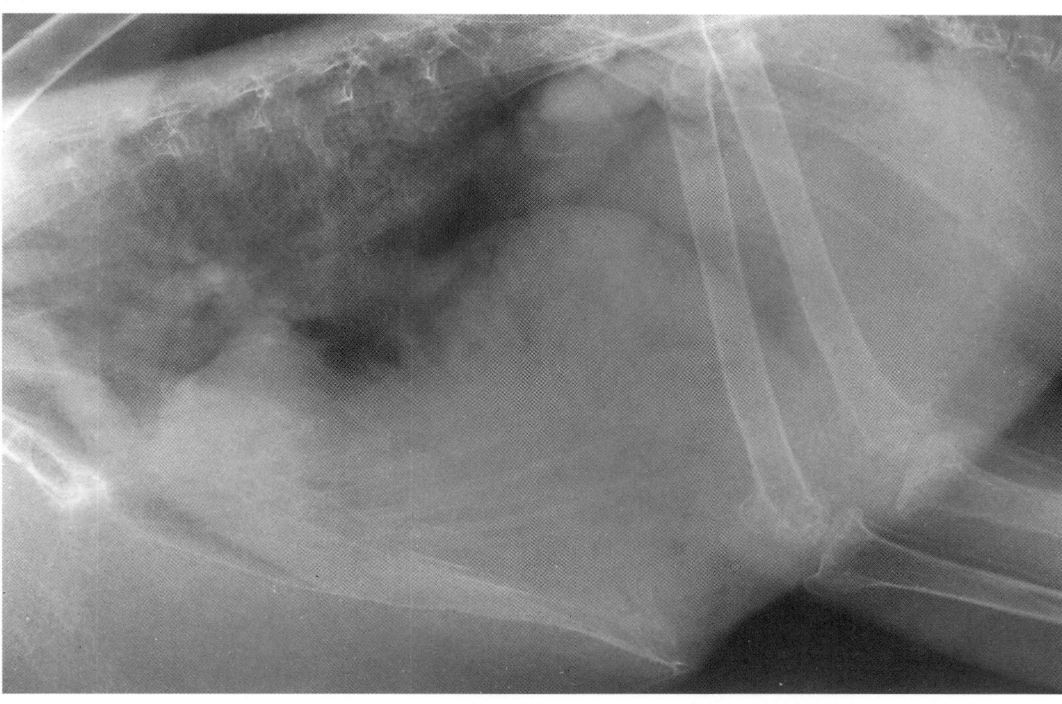

56

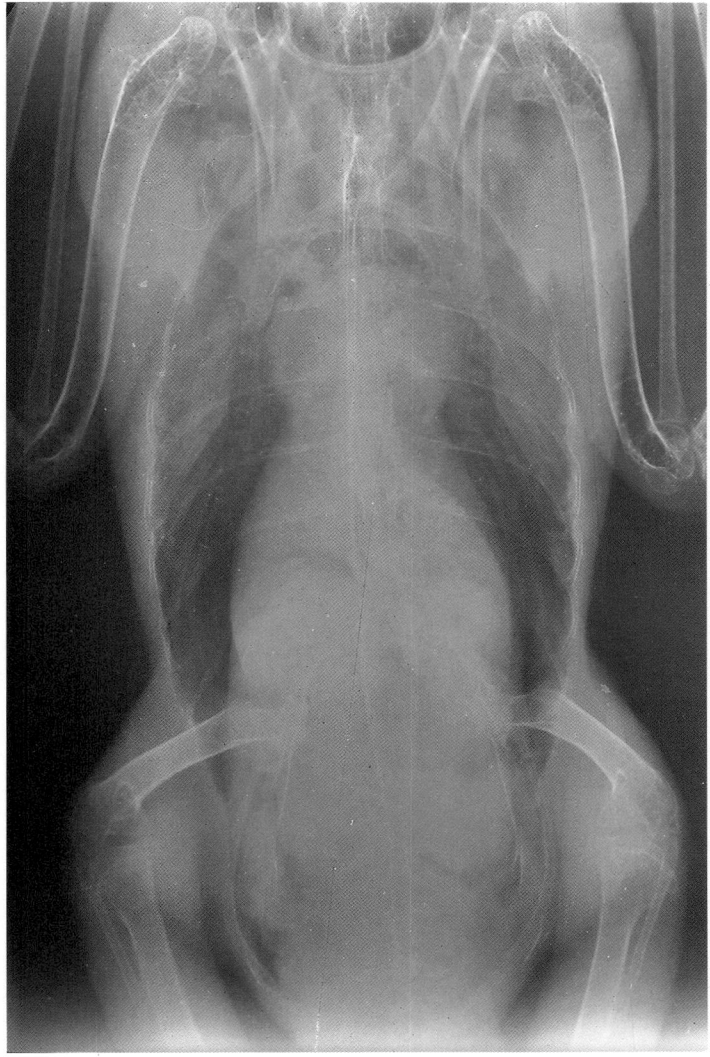

55/56 Intestinal Tuberculosis.

Mealy Amazon *(Amazona farinosa)*, adult.

Some of the changes on these radiographs are difficult to see. On the lateral radiograph, the enlarged proventriculus can be seen clearly. Superimposed upon the shadow of the proventriculus the spleen is faintly visible. It is of normal size. Cardiac and liver shadows look normal; the waist of the "hourglass" is not widened. The intestines, especially in the caudal part of the celomic cavity, are very dense and extend dorsally in the region of the cranial lobes of the kidneys. Some of the enlarged intestinal loops can be seen in both projections. On the lateral radiograph, they are superimposed by the proventriculus.

Note: The striking density of the intestinal loops due to increased thickness of the intestinal walls favors a diagnosis of intestinal Mycobacterium-infection. This tentative diagnosis could be confirmed later.

57

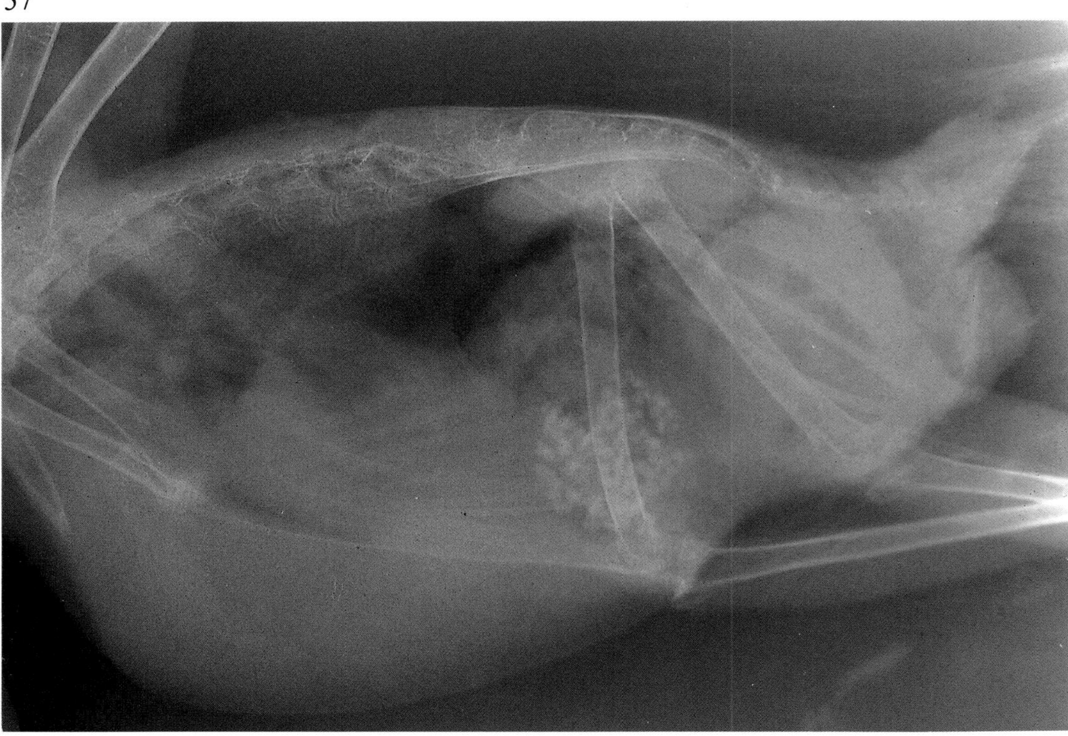

58

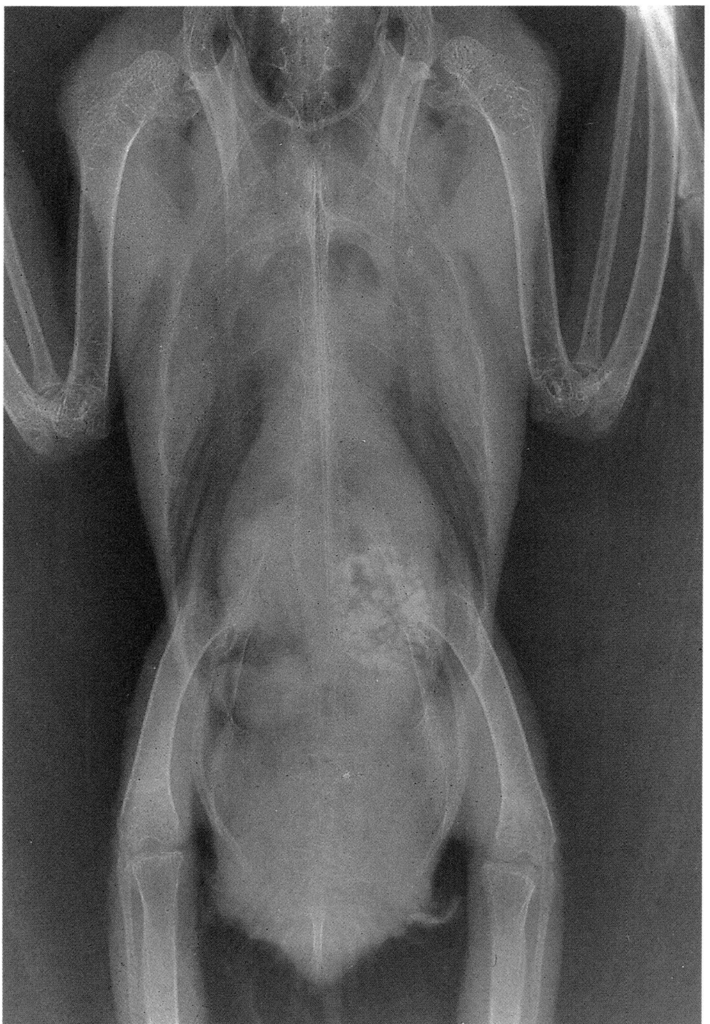

57/58 Cloacitis.

Senegal Parrot *(Poicephalus s. senegalus)*, adult.

Although positioning on the lateral radiograph is not optimal, a round soft tissue density can be seen in the cloacal region. On the ventrodorsal radiograph, this density is more difficult to define. The ventriculus is displaced cranially. Chronic cloacitis with wall-thickening was diagnosed.

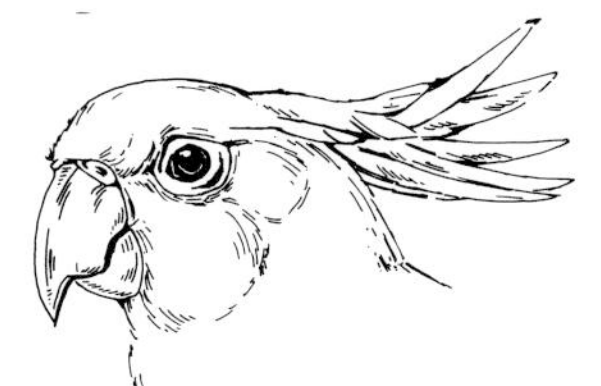

59

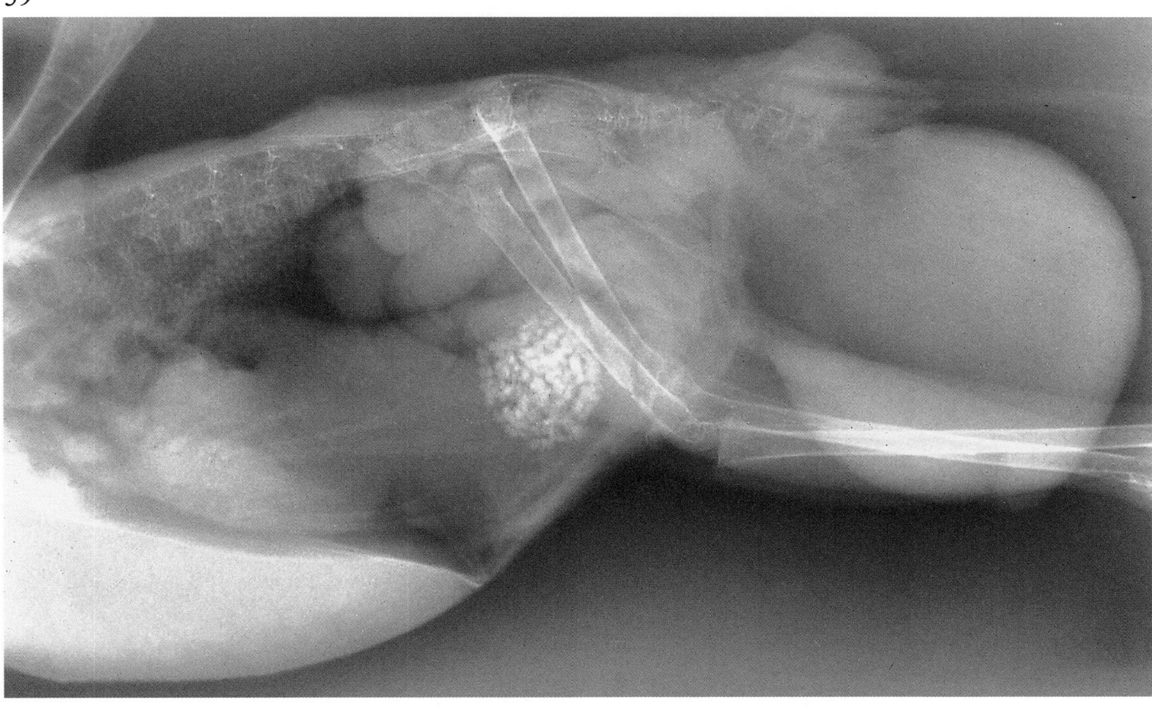

60

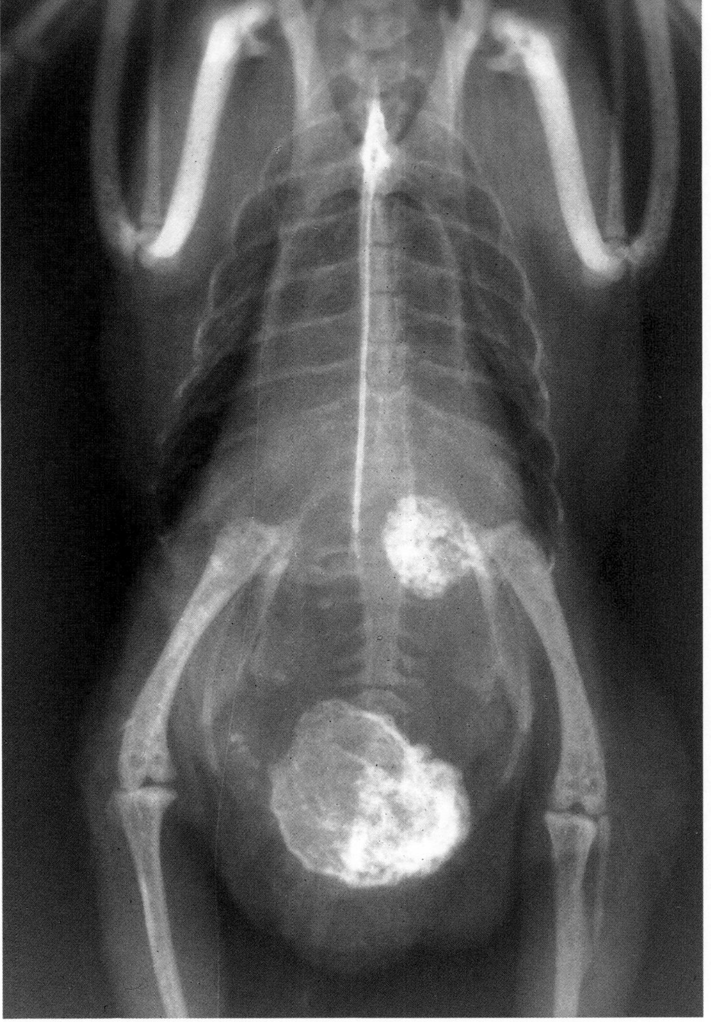

59 Cloacal Edema.

Black Parrot *(Coracopsis nigra)*, male.

A distinctly delineated homogeneous round soft tissue mass occupies the region of the cloaca. Several intestinal loops are unusually well visible in the caudal celom. These findings suggest edematous changes of the intestines and cloaca.

Note: In Coracopsis birds, these edemas are physiologic during the breeding season. Both sexes exhibit these symptoms. In this bird, the testes can clearly be seen permitting sex determination radiographically.

60 Enterolithiasis.

Fischer's Lovebird *(Agapornis p. fischeri)*, female.

The stone in the cloaca cannot be overlooked. As a differential diagnosis, egg binding should be considered. However, in this case it can be excluded because of the architecture of the mass. The ventriculus is displaced cranially, and the "hourglass"-shaped waist sign has disappeared. Osteosclerosis of the long bones is also present.

Note: Dorsal to this cloacal stone an ovarian tumor was found. In this case, the tumor interfered with defecation resulting in stone formation. Osteosclerosis is a common finding with ovarian tumors.

61

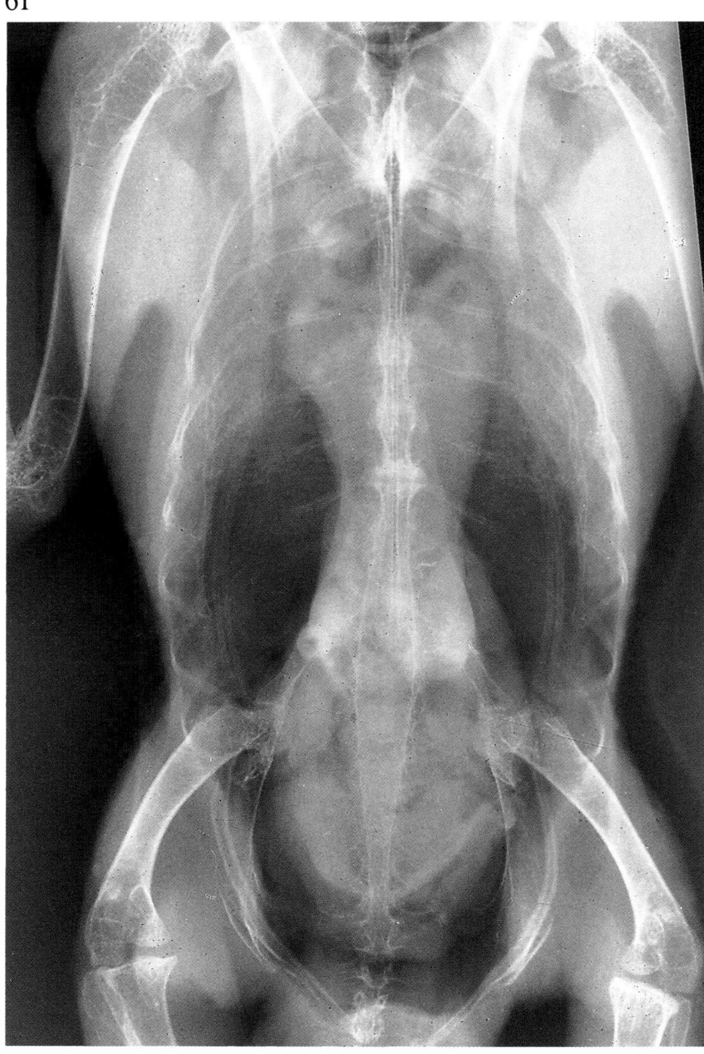

62

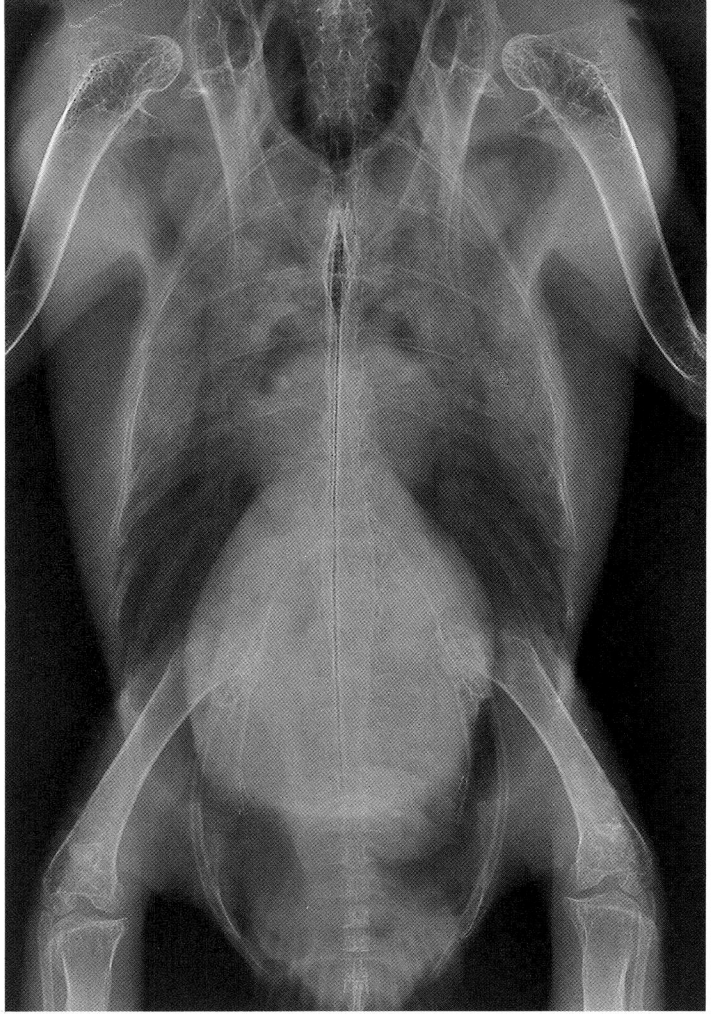

61 Cirrhosis.

Eclectus Parrot *(Eclectus roratus)*, adult.

The waist of the "hourglass" shadow in this parrot is lengthened and narrowed and it does not blend into the liver shadow. On the left side, the proventriculus that is normal in size extends beyond the liver border. The liver shadow is reduced to one half of its normal size and has an increased density. The left and right lobe can be determined. Biopsy confirmed the diagnosis of liver cirrhosis.

62 Hepatomegaly.

Grey Parrot *(Psittacus e. erithacus)*, adult.

The liver shadow is enlarged and very dense. The cranial liver outlines are more convex than usual. The caudal outlines, usually blending into the shadow of the intestinal tract, are distinctly visible. These findings are suggestive for liver disease. Liver biopsy provided a diagnosis of hemochromatosis.

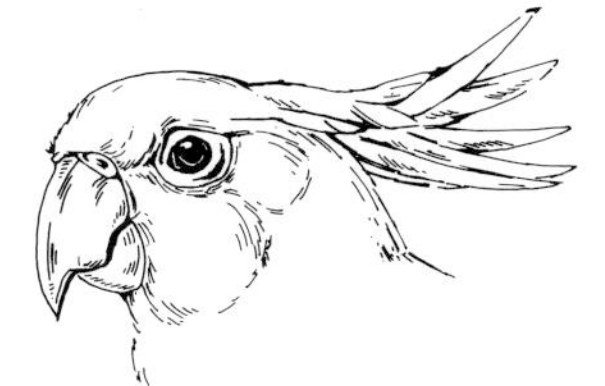

63

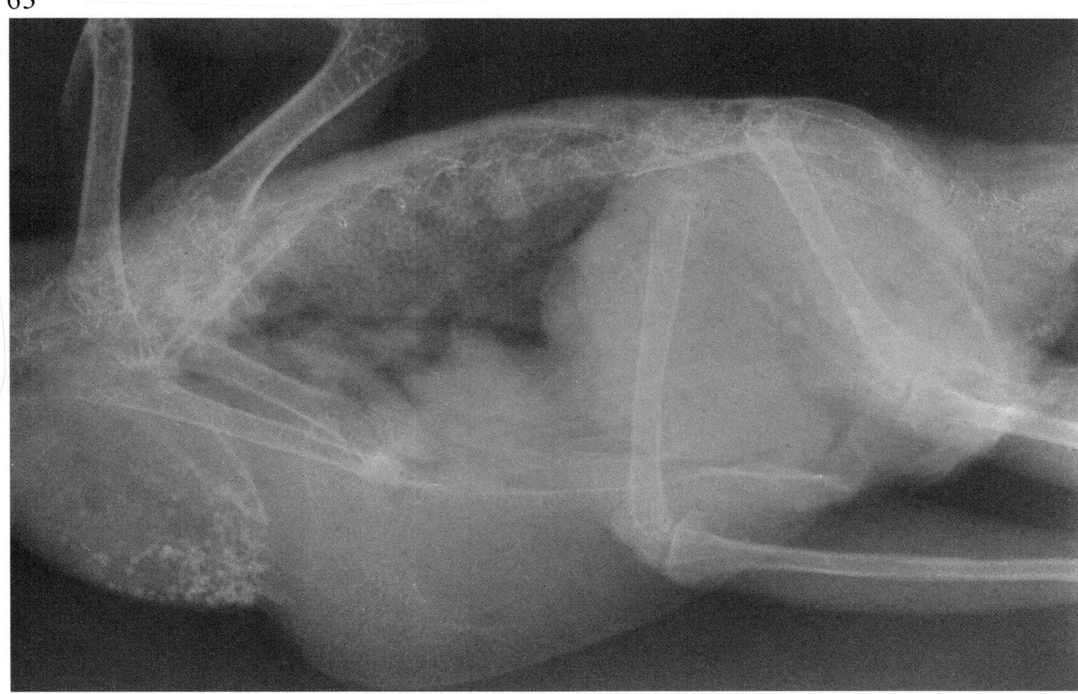

64

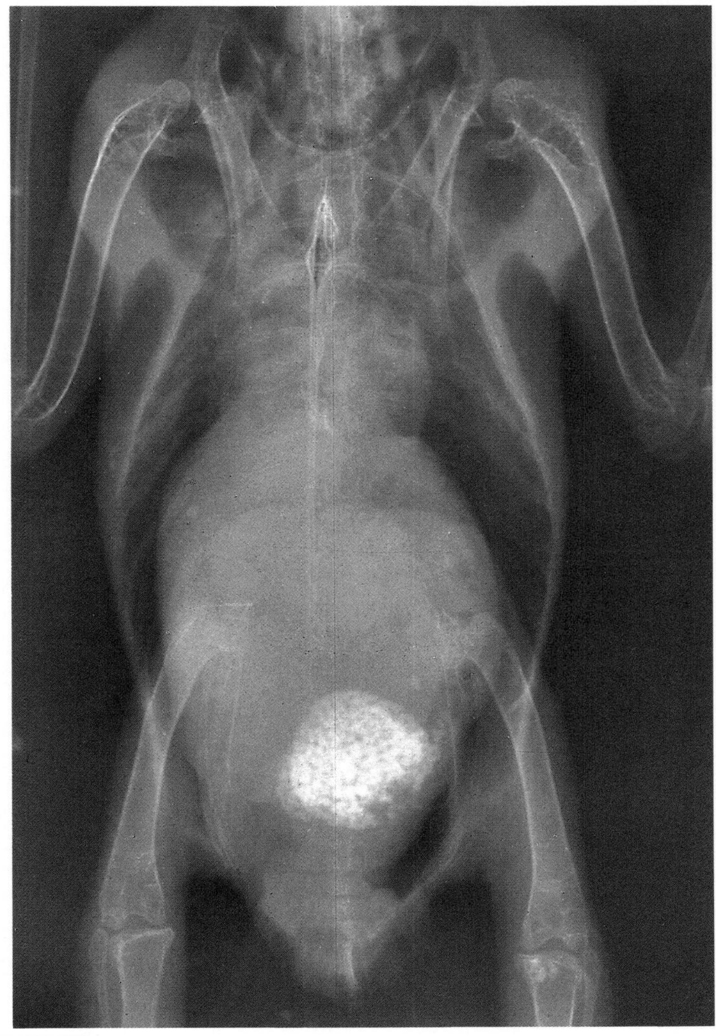

63 Liver Tumor.

White-fronted Amazon *(Amazona a. albifrons)*, 15 years.

The liver is enlarged, swollen and distinctly outlined. It extends far into the air sacs which are compressed and displaced. This liver mass proved to be a bile duct adenocarcinoma.

64 Hepatomegaly.

White-fronted Amazon *(Amazona albifrons)*, adult.

The liver shadow is tremendously enlarged. The gravel-filled ventriculus is displaced far caudally. Necropsy revealed a granulomatous hepatitis due to Mucor sp. infection.

65

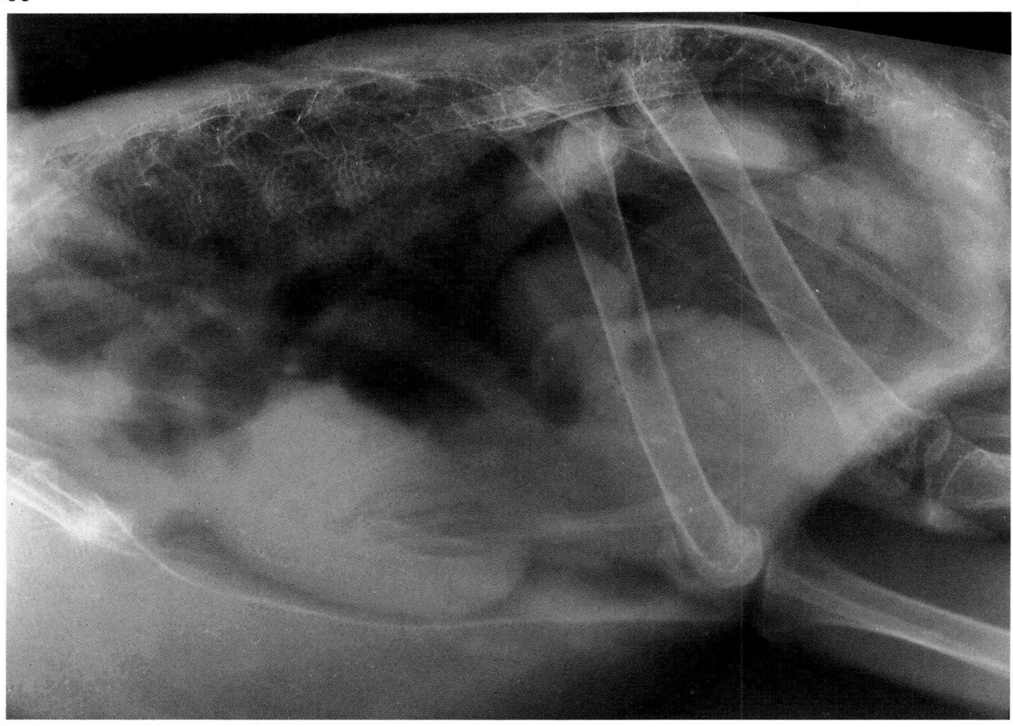

65 Splenomegaly.

Hyazinth-Macaw *(Anordorhynchus hyazinthinus)*, adult.

In this macaw, the spleen is about three times the size of a normal spleen. It is visible as a large round opacity. It is superimposed ventrally by the proventriculus, and caudally by the femur and intestinal loops. Splenomegaly may be seen with infectious, neoplastic or metabolic diseases. A tremendous increase in size is often found with mycobacterial or chlamydial infections, as in this case.

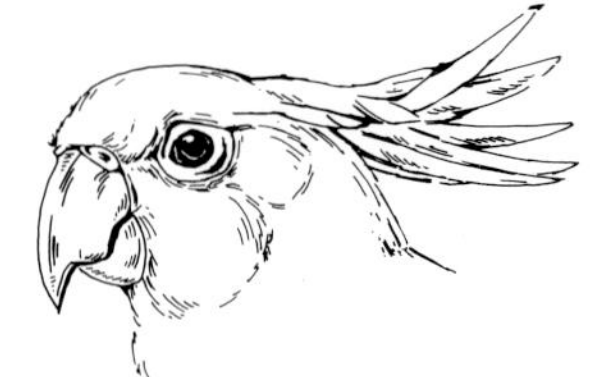

66

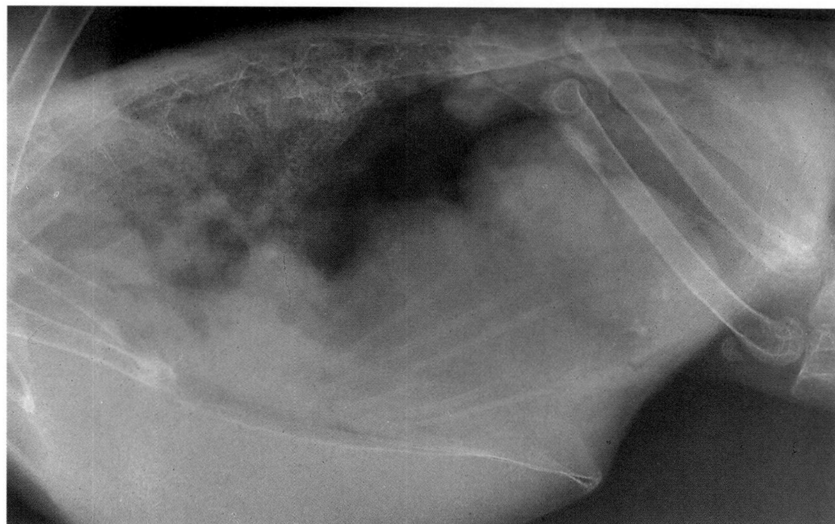

67

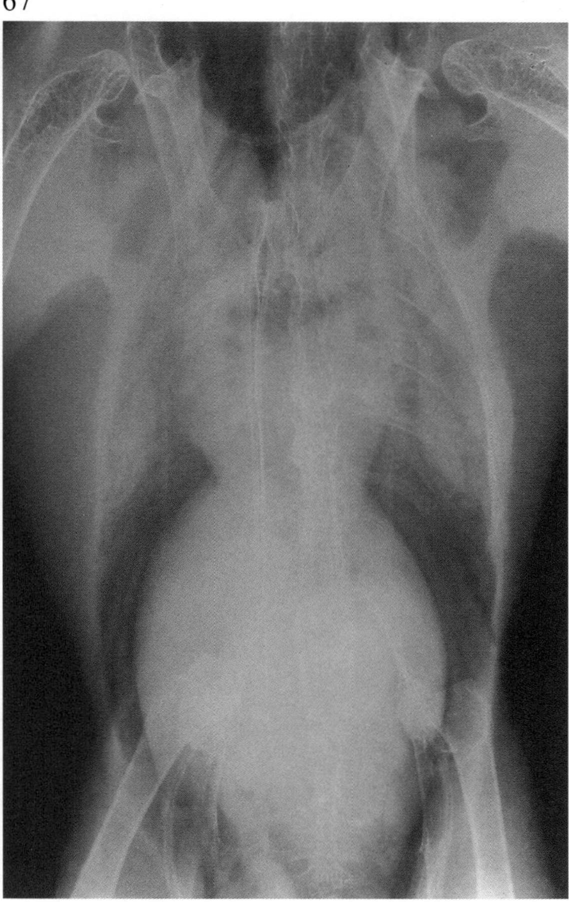

66 A

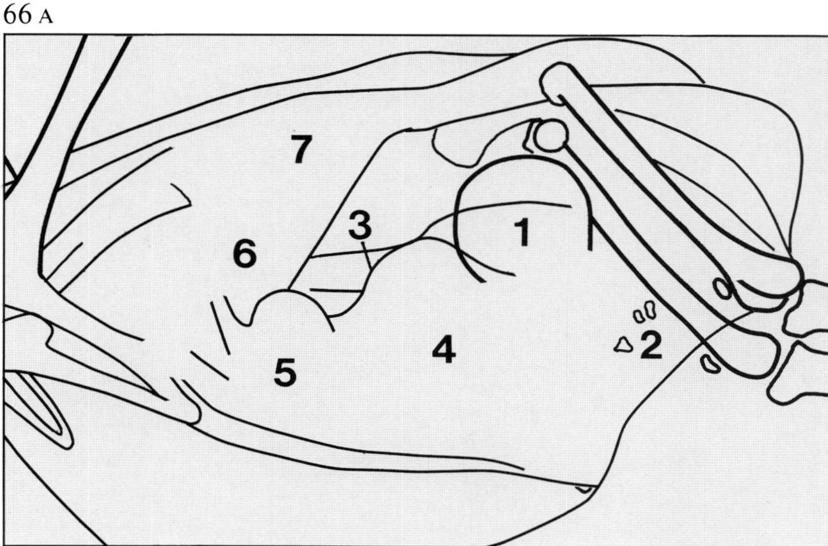

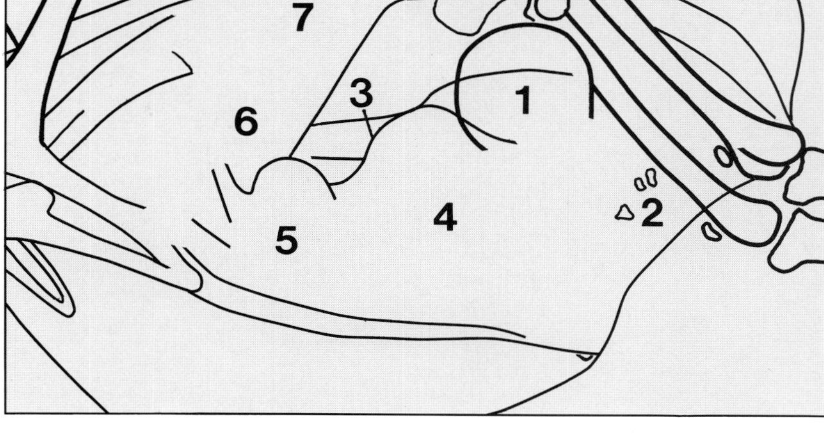

67 A

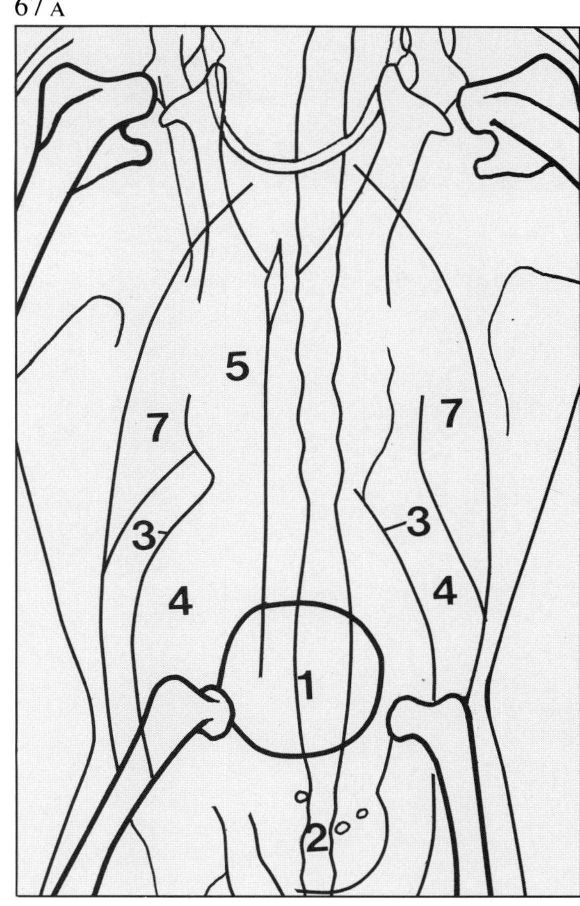

66/66A/67/67A Splenomegaly.

Grey parrot *(Psittacus e. erithacus)*, adult.

The spleen (**1**) is extremely enlarged. The ventriculus (**2**) is displaced caudally. The cranial liver borders (**3**) are well rounded, and the liver itself (**4**) is enlarged in both projections. On the lateral radiograph, the liver cannot be seen as a separate organ because it blends with the neighbouring organs. Its size, however, can be estimated based on the position of the heart (**5**) and of the ventriculus (**2**). A tentative diagnosis of avian tuberculosis was proven by liver biopsy.

Note: The opacities in the hilar region (**6**) and the radiodense lungs (**7**) are signs of a secondary respiratory infection.

68

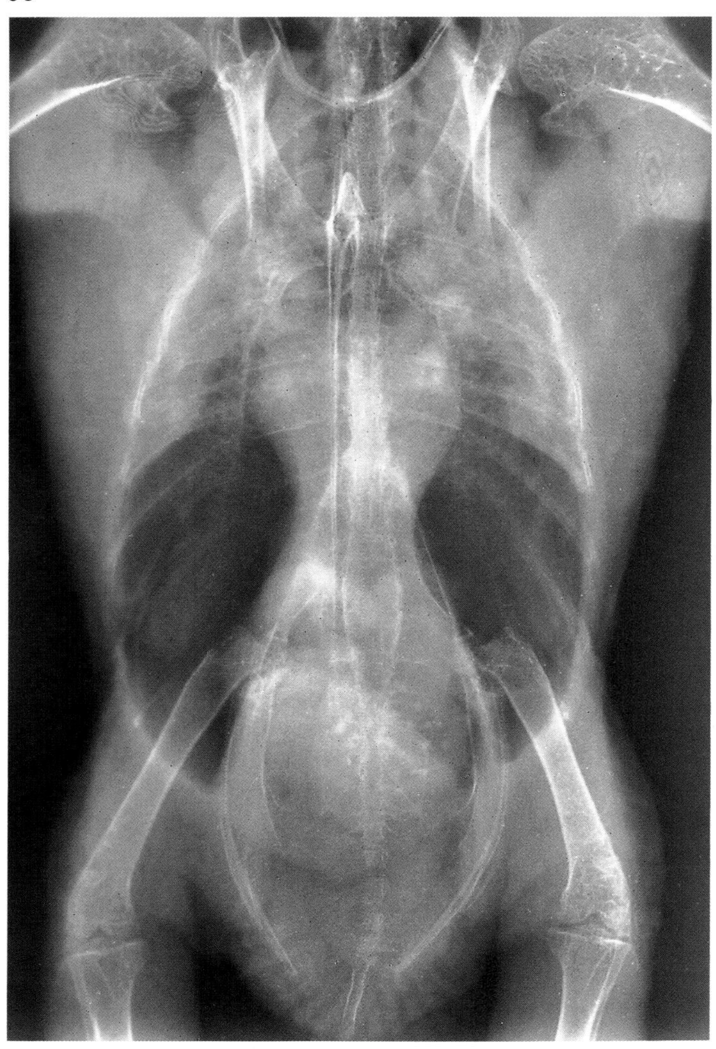

68 A

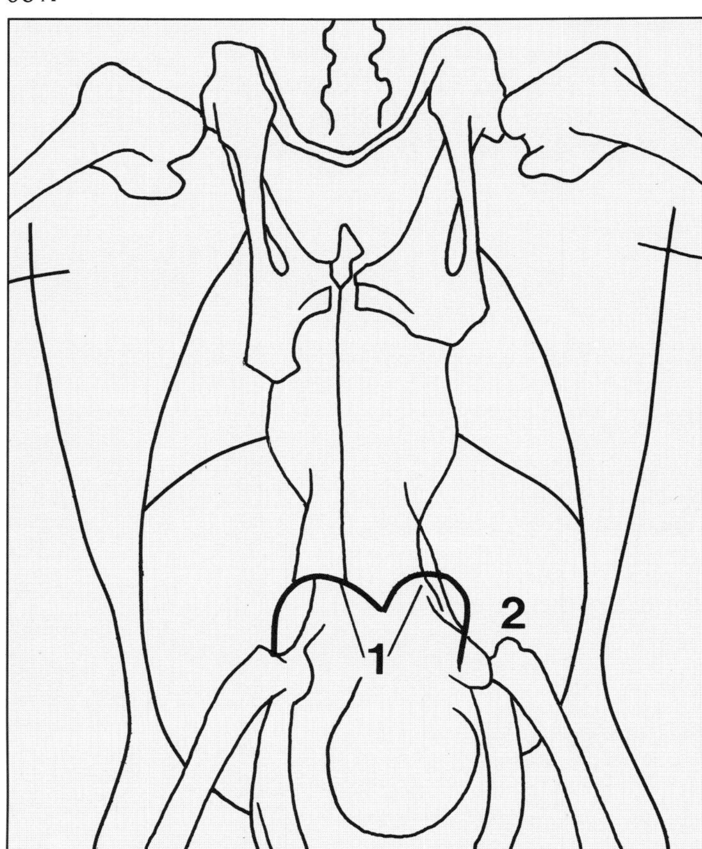

68/68A Nephromegaly.

Mealy Amazon *(Amazona farinosa)*, adult.

Both kidneys are enlarged. If only the kidneys are enlarged without concomitant changes in other organs, the cranial kidney lobes present as semicircular densities (**1**) that, partly superimposed by the liver shadow, extend cranial to the imaginary line connecting the acetabula. The lobe of the left kidney extends into the radiolucent air sac (**2**).

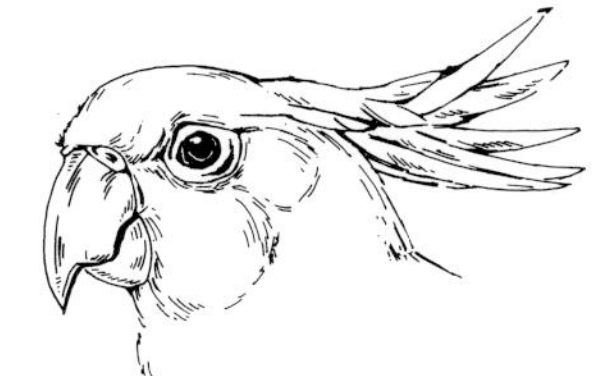

69

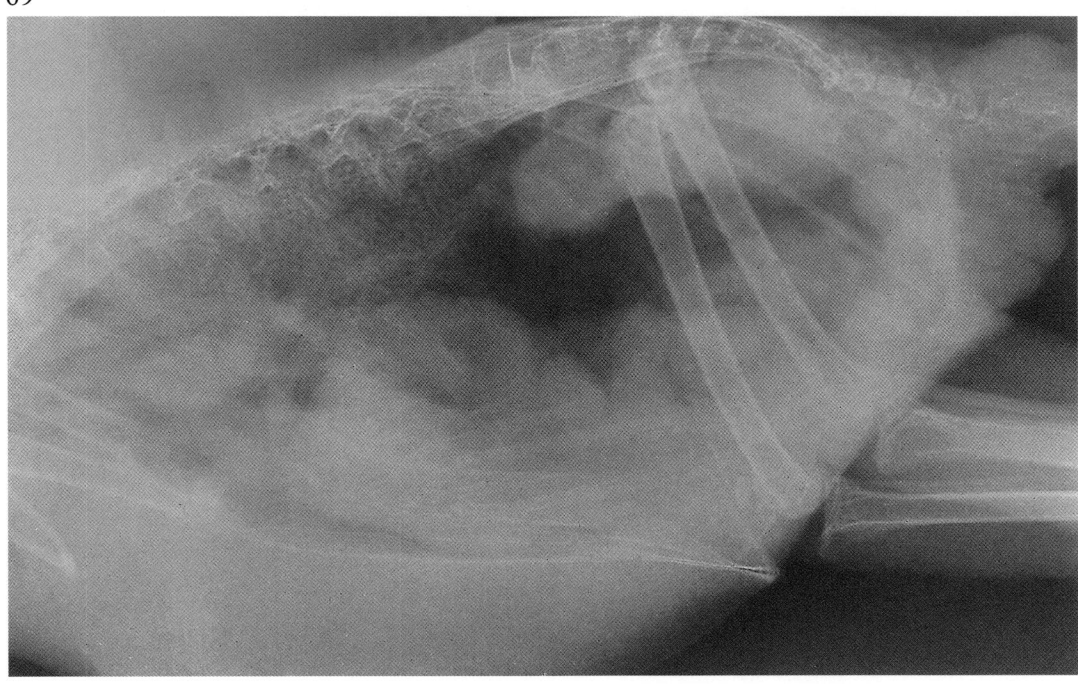

70

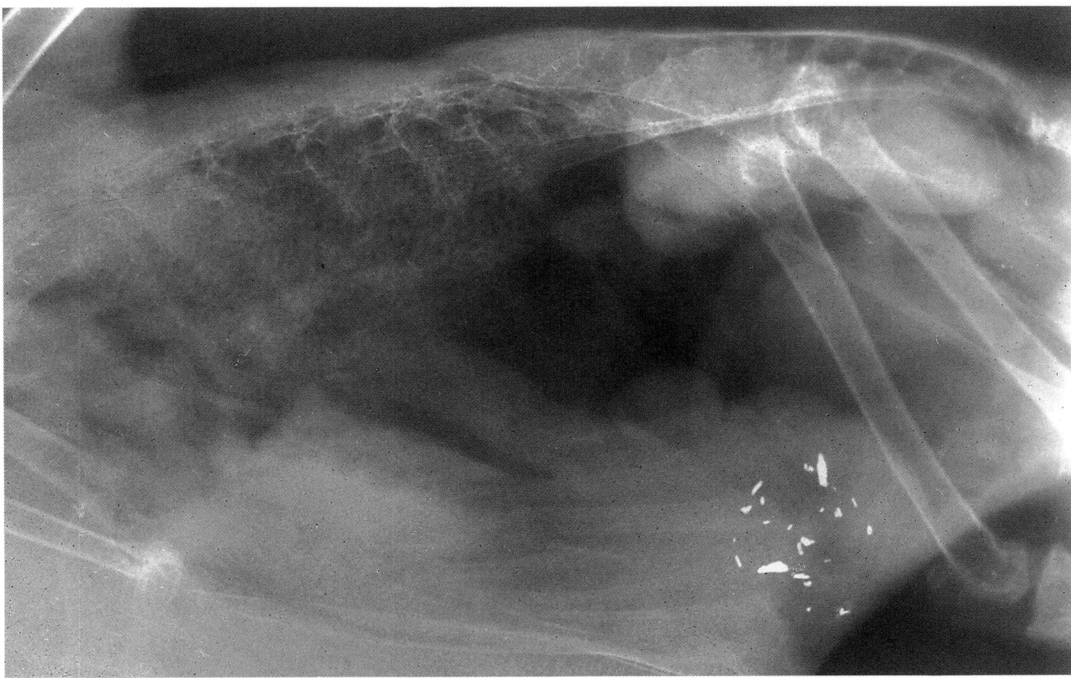

69 Nephromegaly.

Grey Parrot *(Psittacus e. erithacus)* , adult.

The enlarged, radiodense kidneys are clearly visible.

Note: This bird presented with the symptoms of polyuria and polydipsia. It had been treated with large doses of corticosteroids, which caused an intoxication resulting in nephromegaly.

70 Nephromegaly / Lead Poisoning.

Yellow-crowned Amazon *(Amazona ochrocephala panamensis)*, male, 12 years.

Both kidneys show an increased density and are enlarged. In the ventriculus, multiple lead fragments are present. Nephromegaly is a common sign in chronic lead intoxication.

71

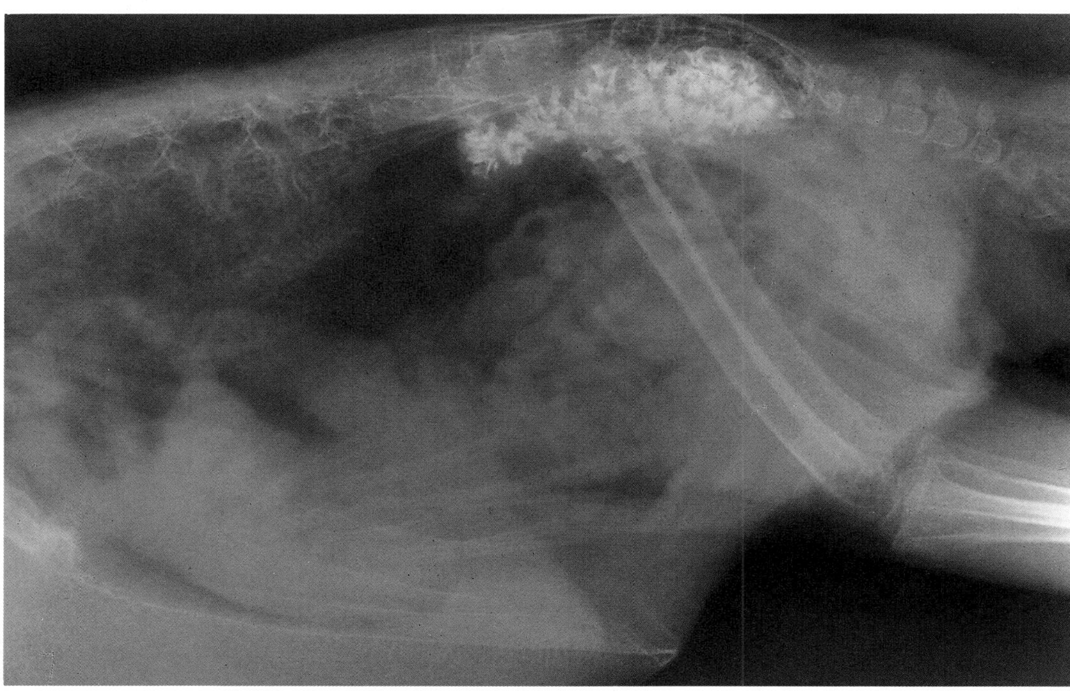

72

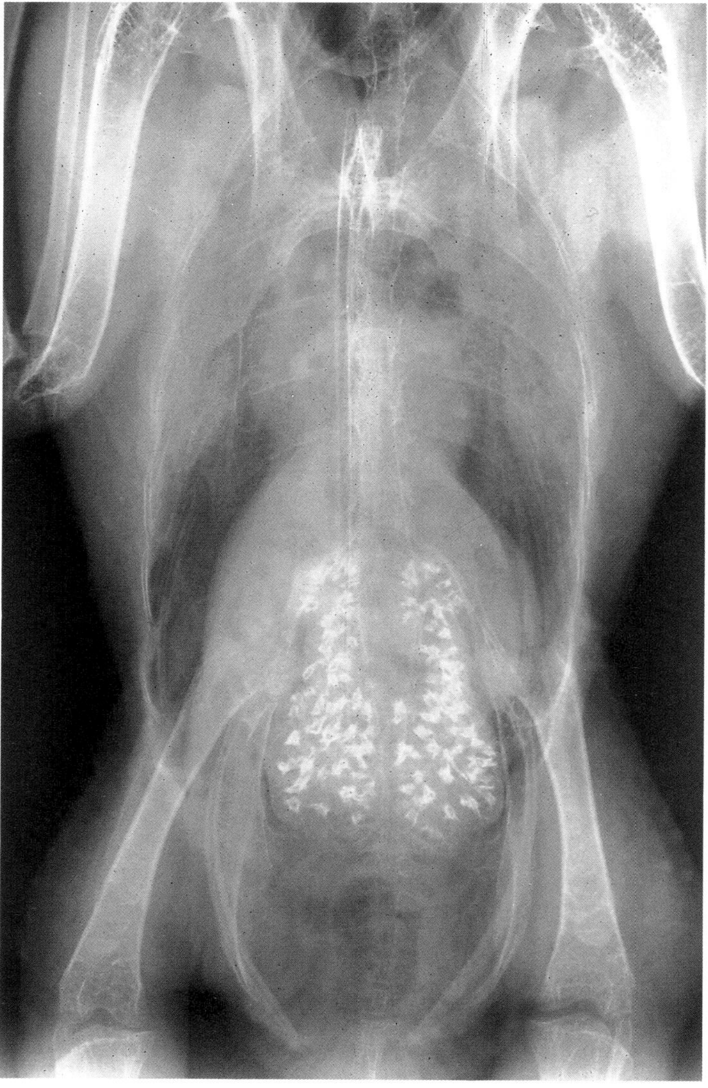

71/72 Kidney-Calcinosis.

Grey Parrot *(Psittacus e. erithacus)*, adult.

Because of deposition of calcium-containing crystals in the renal tissues, the kidneys can be seen completely. The pathophysiology of this type of nephrosis in psittacines is still unknown.

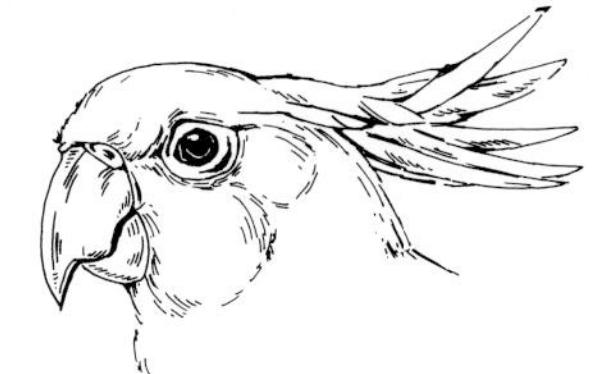

73

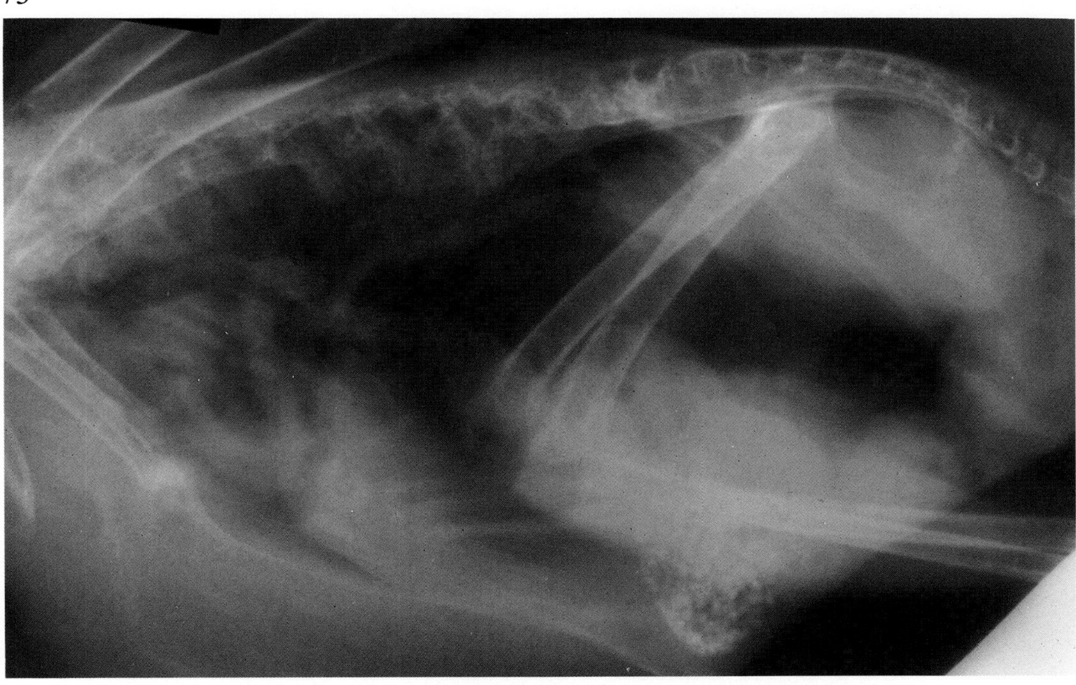

73 Kidney Tumor.

Yellow-faced Amazon *(Amazona xanthops)*, male, 12 years.

One of the caudal lobes of the kidneys is extremely enlarged. A renal adenocarcinoma was diagnosed. This is a common tumor in psittacines, especially in budgerigars.

74

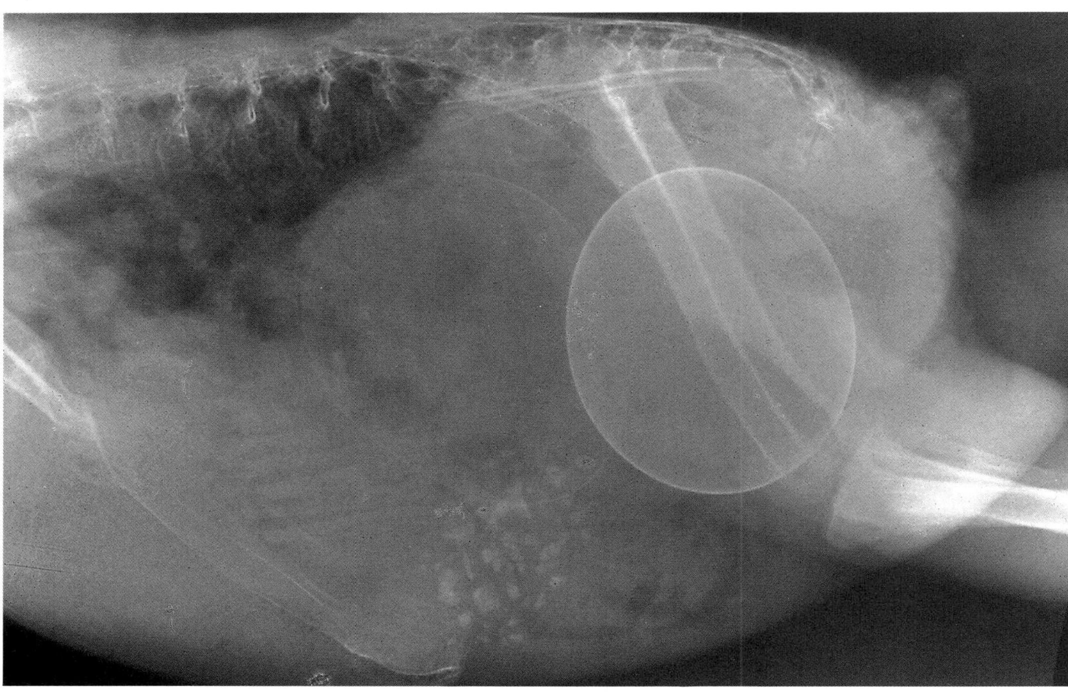

75

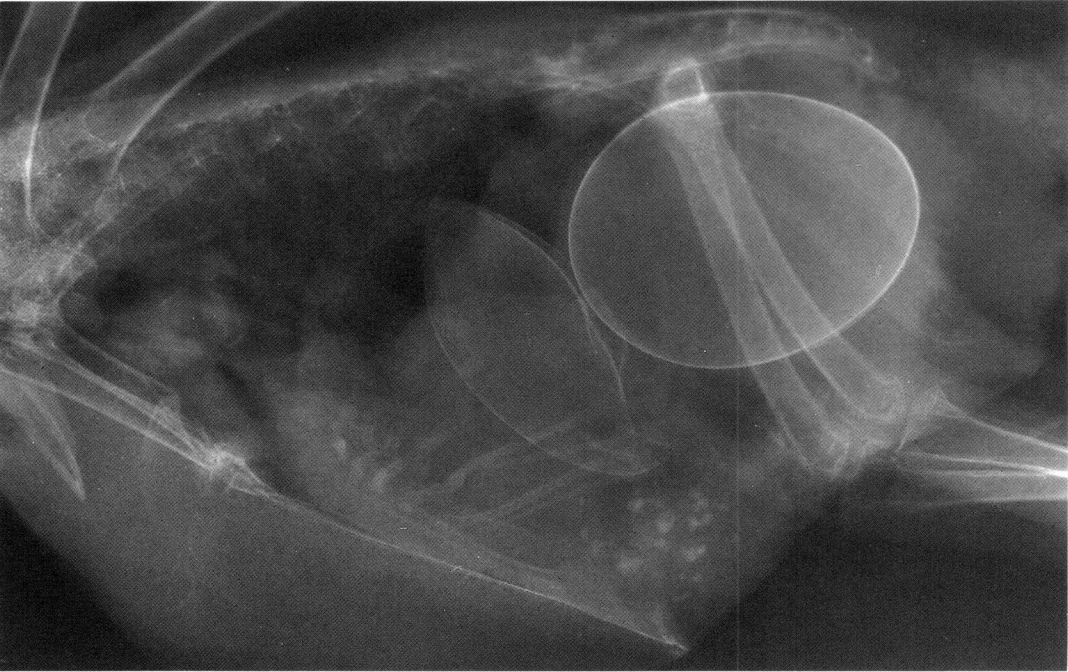

74 Egg Binding.

Mealy Amazon *(Amazona farinosa)*, female, adult.

In the caudal celom, an egg with a completely calcified shell is visible. The long axis of the egg is oriented vertical to the body axis preventing normal delivery. The abnormal position of this egg is caused by a second egg, with a thin shell, that lies partly beneath the first egg and puts pressure on it. The large ventriculus is displaced ventrally and to the left. As a result, this bird is egg bound. Due to compression of the air sacs, birds with egg binding often present with respiratory distress.

75 Rupture of the Salpinx.

Grey Parrot *(Psittacus e. erithacus)*, female, 8 years.

Next to the first egg, a second egg has already been formed. The folded shell of this second egg proves that it has been damaged. The leaking contents of the egg should have resulted in an increase in size and density of the salpinx. However, this is not visible. On surgical exploration a rupture of the salpinx was found. The contents of the collapsed egg had spelled into the celomic cavity.

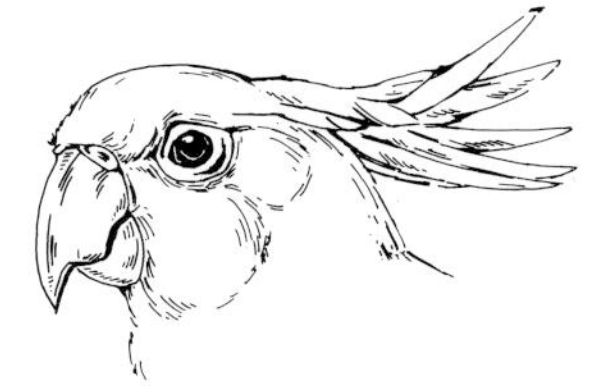

76

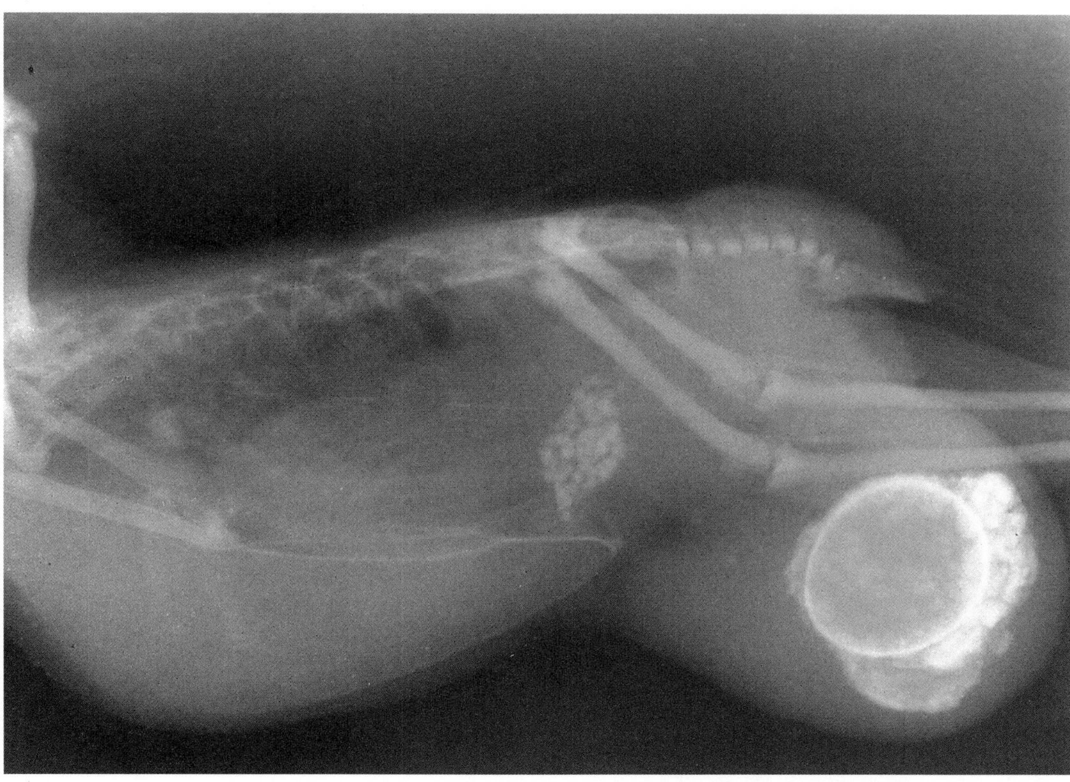

77

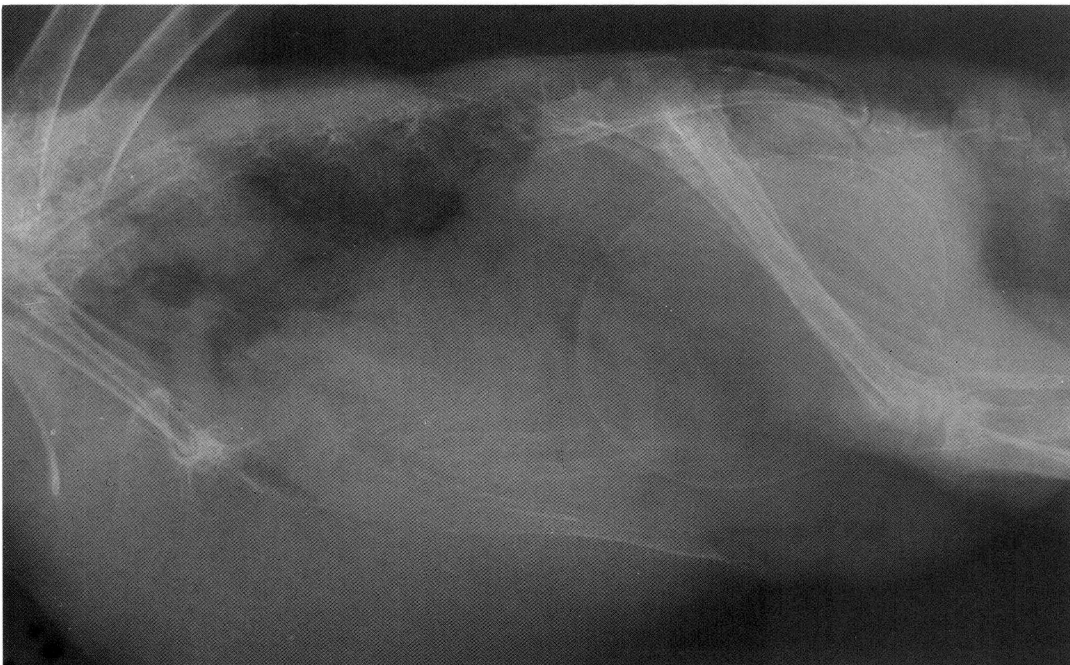

76 Hernia Ventralis with Egg Binding.

Budgerigar *(Melopsittacus undulatus)*, female, 8 years.

In the ventral hernia, an egg can be seen with large crusty calcifications on the shell. In spite of the hernia, still the caudal celom is overfilled and the ventriculus displaced cranioventrally. This suggests the presence of a soft tissue mass. The bones of the budgerigar show osteosclerosis.

Note: This budgerigar had cystic ovarian degeneration. The hernia hindered normal delivery of the egg that remained intracelomic for a long time.

77 Softshell Egg.

Hawk-headed Parrot *(Deroptyus accipitrinus fuscifrons)*, adult.

The shell of the egg can hardly be distinguished. The top of the egg points towards the tail. An abnormally positioned egg like this results in egg binding.

78

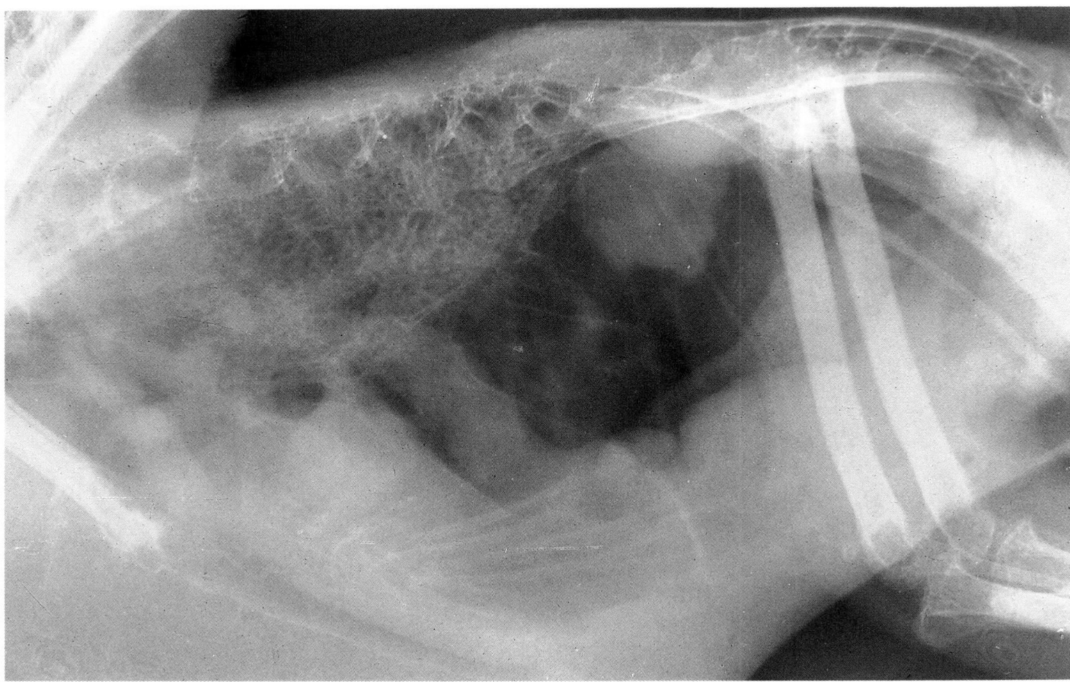

79

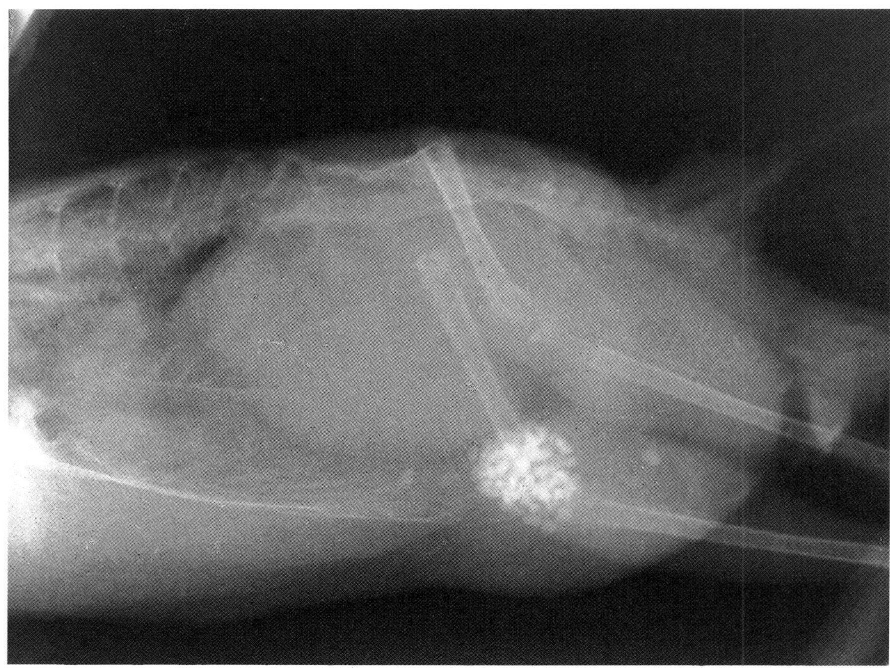

78 Ovarian Tumor.

Yellow-crowned Amazon *(Amazona ochrocephala)*, female, adult.

Ventral to the cranial kidney lobe, a round nodular shadow is present suggesting abnormal enlargement of the gonads. The long bones have an increased opacity of the medullary cavity. Biopsy of this celomic mass revealed an ovarian tumor. Osteosclerosis is often associated with ovarian abnormalities.

79 Tumor of the Testis.

Budgerigar *(Melopsittacus undulatus)*, male, adult.

The dorsal celom is filled by a soft tissue mass that expands ventrally to the ventriculus and cranially to the heart base. The ventriculus itself is displaced ventrally, distending the abdominal wall.

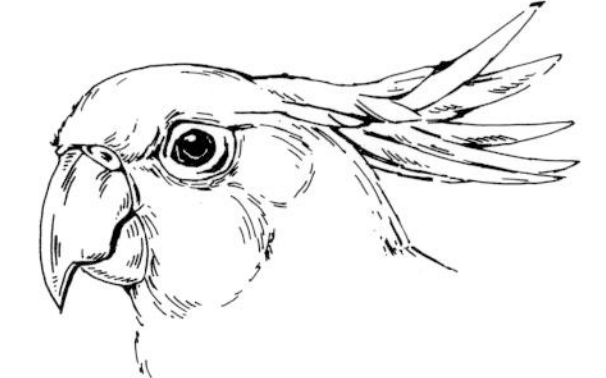

80

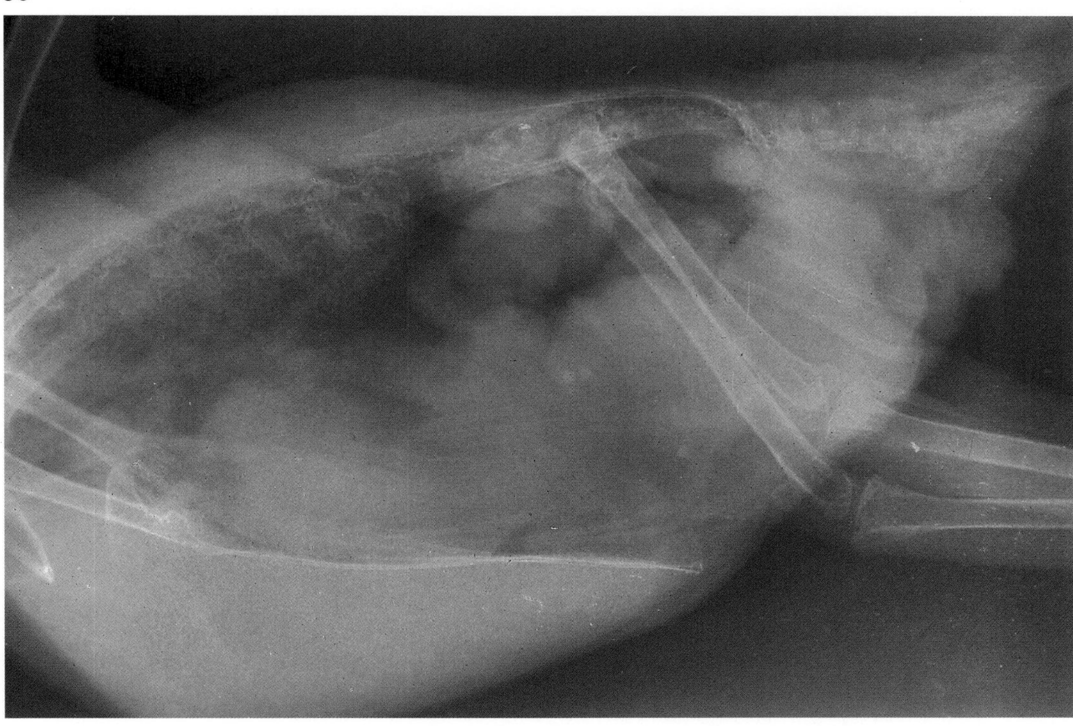

81

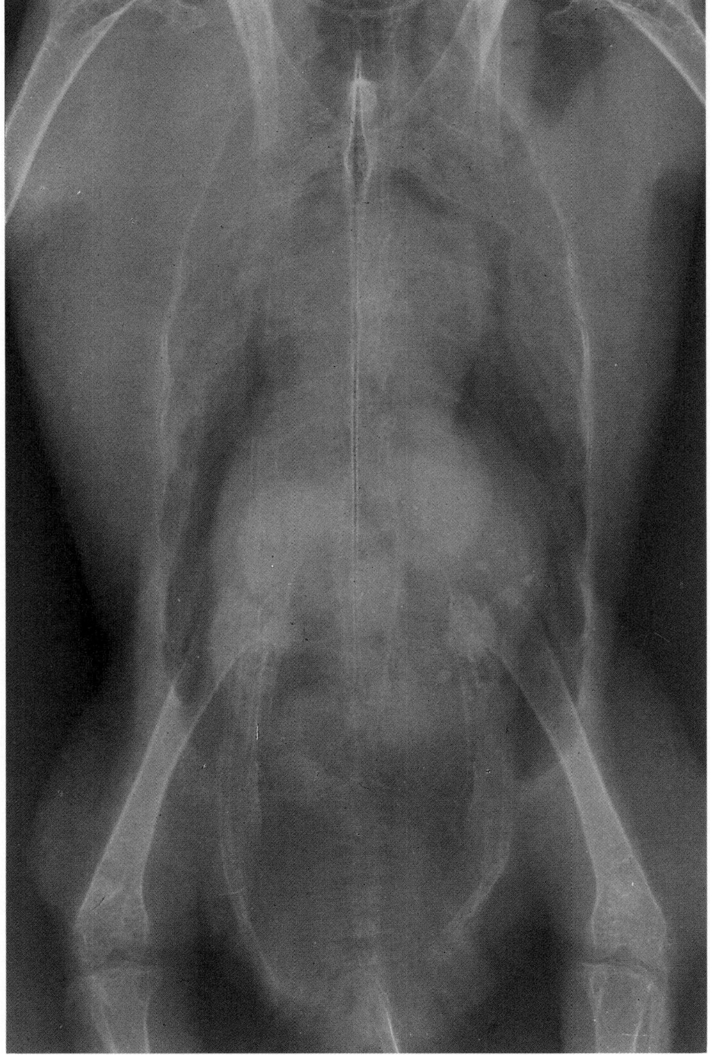

80/81 Visible Testes.

Alexandrine Parakeet *(Psittacula e. eupatria)*, male, adult.

Both testes are clearly visibile in both projections.

The left testis is positioned more cranially than the right one.

Note: In some species of psittacines, for example the parakeets, the testes can be identified on radiographs. They are best visible during the breeding season, when size reaches to a maximum. Then, they can easily be confused with tumors.

82

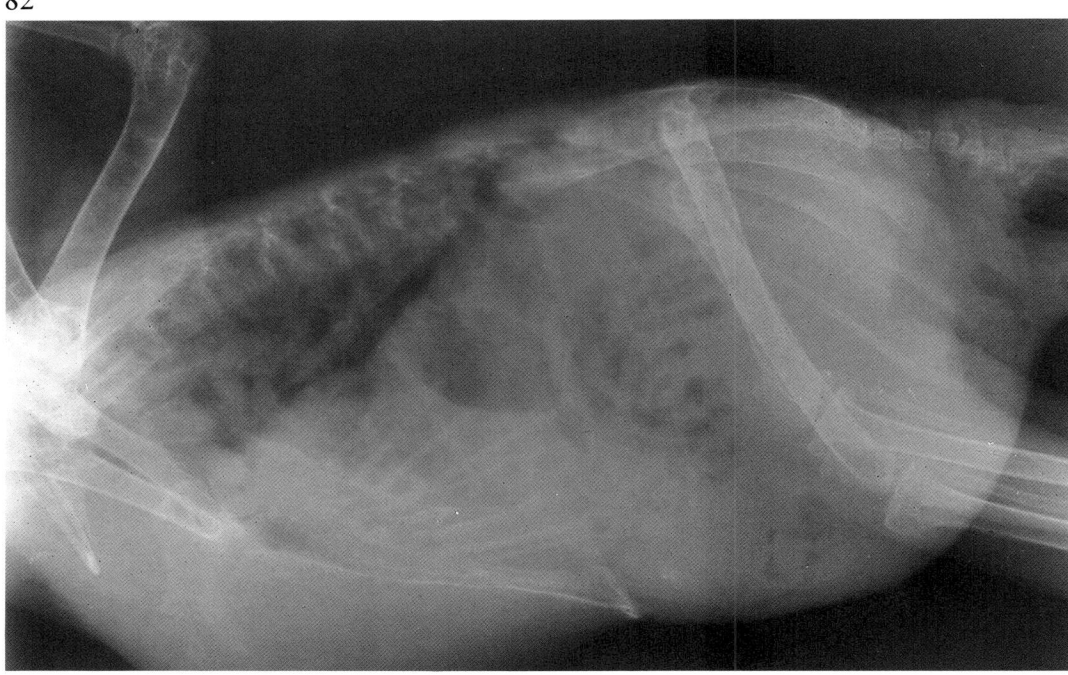

83

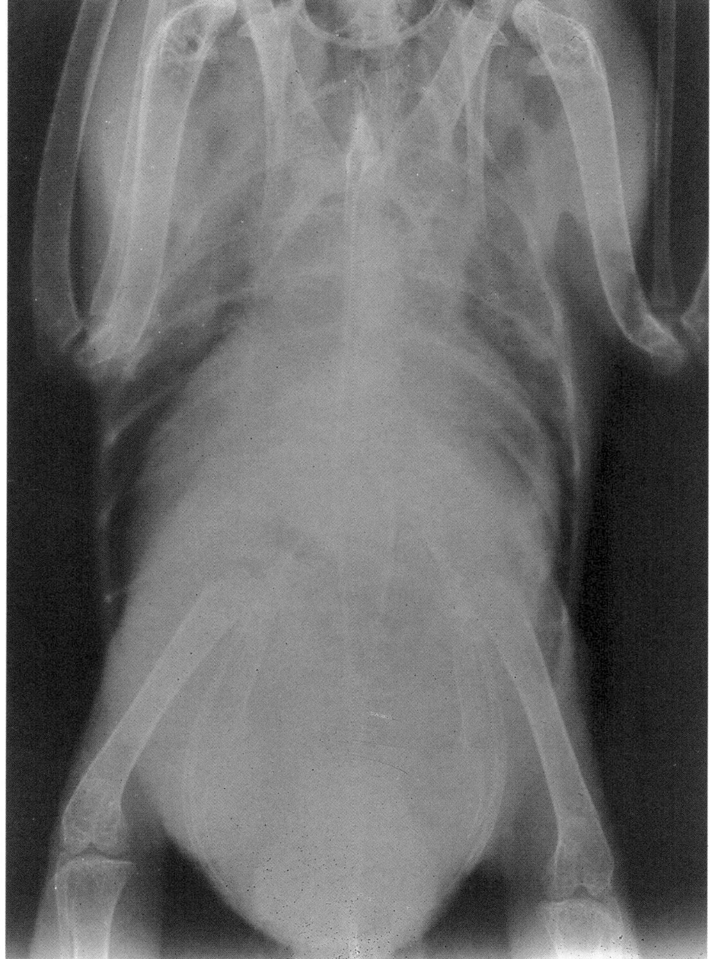

82/83 Ascites.

Blue-fronted Amazon *(Amazona aestiva)*, adult.

The celom has a homogeneous ground-glass density. This indicates the presence of fluid. Several gas-filled intestinal loops can be recognized within the fluid. The reticular pattern of the lungs is more dense than normal. The "hourglass"-shaped celomic shadow has disappeared because of lack of air in the surrounding air sacs. The ascites was due to liver cirrhosis.

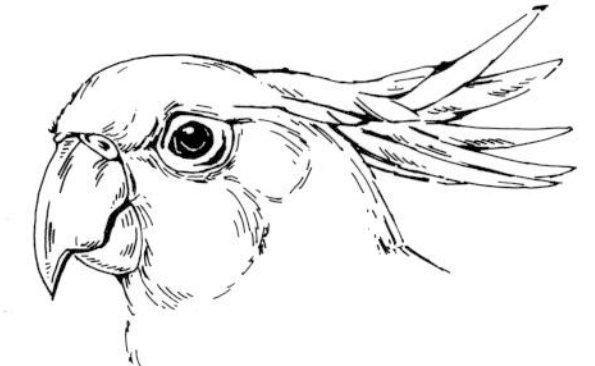

84

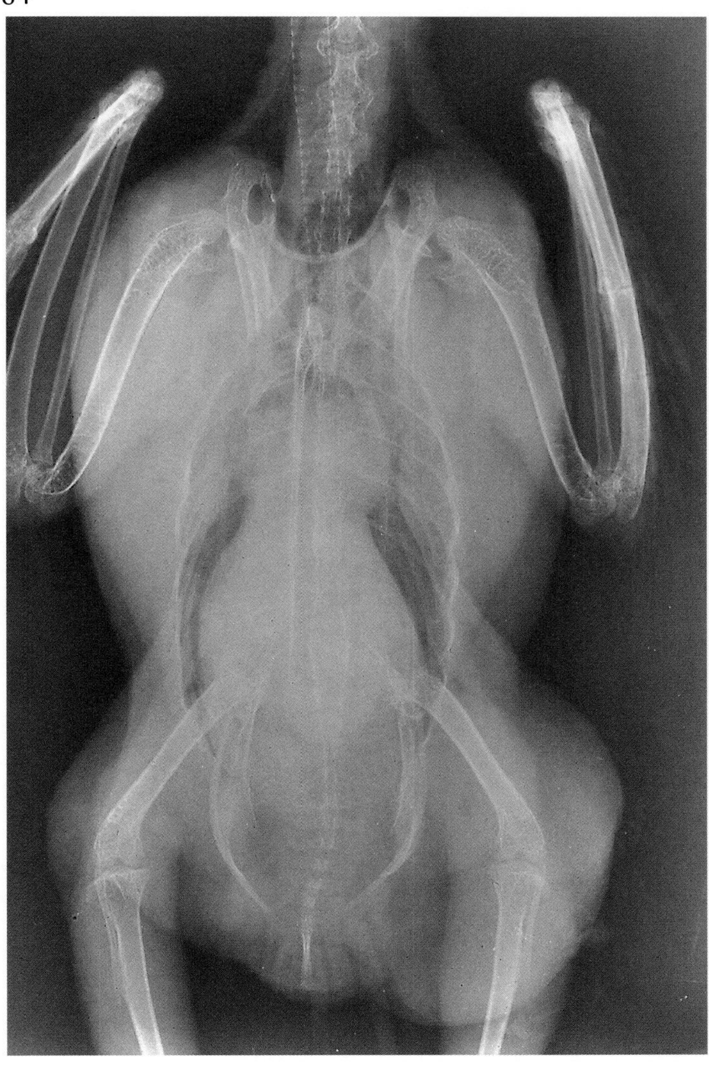

85

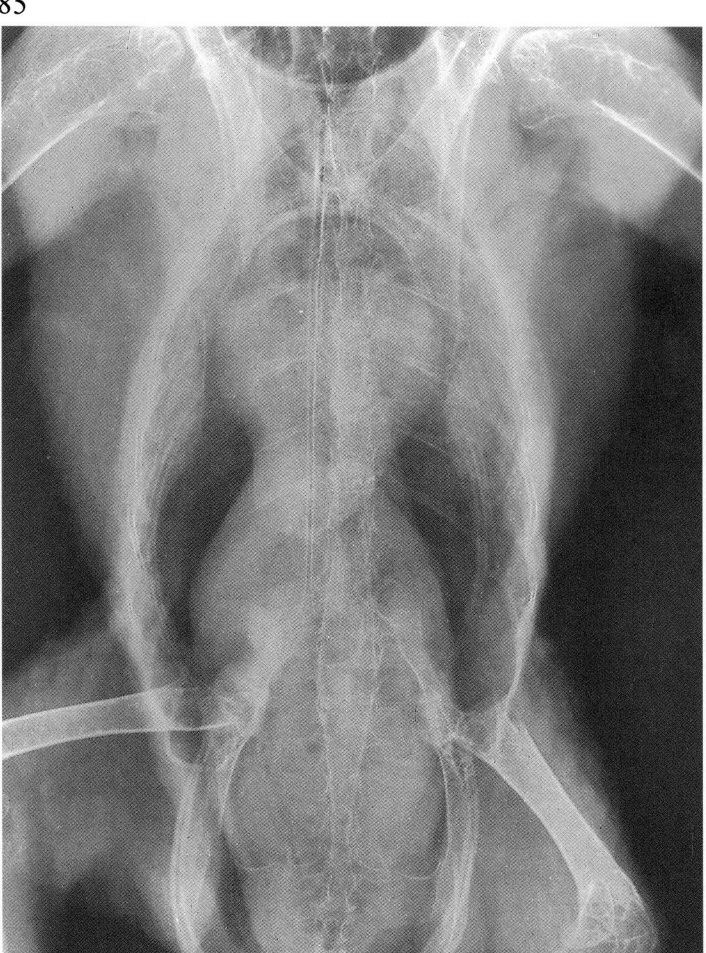

84 Lipidosis.

Yellow-crowned Amazon *(Amazona ochrocephala oratrix)*, adult.

In addition to the large fat deposits in the flanks and around the thighs, also the shadows of the internal organs are enlarged due to fat deposition.

85 Visceral Gout.

Salmon-crested Cockatoo *(Cacatua moluccensis)*, female, 4 years.

In cockatoos, normally the internal organs are very well-defined radiographically. However, in this cockatoo the cardiac shadow has an increased density with sharply defined borders. At necropsy, visceral gout was diagnosed. The pericardium was covered by uric acid depositions.

86

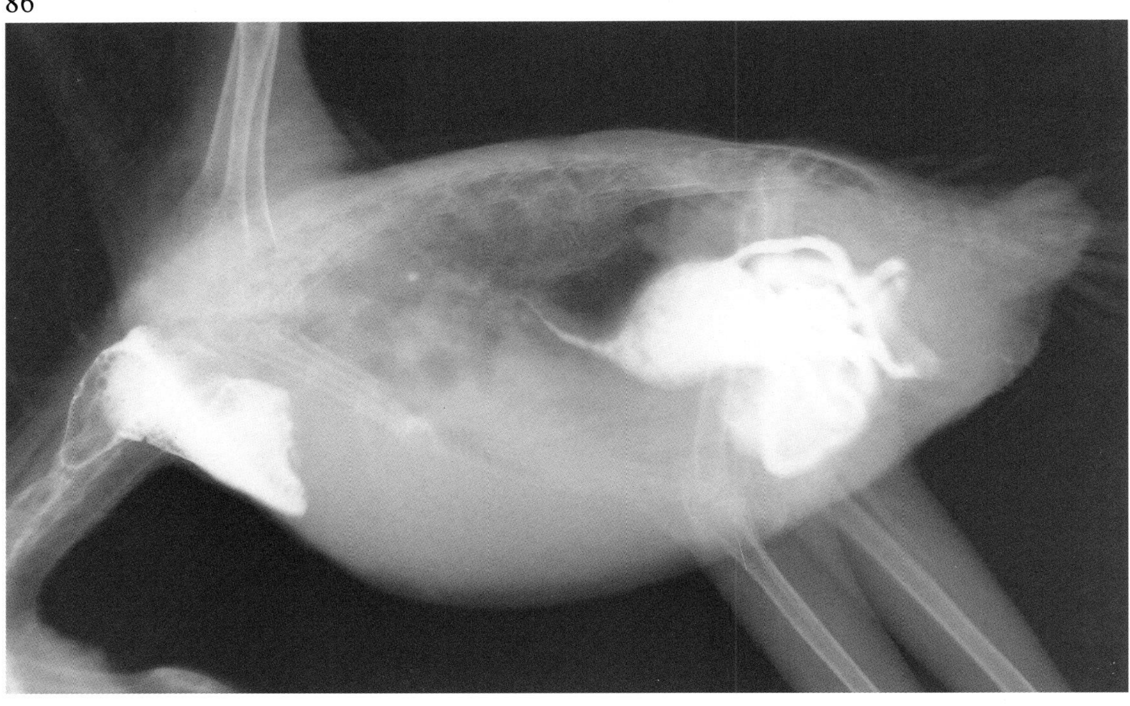

87

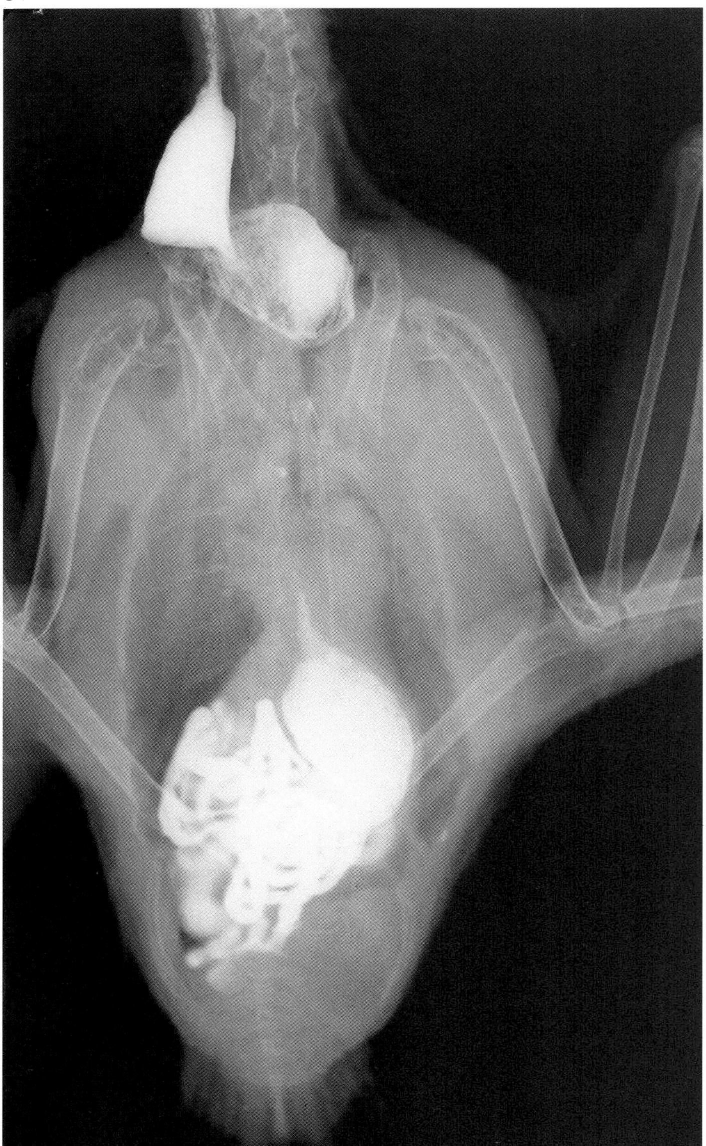

86/87 Tumor in the Cloacal Wall, contrast study.

Yellow-crowned Amazon *(Amazona ochrocephala)*, adult.

At the end of a contrast study there is no filling of the cloaca with contrast medium. Furthermore, the intestines seem to be compressed and displaced cranially. A walnut-sized tumor of the left cloacal wall with obstruction of its lumen was found.

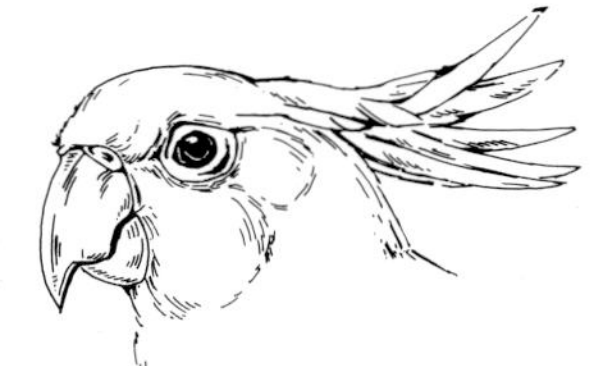

88

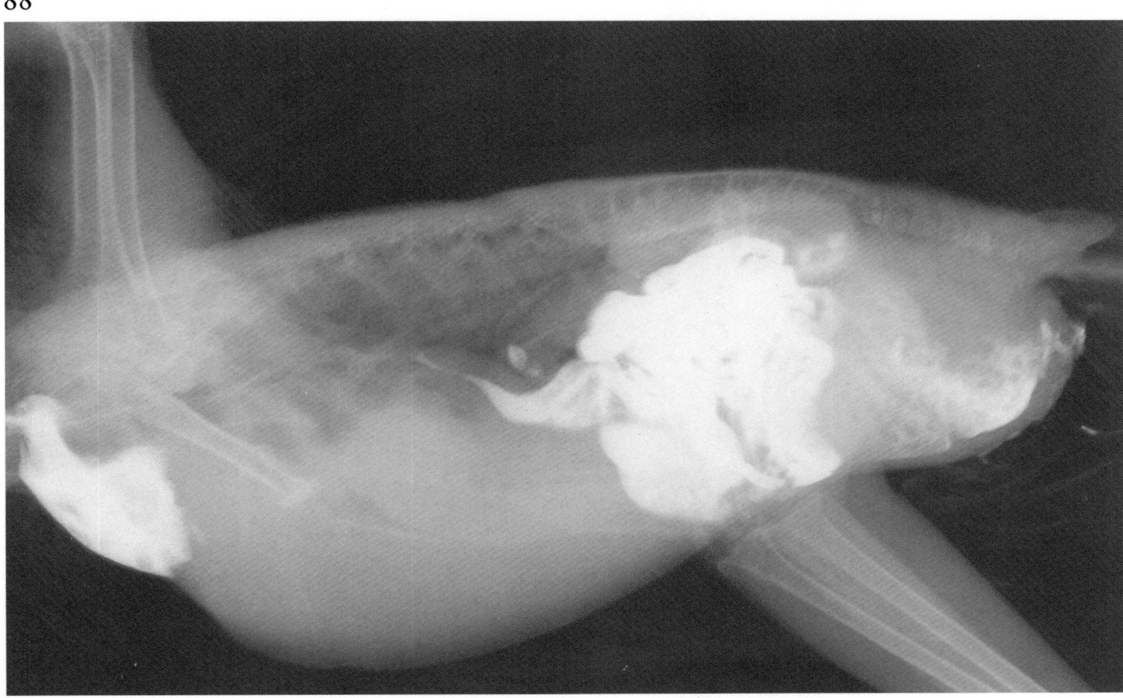

89

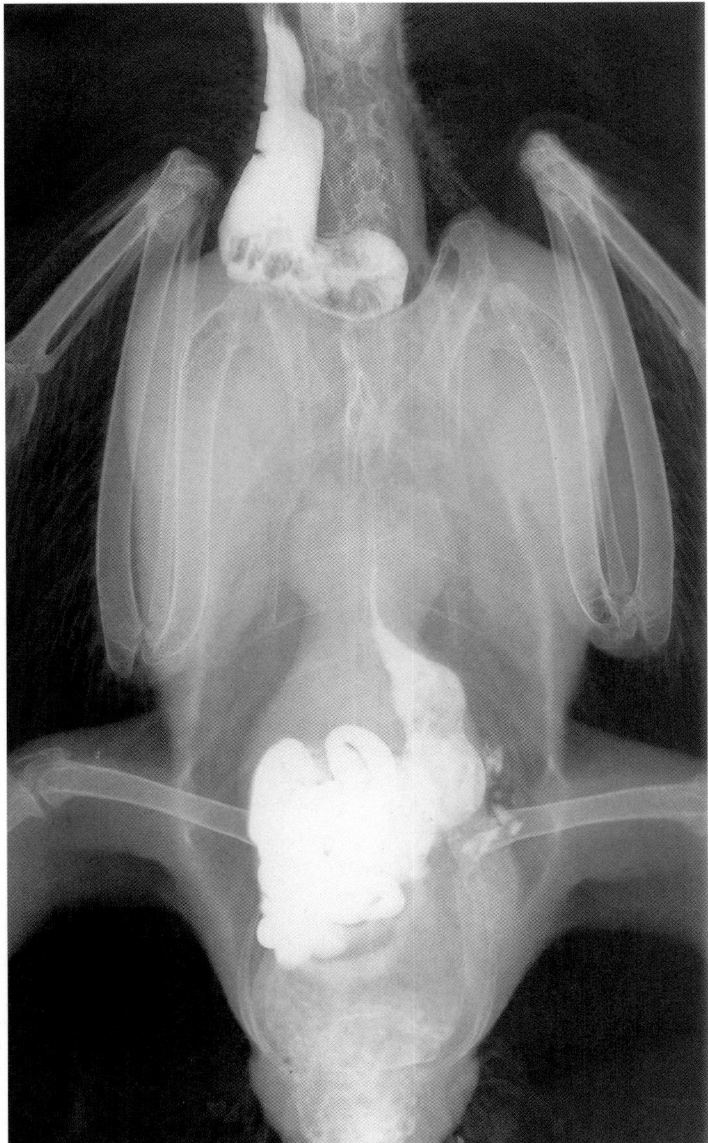

88/89 Cloacal Stone, contrast study.

Orange-winged Amazon *(Amazona amazonica)*, adult.

The contrast study reveals a space-occupying mass in the caudal celom displacing the intestines cranially.

A small amount of contrast medium covers the wall of the cloaca and passes towards the outlet. A cherry-sized urate stone caused massive coprostasis.

90

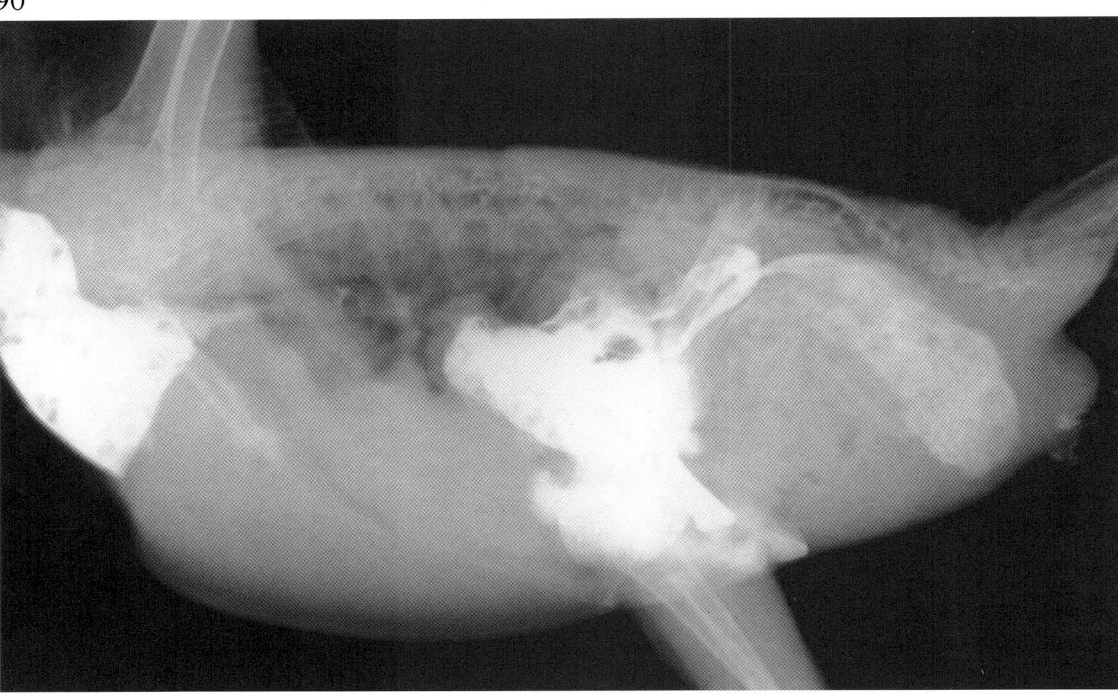

91

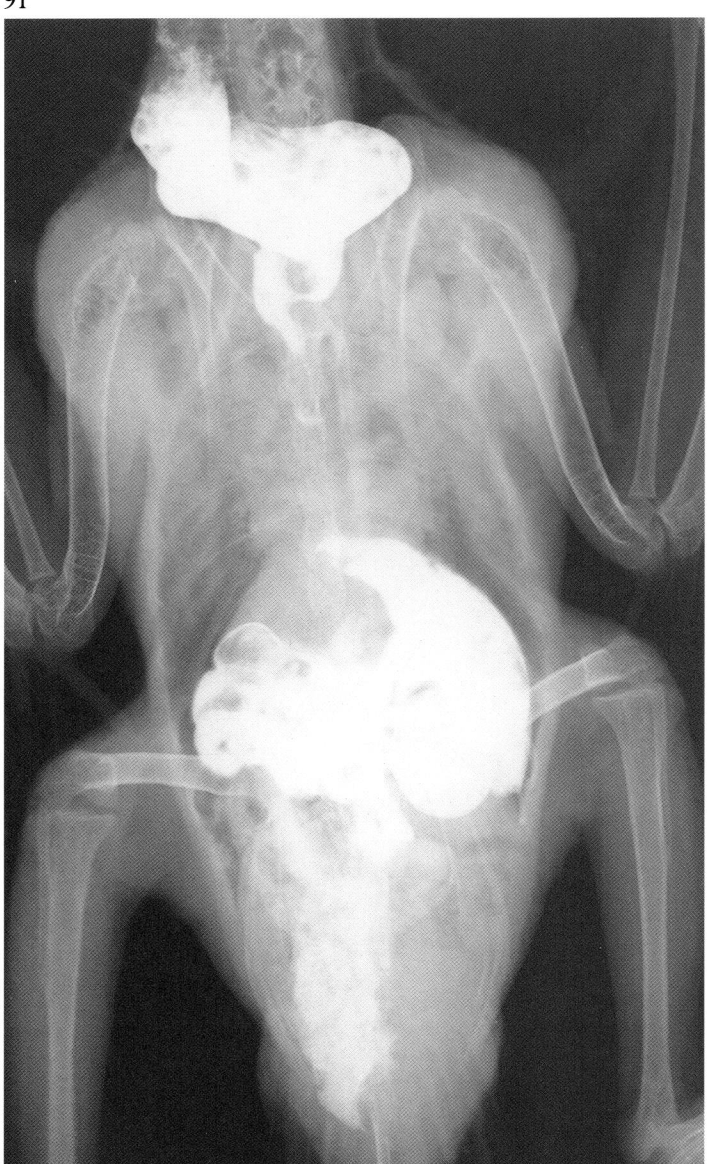

90 Concrements in the Oviduct, contrast study.

Blue and Yellow Macaw *(Ara ararauna)*, adult.

The oviduct, that is filled with egg concrements is pushing the intestines cranially. The contrast medium coats the wall of the cloaca with a thin film.

91 Dilatation of the Proventriculus, contrast study.

Yellow-crowned Amazon *(Amazona ochrocephala)*, adult.

Due to dilatation of the proventriculus the passage of contrast medium is delayed.

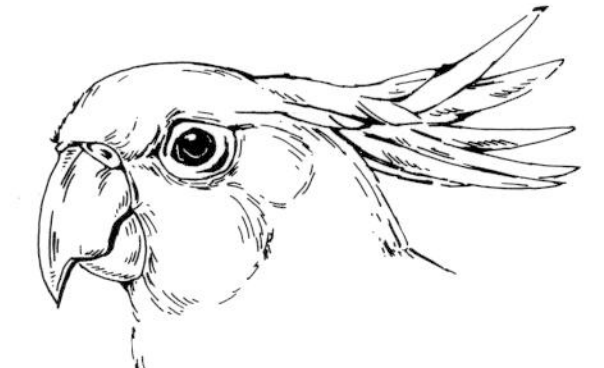

92

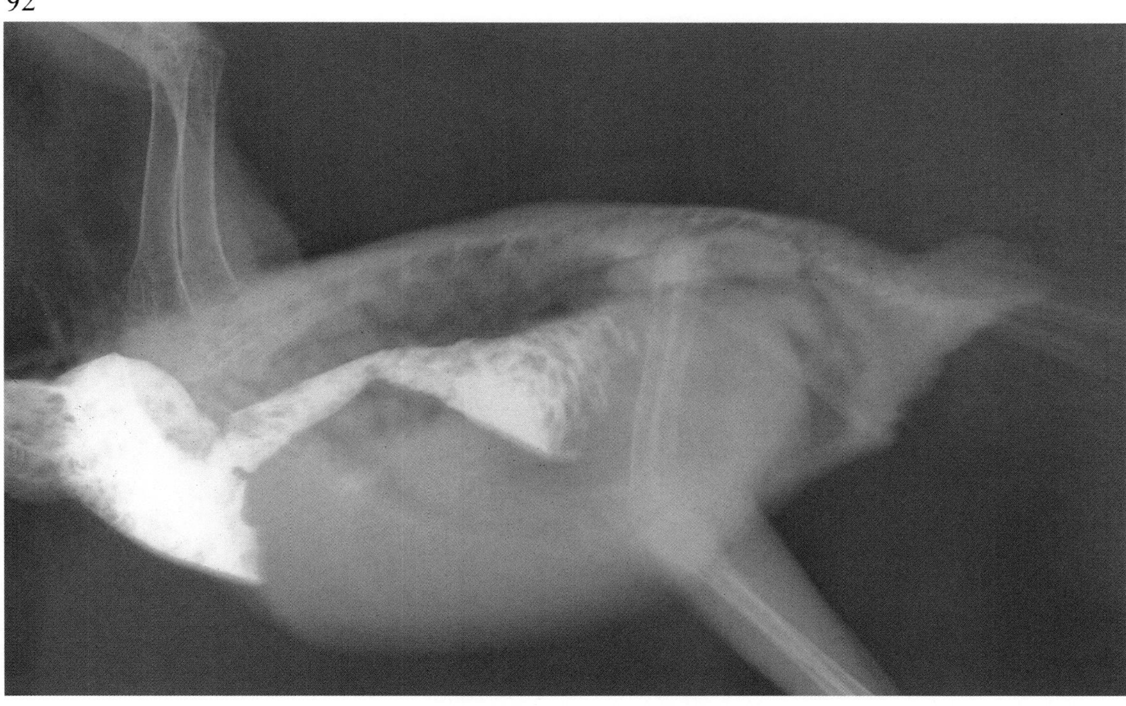

93

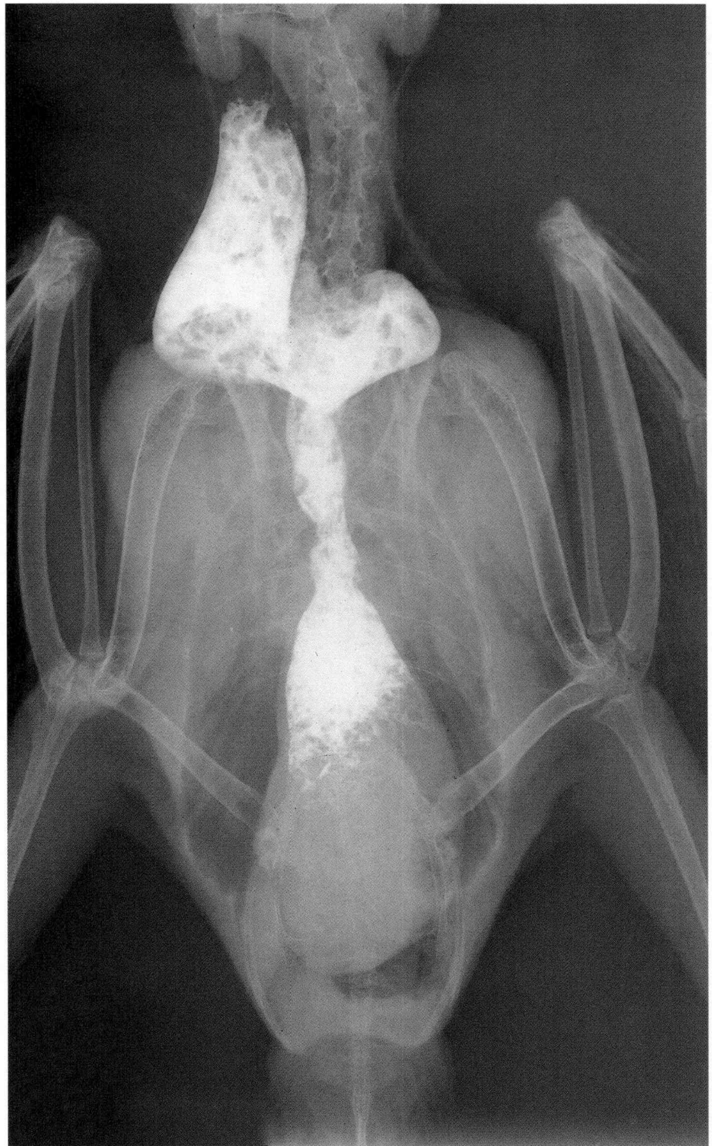

92/93 Macaw wasting disease, contrast study.

Blue-fronted Amazon *(Amazona aestiva)*, adult.

Passage of contrast medium is obstructed and delayed by dilatation of a fluid-filled proventriculus. These are common findings with "Macaw-wasting-disease".

94

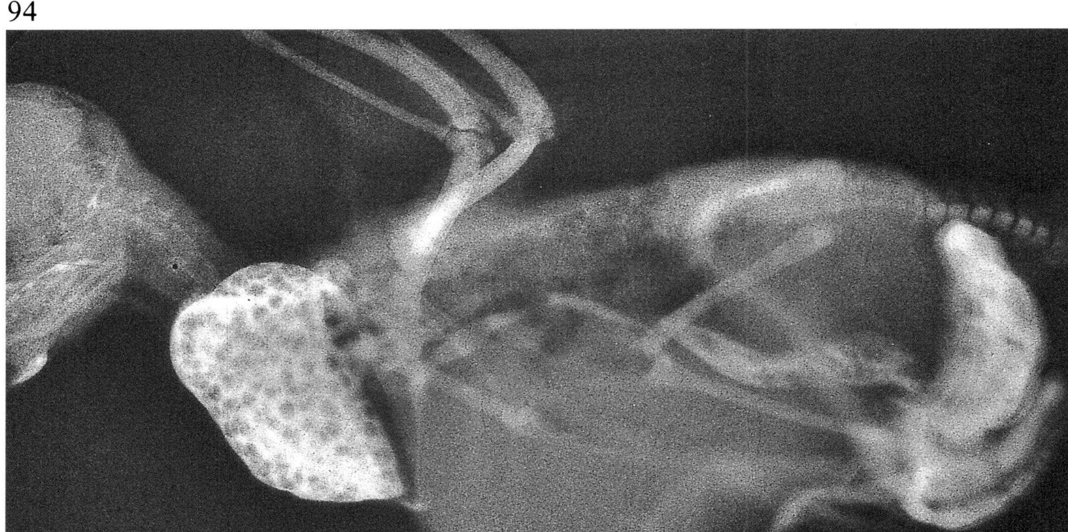

95

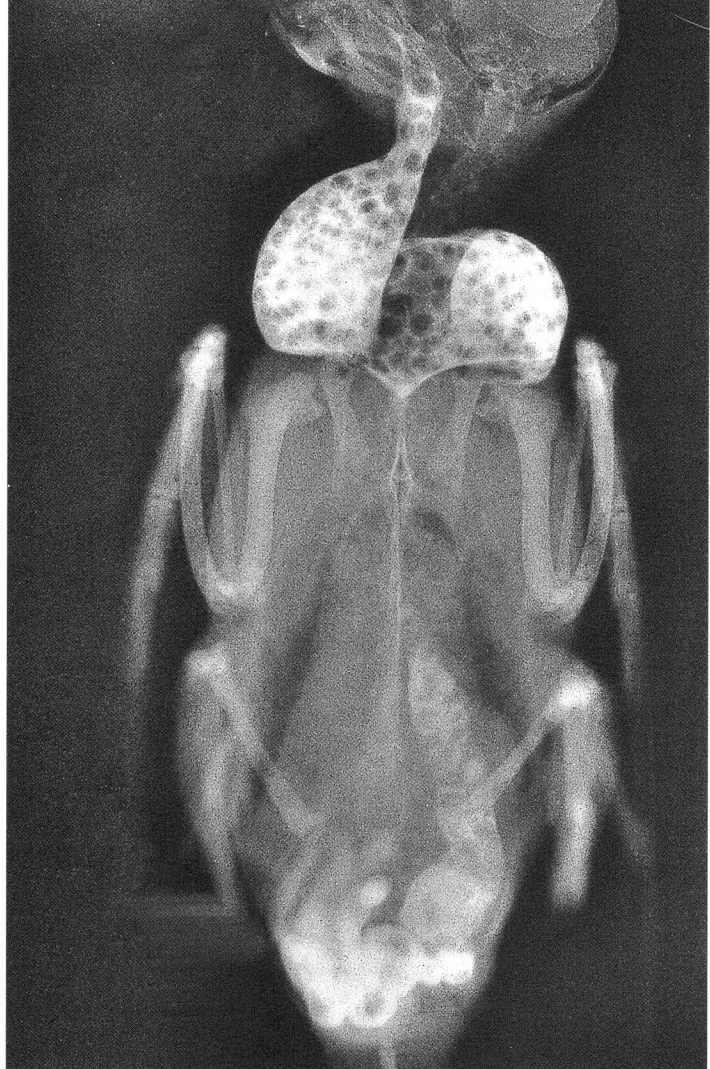

94/95 Testicular Tumor, contrast study.

Budgerigar *(Melopsittacus undulatus)*, male, adult.

The lateral view shows a space-occupying mass in the gonadal area. On the ventrodorsal radiograph, displacement of the proventriculus to the left is visible. Osteosclerosis of the bones is present. Based on these signs, a tumor of the gonads was suspected and confirmed at necropsy.

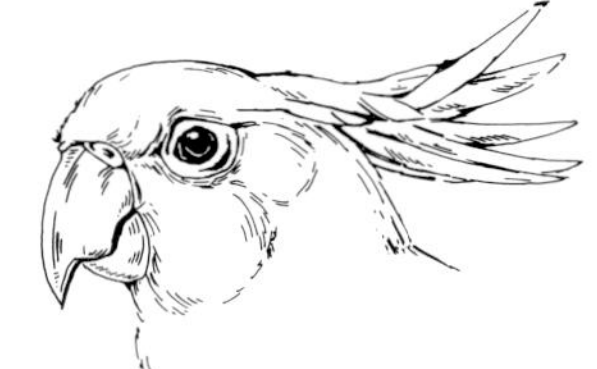

96

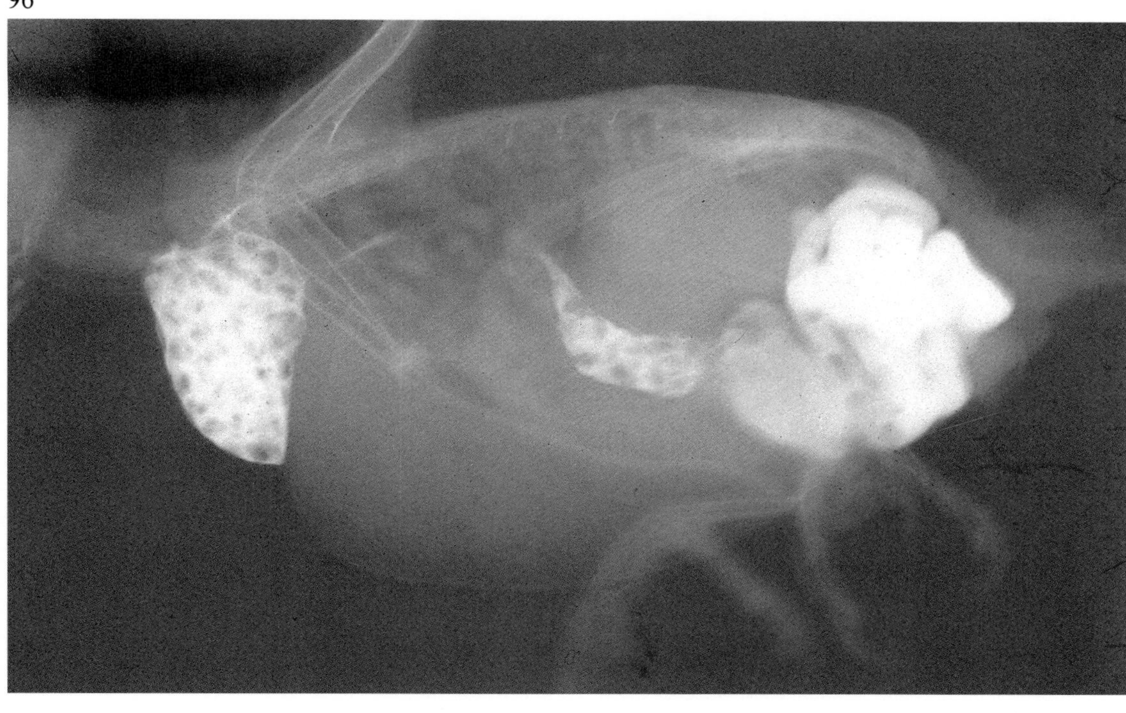

97

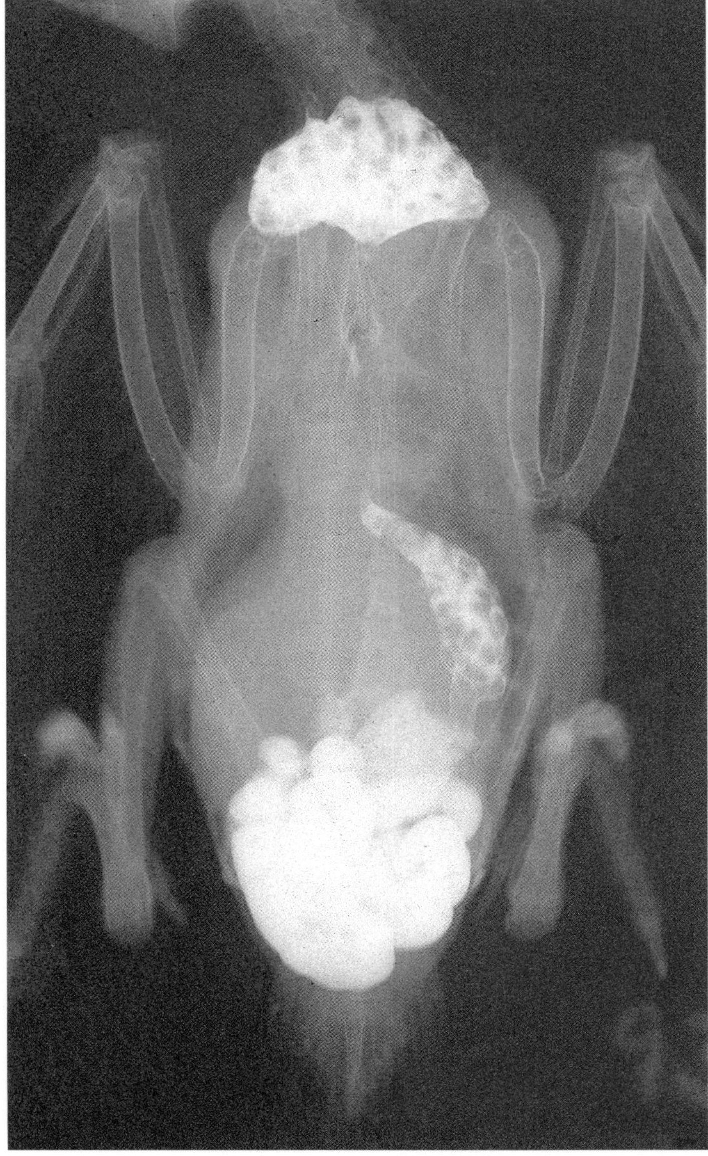

96/97 Renal Tumor, contrast study.

Budgerigar *(Melopsittacus undulatus)*, adult.

On the lateral radiograph, a soft tissue mass in the sublumbar area is visible. On the ventrodorsal radiograph, the proventriculus and ventriculus are displaced to the left, and the intestines are shifted to a caudal position. There are no signs of osteosclerosis. These radiographic signs are compatible with a renal mass. In this bird, a tumor of the right kidney was found at necropsy.

98

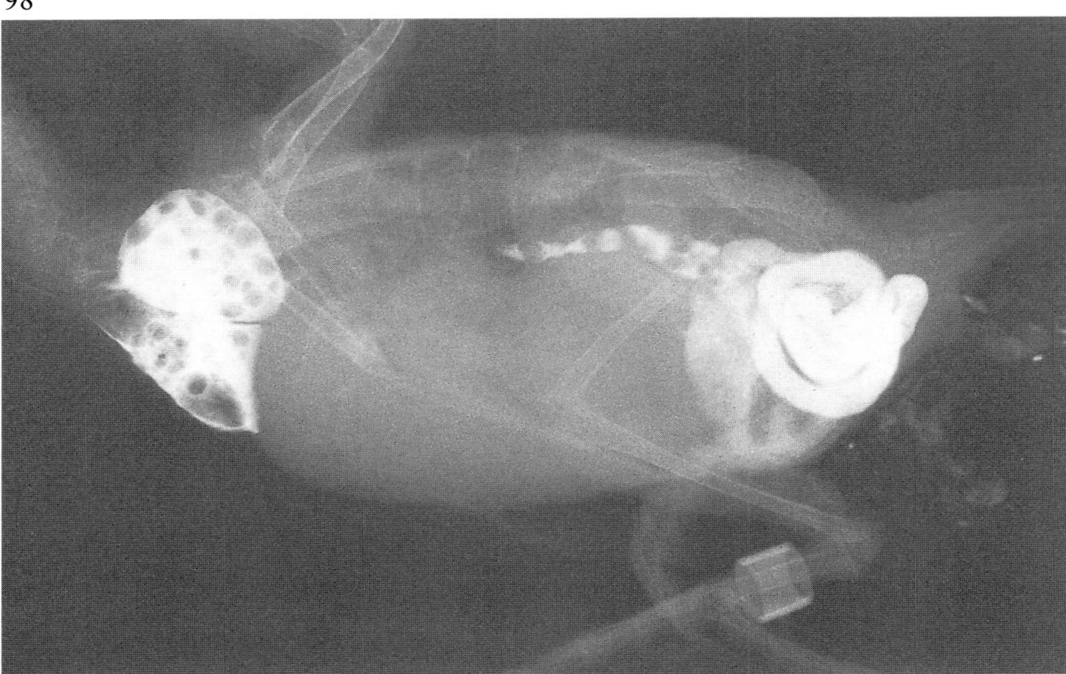

99

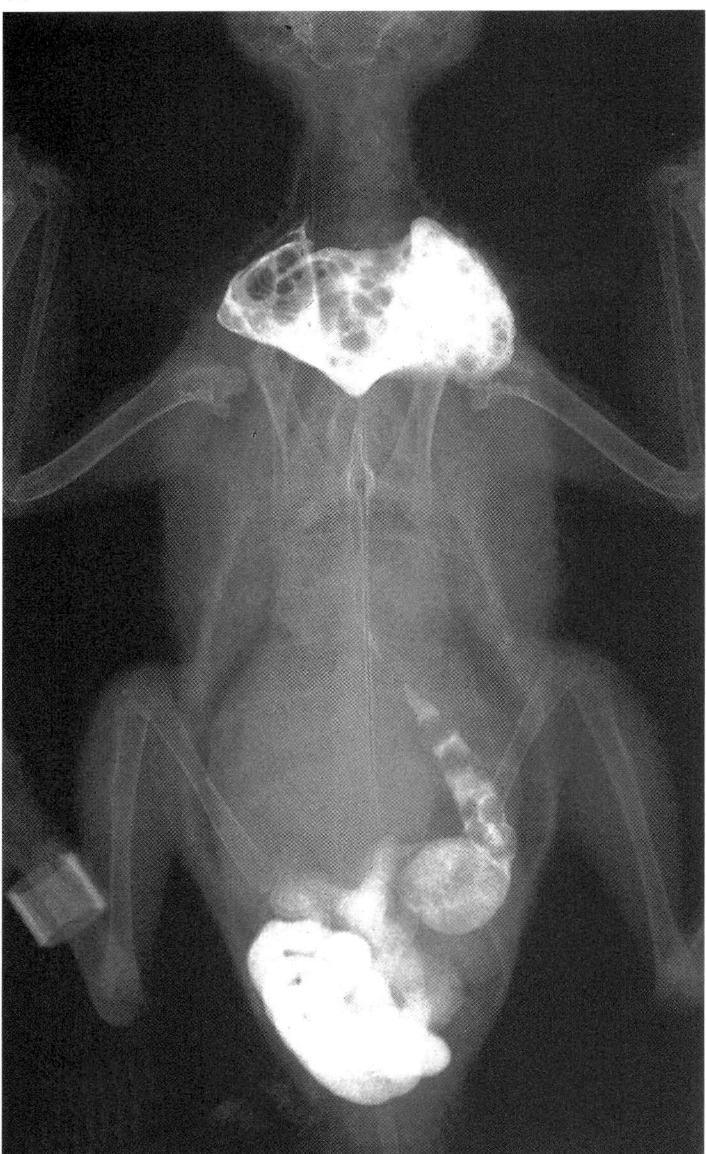

98/99 Liver Tumor, contrast study.

Budgerigar *(Melopsittacus undulatus)*, adult.

A large mass displaces the proventriculus dorsally and laterally, and the intestines caudally. The pattern of dislocations by this mass is typical of a liver mass.

In this case, a cherry-sized tumor of the liver was found.

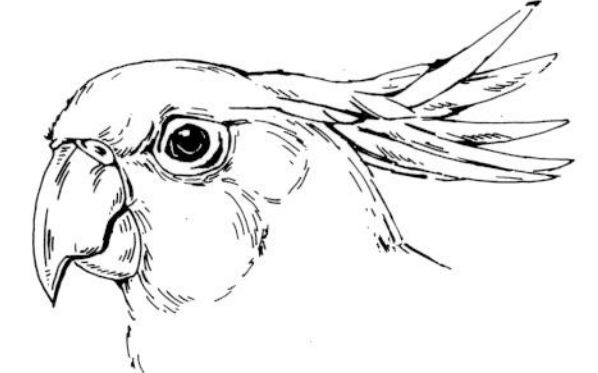

100

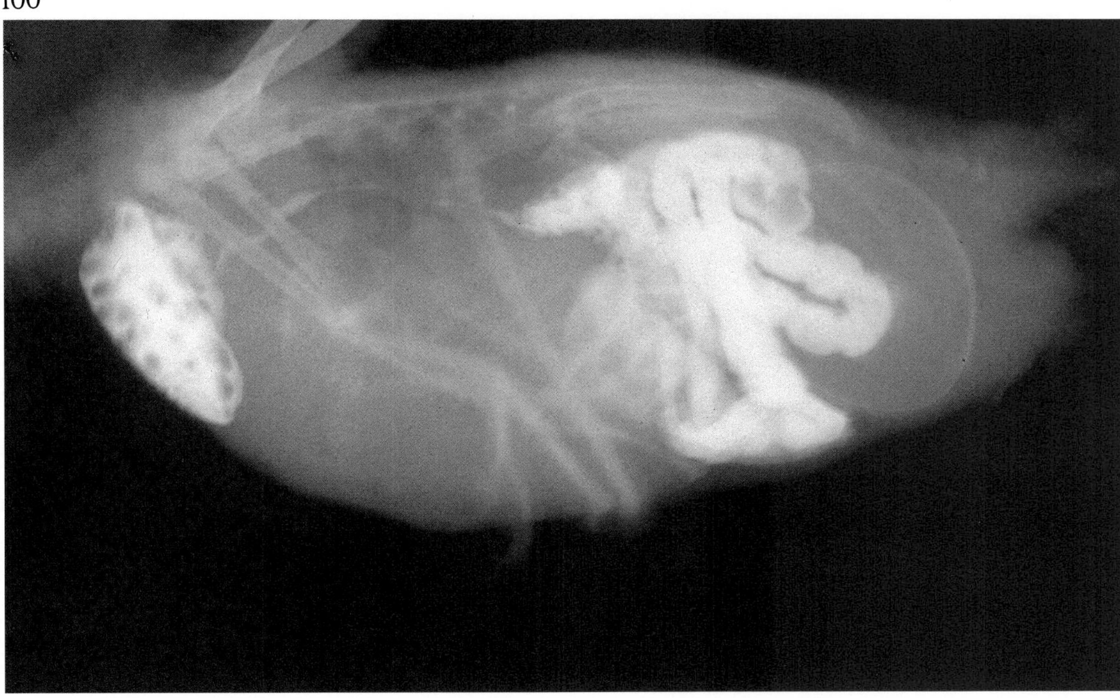

101

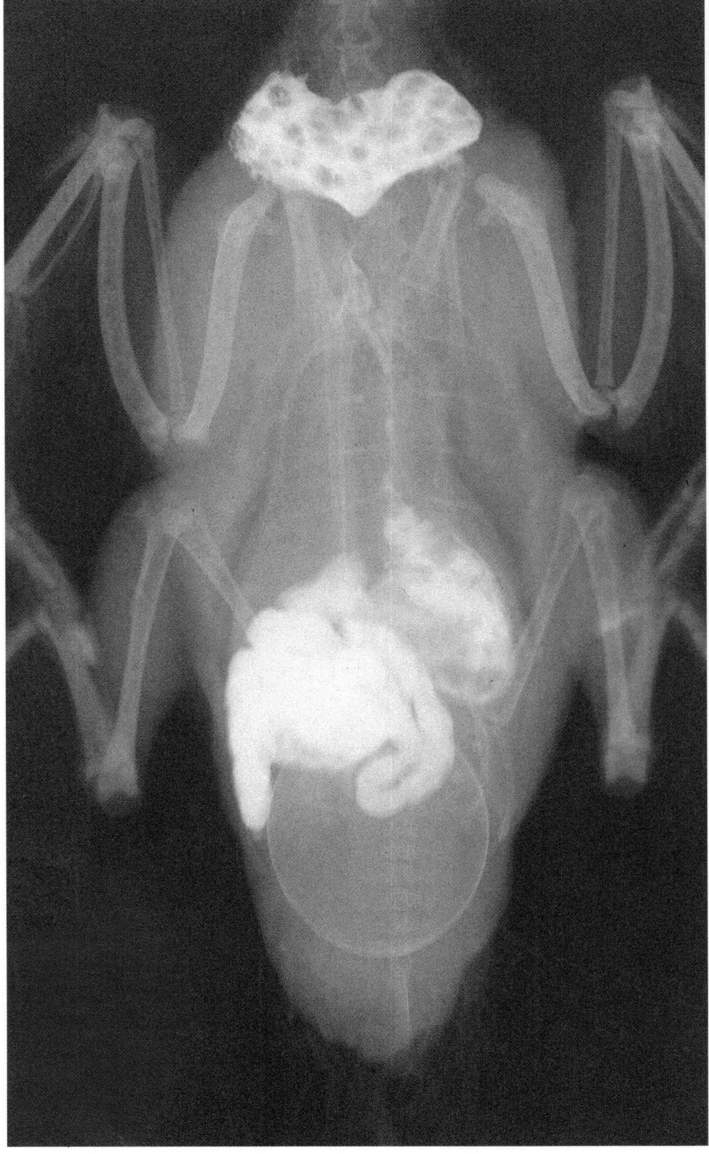

100/101 Egg Binding, contrast study.

Budgerigar *(Melopsittacus undulatus)*.

The caudal celom is occupied by a large egg. The other celomic viscera are displaced cranially by the egg.

102

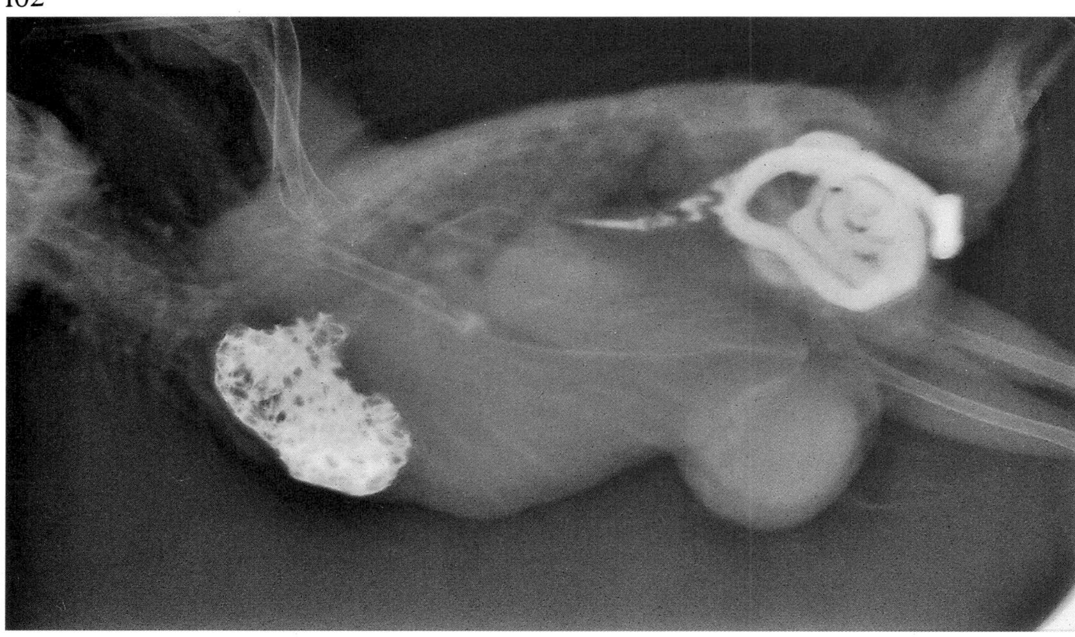

103

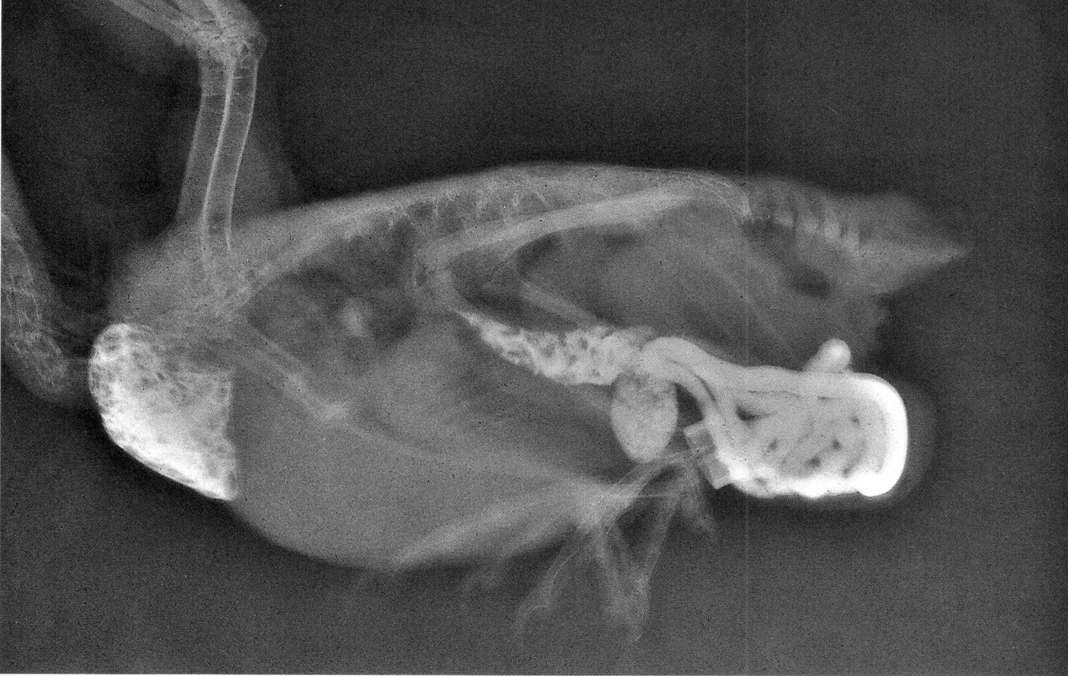

102 Lipoma, contrast study.

Budgerigar *(Melopsittacus undulatus)*, adult.

A cherry-sized soft tissue mass extends from the ventral body wall. The contrast study shows no intestinal prolapse into the mass. Because of this finding, herniation is very unlikely. The mass proved to be a lipoma.

103 Hernia ventralis, contrast study.

Cockatiel *(Nymphicus hollandicus)*, adult.

The contrast medium clearly defines a ventral hernia with prolapse of the intestines. Notice the enlarged kidneys that compress the intestines ventrally probably inducing the herniation. A kidney tumor was found.

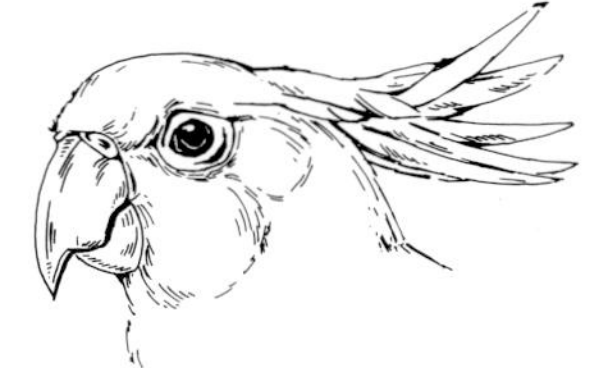

104

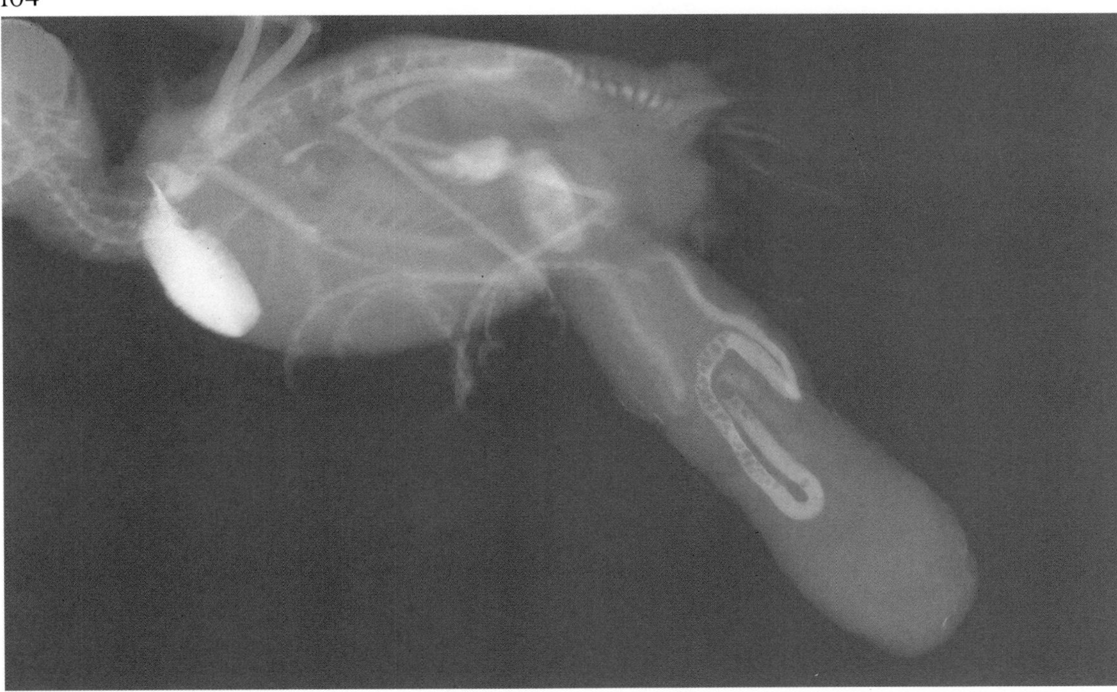

105

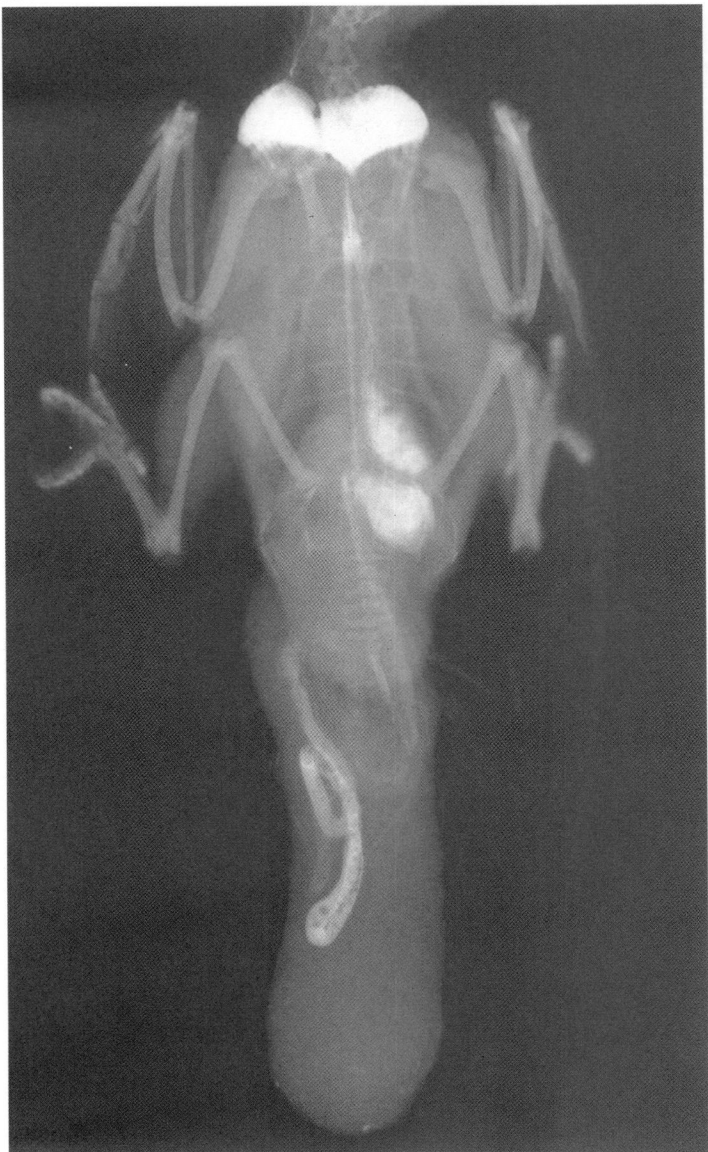

104/105 Hernia ventralis, contrast study.

Budgerigar *(Melopsittacus undulatus)*, adult.

In most cases, a ventral hernia is filled with parts of the oviduct, often accompanied by intestinal loops. The latter can easily be delineated with contrast medium. This bird required a resection of the oviduct, reposition of the intestine, closing of the open abdominal wall, and resection of excessive skin.

106

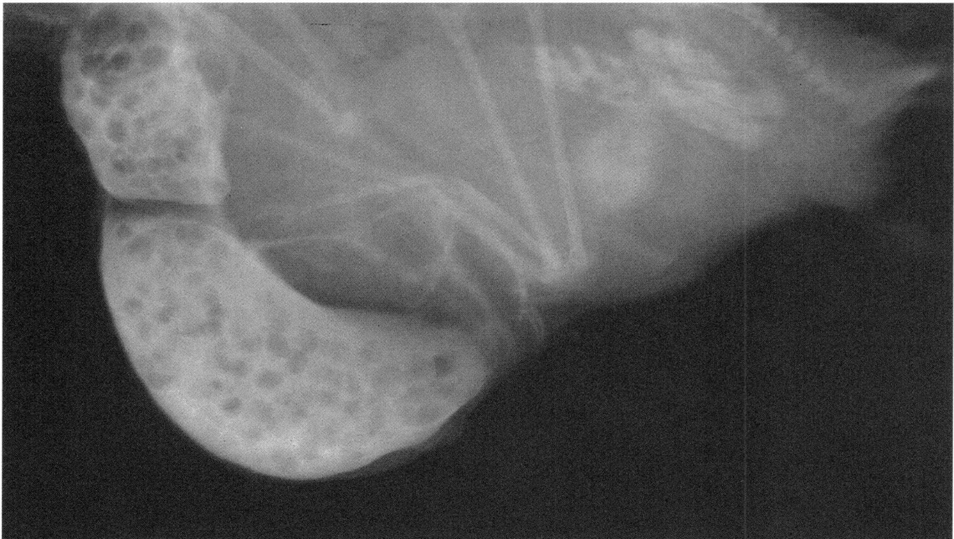

107

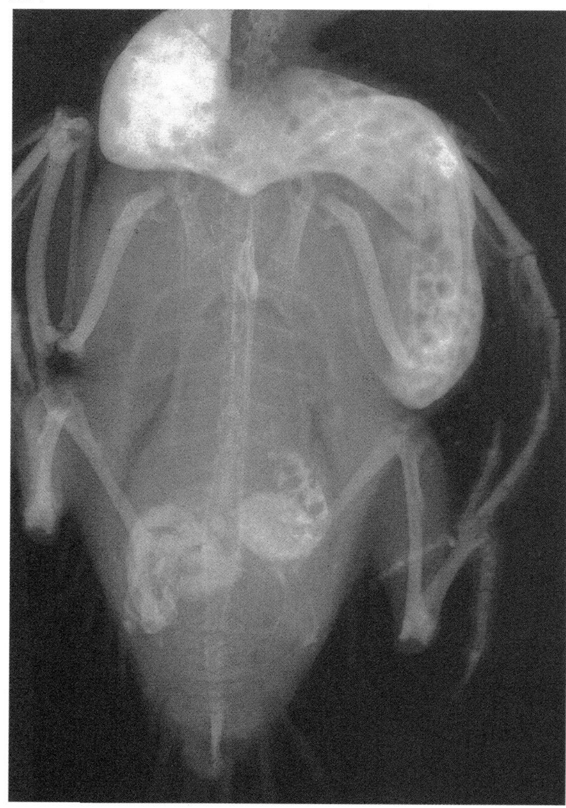

106/107 Crop Dilatation, contrast study.

Budgerigar *(Melopsittacus undulatus)*, adult.

In cases of dilatation of the crop, the passage-time of contrast medium is prolonged. In this bird, contrast medium has reached the duodenal loop after two and a half hours. This indicates a severely prolonged passage-time.

108

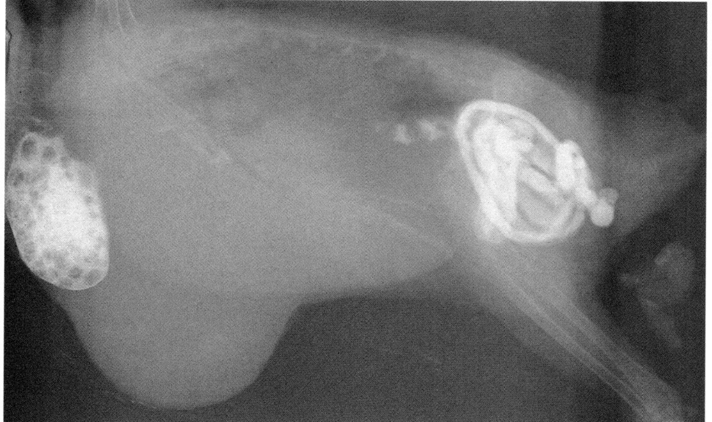

108 Lipoma in the Crop Area, contrast study.

Budgerigar *(Melopsittacus undulatus)*, adult.

Lipomas in the region of the crop can be differentiated from crop dilatation by marking its lumen with contrast medium.

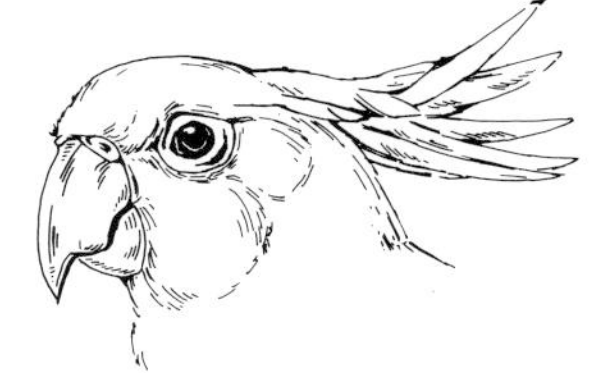

109

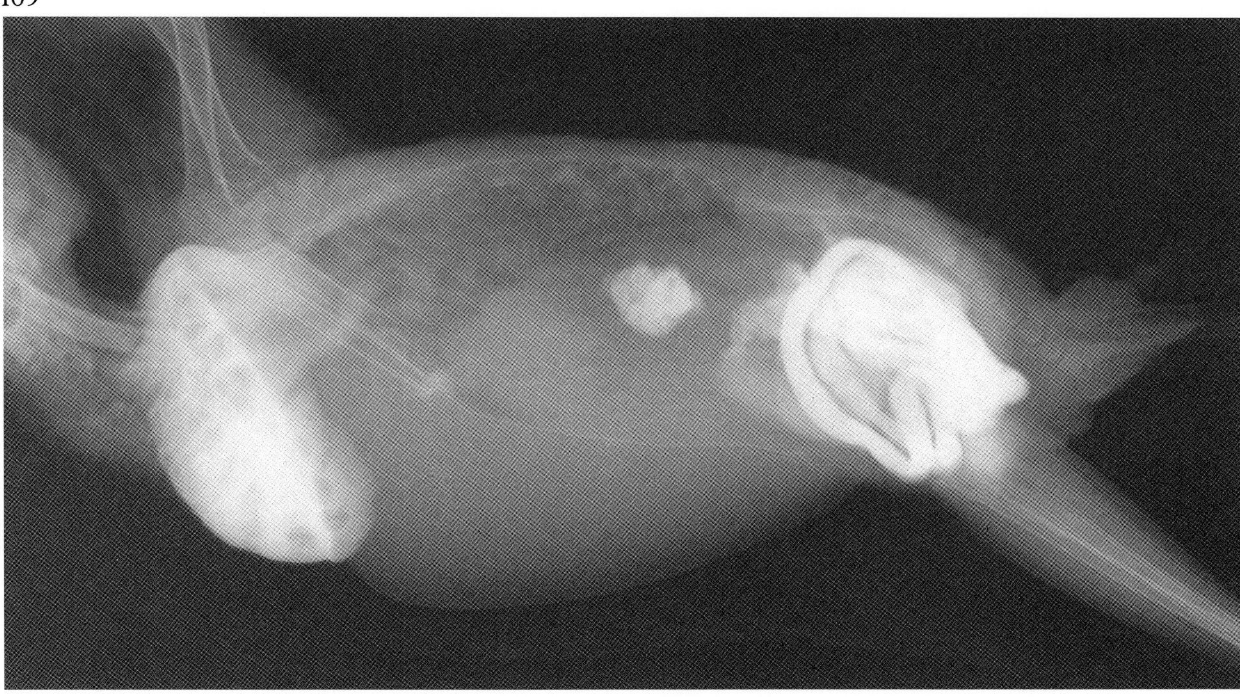

110

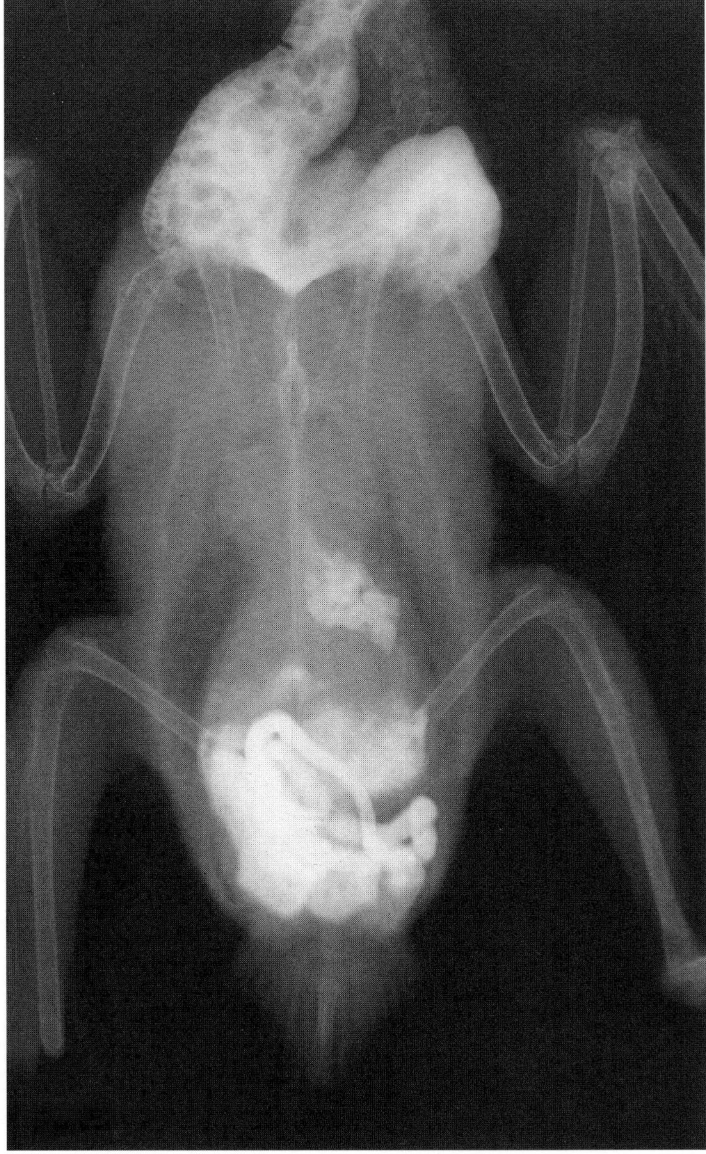

109/110 "Going Light Syndrome", contrast study.

Budgerigar *(Melopsittacus undulatus)*, adult.

Contrast medium is present in the crop and in the intestines. However, the esophagus and proventriculus are not filled. This indicates abnormal contractions of these organs due to severe irritation resulting in the "Going light syndrome" in budgerigars. Megabacteria that can be isolated from the feces of these budgerigars seem to cause these irritations.

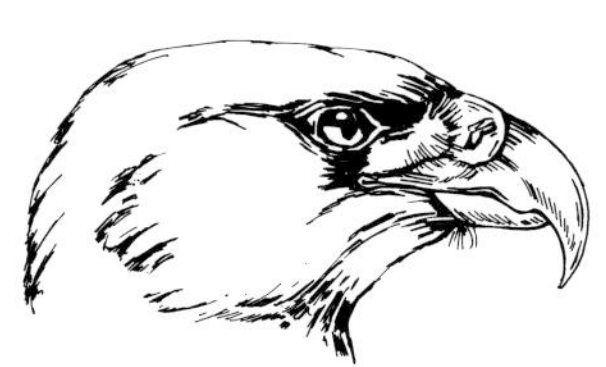

Birds: Raptors

Radiographic Anatomy
Internal Organs

111

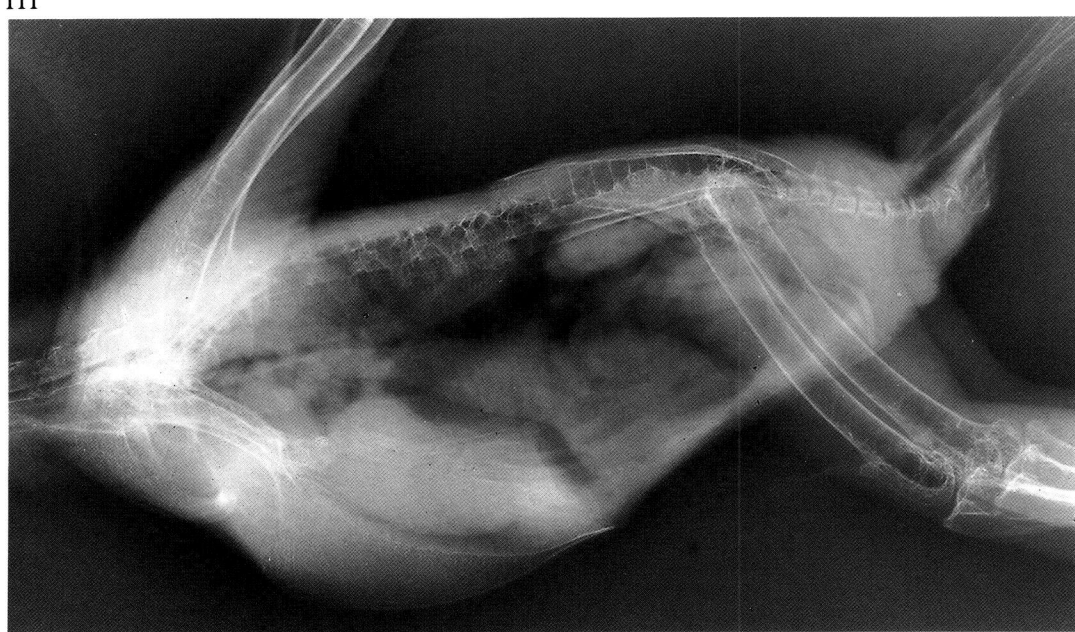

111 A

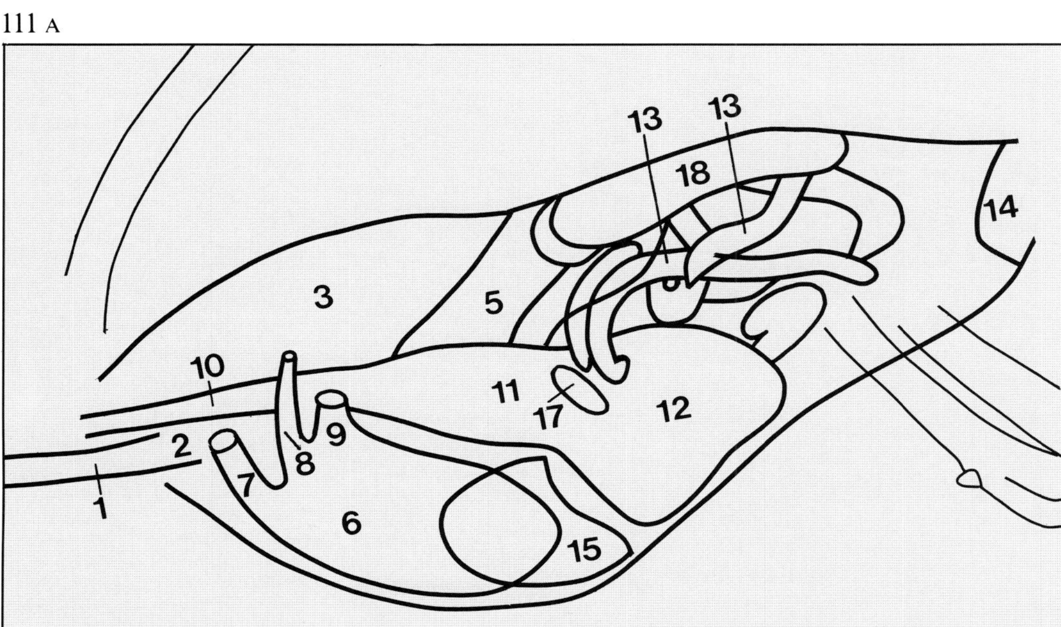

111/111A/112/112A Internal Organs: Normal Radiographic Appearance,
lateral and ventrodorsal.

Common Buzzard *(Buteo buteo)*, adult.

Respiratory Organs

The trachea (**1**) can be followed ventral to the spine from the mandible to the syrinx. The syrinx (**2**) is usually superimposed by bony structures and lies craniodorsal to the cardiac shadow. The central parts of the lungs and the bronchi, which are superimposed by the same structures on the ventrodorsal radiograph, can be evaluated easily on the lateral radiograph. The lungs (**3**) are characterized by their reticular pattern. They blend into the air sacs that are well defined.

The clavicular air sacs (**4**) are recognizable in the axillary area. The individual air sac walls cannot be seen on normal radiographs. On the ventrodorsal radiograph, the symmetrical thoracic and abdominal air sacs (**5**) can easily be compared and examined.

Heart and Vessels

On the ventrodorsal radiograph, the heart shadow (**6**) forms the cranial part of the "hourglass"-shaped density in the celom. Because of the elongated liver shadow, the "hourglass" of raptors is less distinct than in psittacines. Of the large vessels only the aorta (**7**) that is projected end-on by the parallel beam is visible as a small round shadow. On the lateral radiograph, the aorta (**7**), pulmonary arteries (**8**) and the vena cava caudalis (**9**) are recognizable.

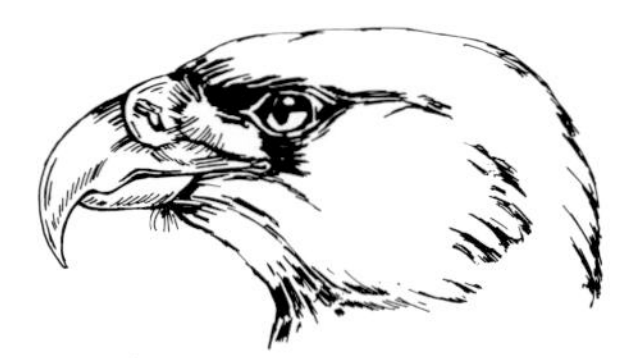

112

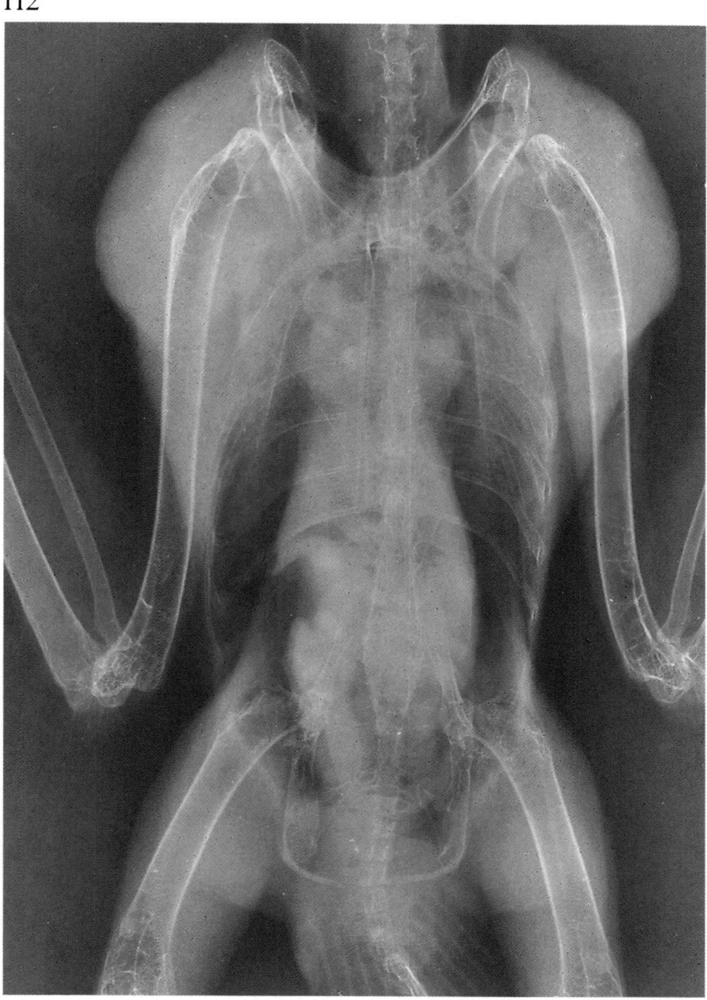

112 A

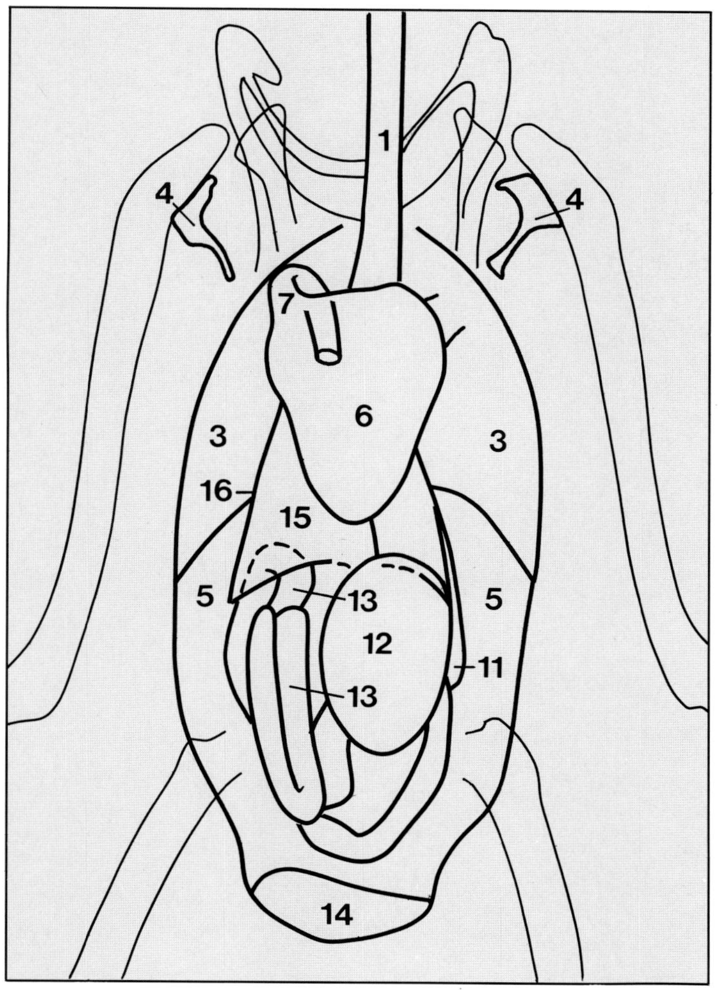

Gastrointestinal Tract

On the lateral radiograph, the esophagus (**10**) and proventriculus (**11**) crossing the air sacs can be evaluated. Depending on the feeding condition, the proventriculus can easily be followed when passing into the ventriculus. On the ventrodorsal radiograph, both the esophagus and proventriculus are not easily detectable due to superimposition by bony structures, heart and liver. In raptors, the ventriculus (**12**) usually is located cranial to an imaginary line that connects the two acetabula. Individual intestinal loops (**13**) can be distinguished, however, it is difficult to differentiate between small and large intestine. The cloaca (**14**) is visible as an oval shadow at the caudal side of the celomic cavity.

Liver

On the lateral radiograph, the cranial part of the liver (**15**) is superimposed by the apex of the heart. On the ventrodorsal radiograph, the cranial liver outline is (**16**) sharply delineated by the air sacs. Caudally, the liver blends into the shadow of the gastrointestinal tract.

Spleen

The spleen (**17**) is only visible on the lateral radiograph. It is an oval-shaped density that is superimposed on the shadows of the proventriculus and ventriculus.

Kidneys

On the ventrodorsal radiograph, the kidneys (**18**) are superimposed by the densities of the gastrointestinal tract. On the lateral radiograph, they can be recognized to their full extension.

Reproductive Tract

Testes and ovaries can only be seen during the breeding season, when they enlarge due to an increased function. They are located dorsally in the celom between lungs and kidneys and are attached to the ventral part of the cranial kidney lobe. The salpinx cannot be demarcated from the shadows of the intestinal tract.

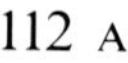

113

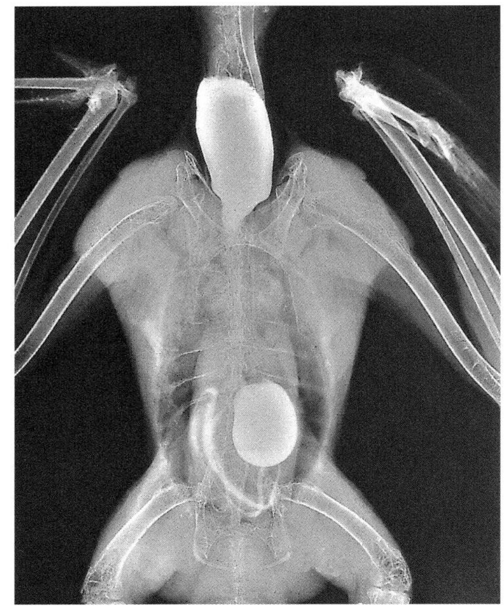

114

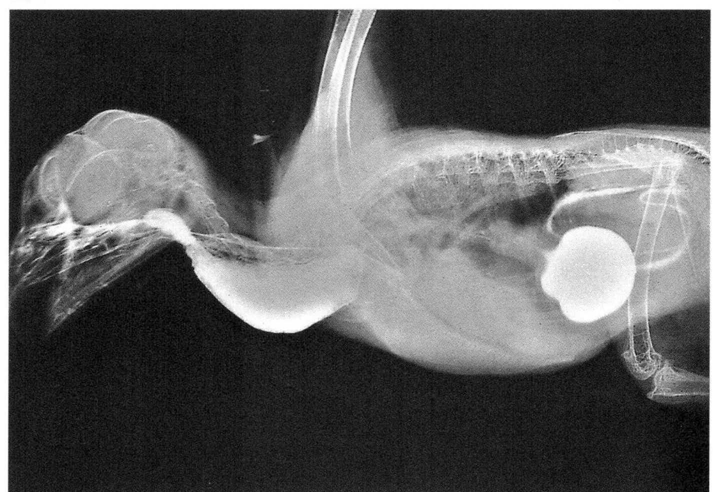

115

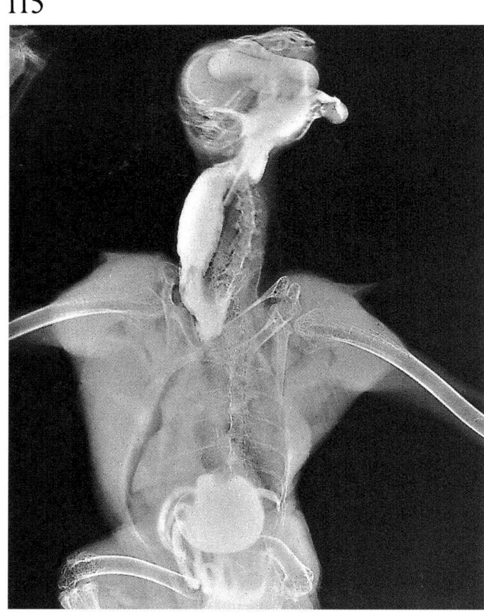

116

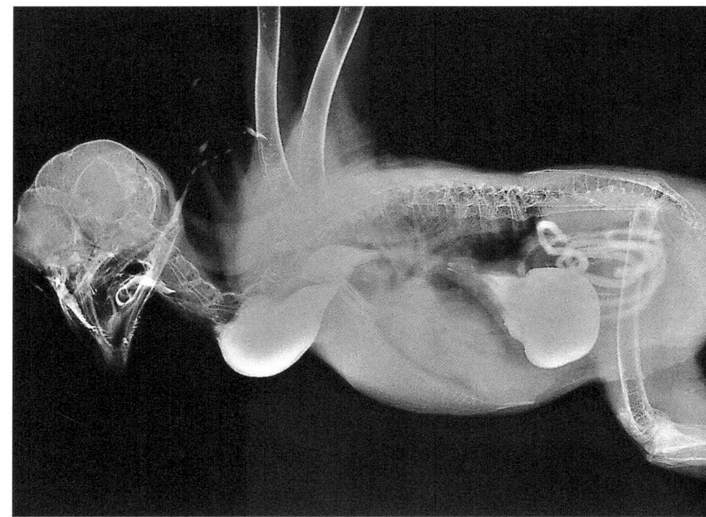

117

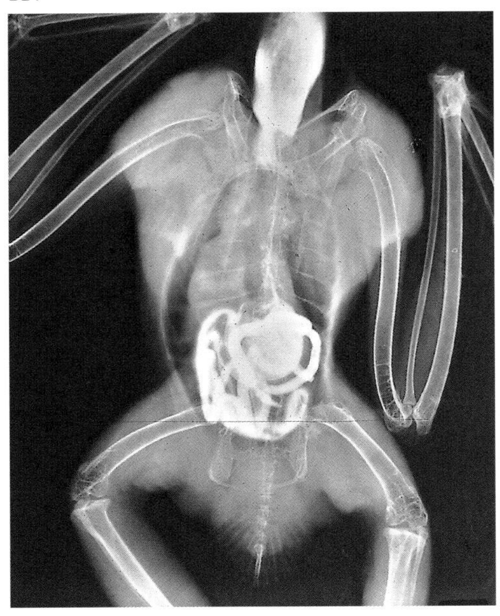

118

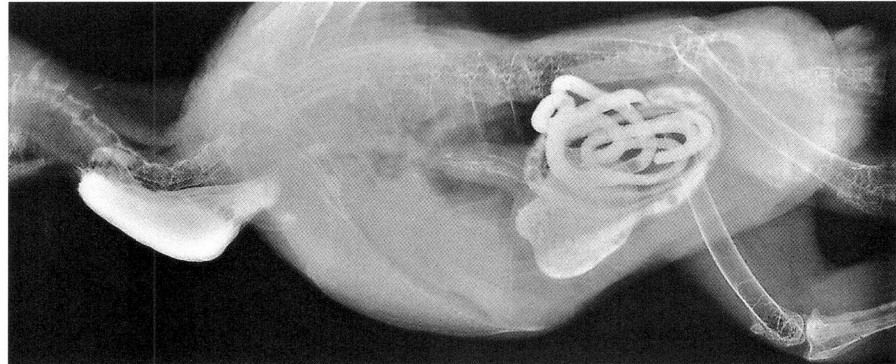

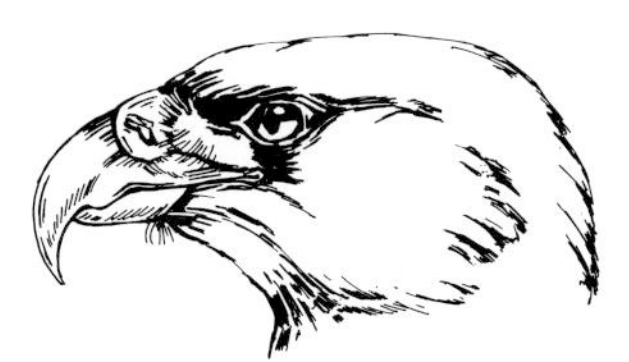

119

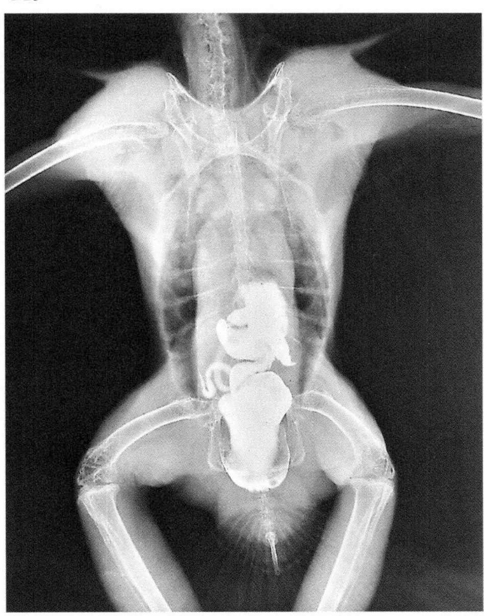

120

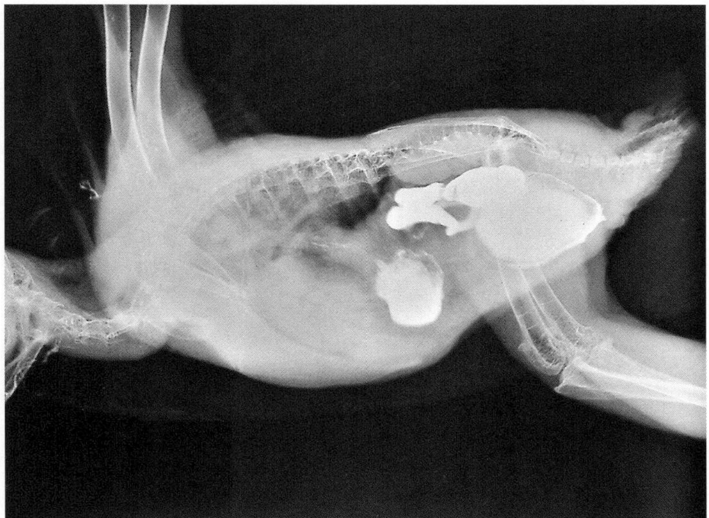

121

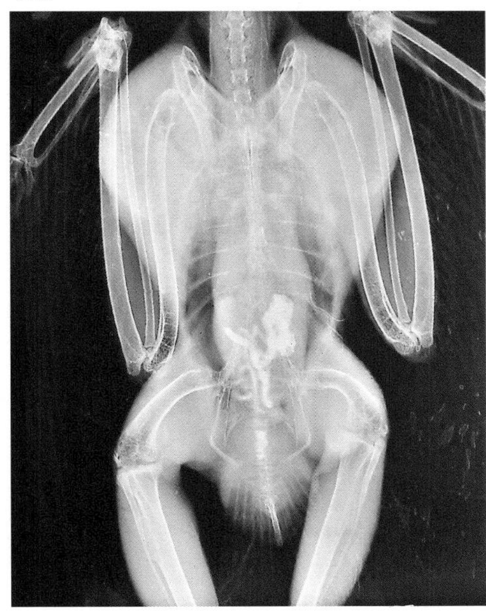

122

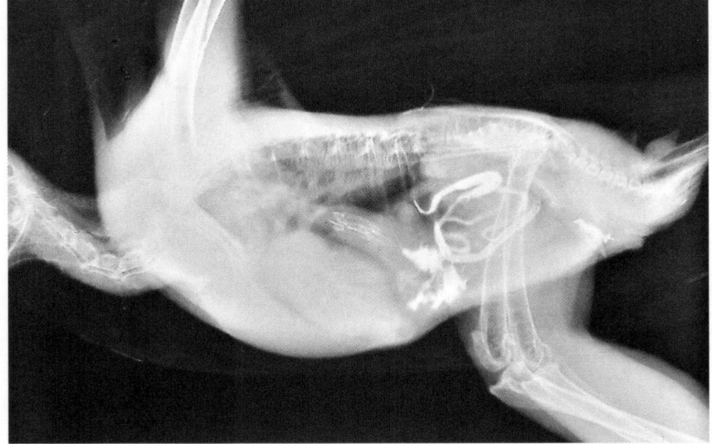

113-122 Normal Radiographic Appearance, lateral and ventrodorsal: contrast study.

Goshawk *(Accipiter gentilis)*, adult.

In birds of prey, the time for the passage of barium sulfate through the intestinal tract is shorter than in psittacine birds. As a result, the entire gastrointestinal tract can be outlined within 2 hours.

This series demonstrates five typical moments during the passage of barium sulfate in a goshawk. FIG. **113/114** were taken 15 minutes, FIG. **115/116** 30 minutes, FIG. **117/118** 60 minutes, FIG. **119/120** 120 minutes and FIG. **121/122** 180 minutes after administration of barium sulfate.

123

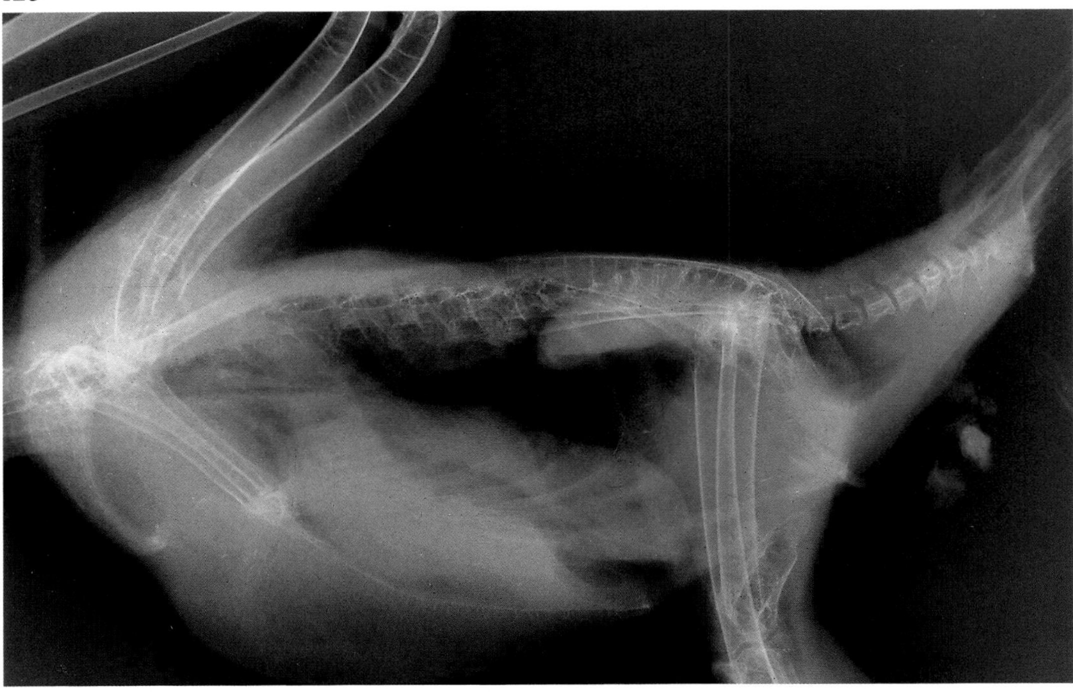

123A

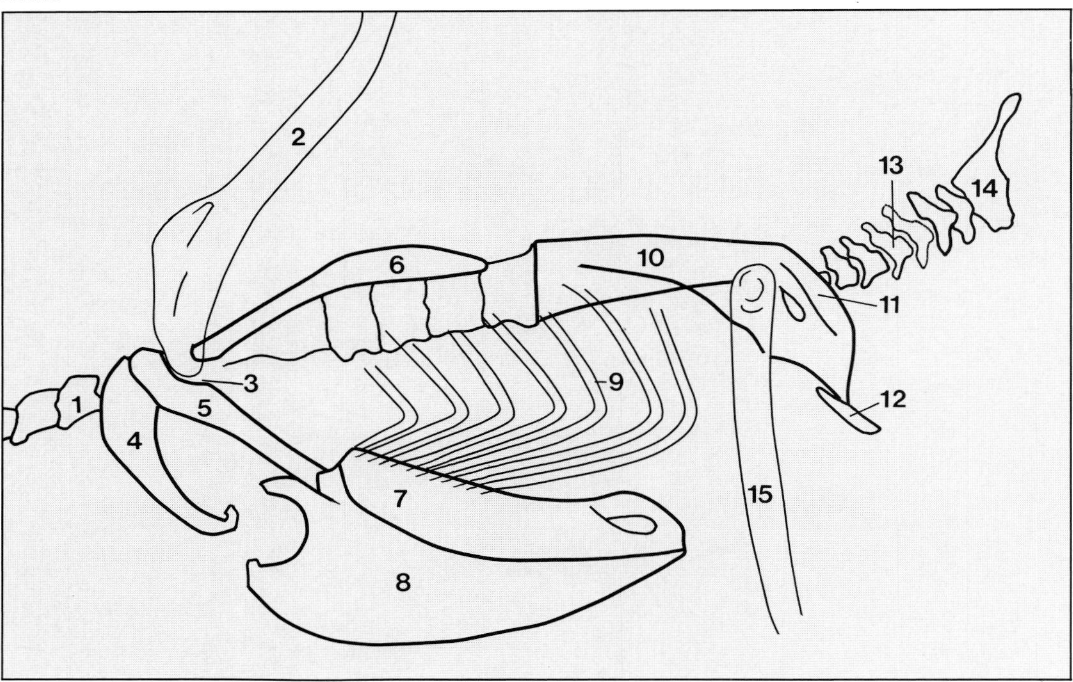

The radiographs published in this atlas allow comparison with pathological radiographs. For reasons of clarity, the bones of only one side have been outlined on the lateral drawing.

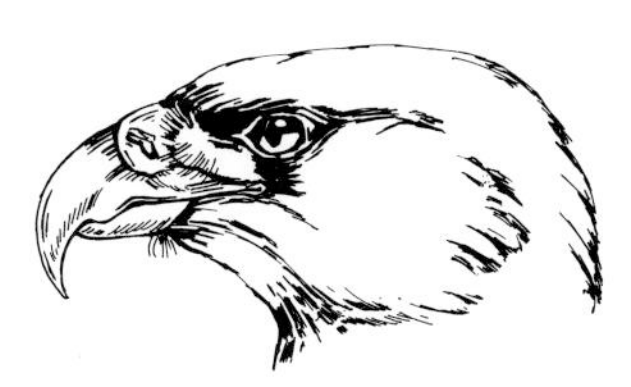

124

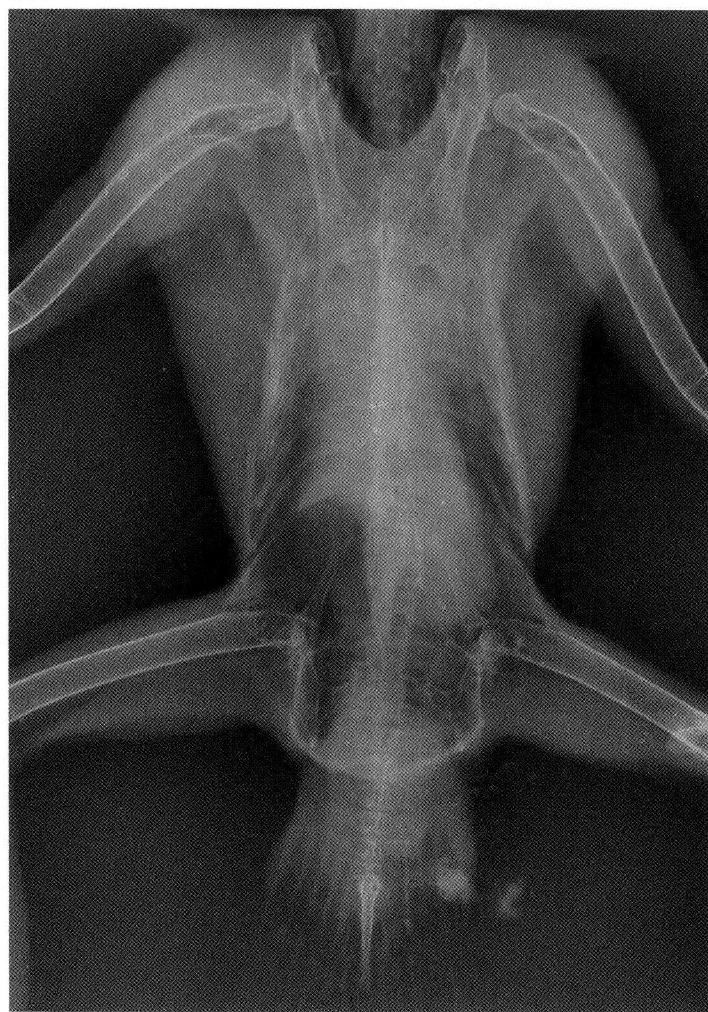

124 A

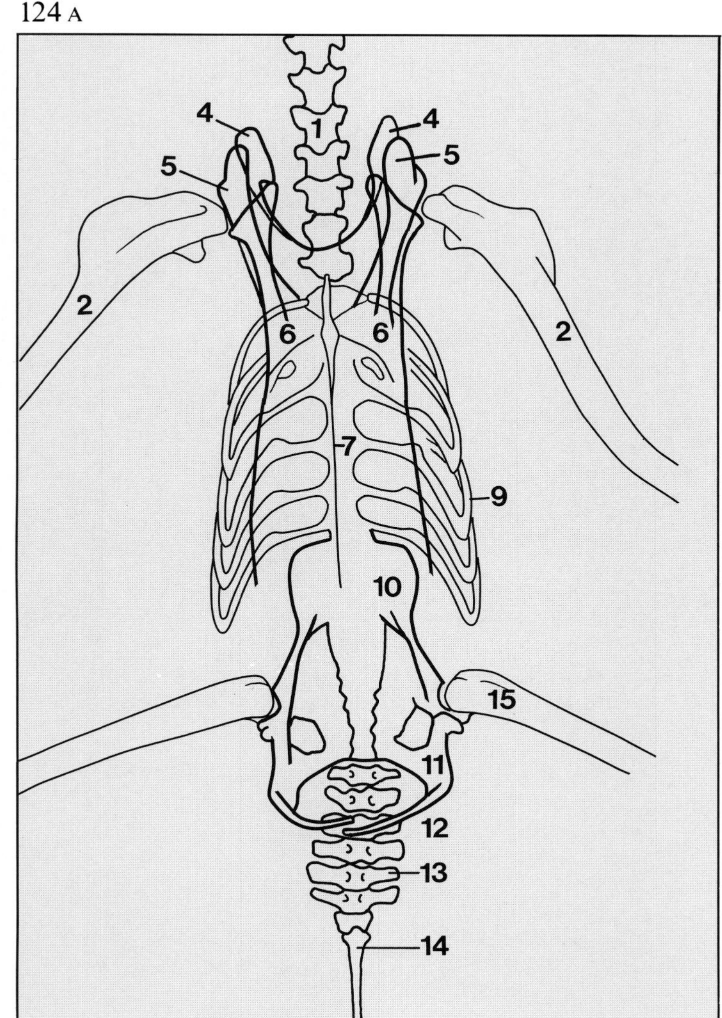

123/123A/124/124A Skeleton: Normal Radiographic Appearance,
lateral and ventrodorsal.

European Sparrow-Hawk *(Accipiter nisus)*, adult.

Cervical vertebrae (**1**); humerus (**2**); glenoid fossa (**3**); clavicle (**4**); coracoid (**5**); scapula (**6**); sternum (**7**); carina sterni (**8**); sternal ribs (**9**); synsacrum formed by the last thoracic and the lumbar vertebrae; ilium (**10**); ischium (**11**) and pubis (**12**); free caudal vertebrae (**13**); pygostyle (**14**); femur (**15**).

Note: A fracture of the femur is also visible.

125

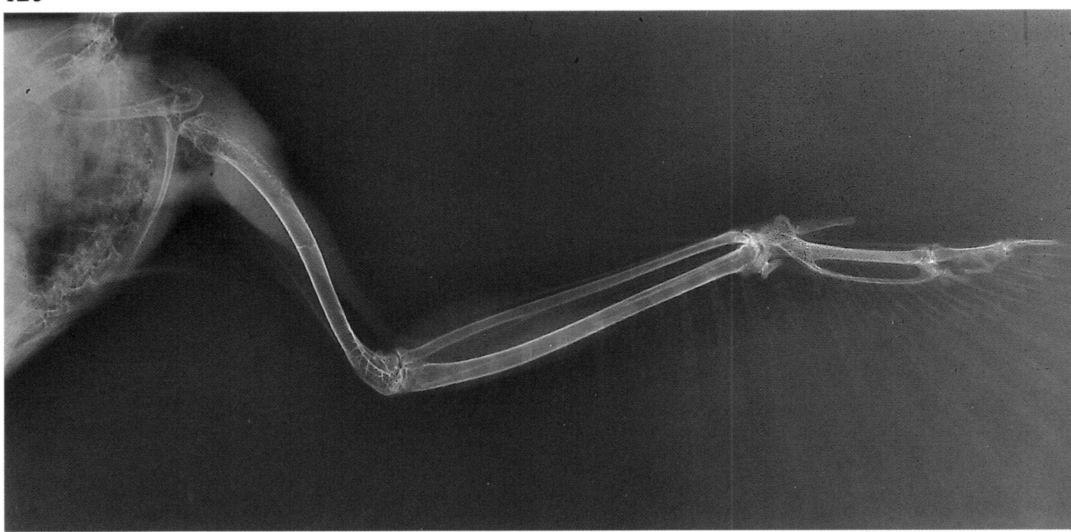

125A

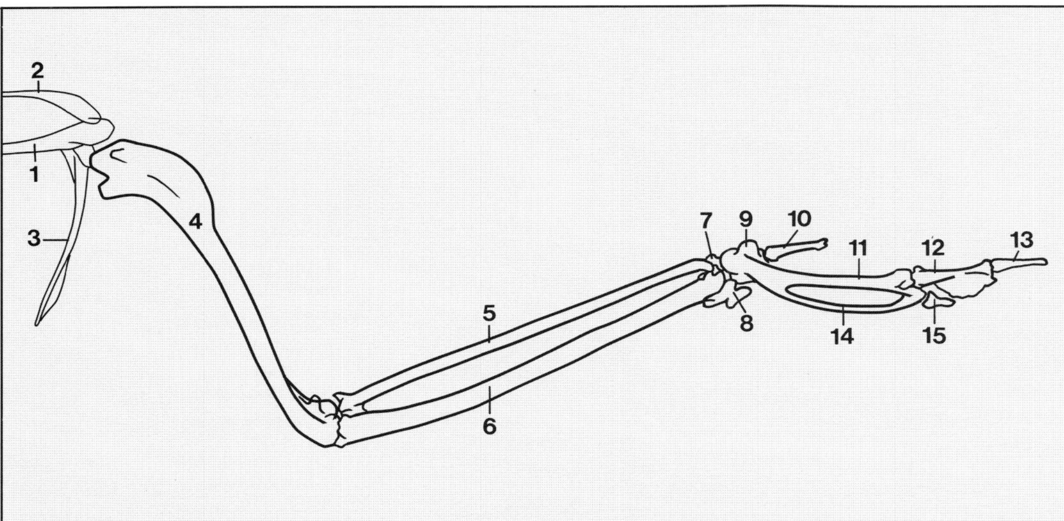

125/125A Wing: Normal Radiographic Appearance, ventrodorsal.

Tawny Owl *(Strix aluco)*, adult.

The axial skeleton is suspended by the bones of the shoulder girdle, the coracoid (**1**), and the clavicle (**2**). The scapula (**3**) together with the coracoid forms the glenoid cavity to fit the head of the humerus (**4**). The humerus is pneumatized.

The ulna (**6**) is larger than the relatively small radius (**5**).

Of the proximal row of the carpal bones only the radial carpal (**7**) and ulnar carpal bones (**8**) are visible separately.

The carpometacarpals are fused. The alular metacarpus (**9**) is integrated in the carpus. It is lengthened by the alula (pollex) (**10**). The other two carpometacarpal bones form the basal support for the primaries. The carpometacarpal II (**11**) is strongly developed and prolonged by the proximal (**12**) and distal (**13**) phalanges of the major digit. The carpometacarpus III (**14**) ends with the minor digit (**15**).

When examining radiographs of limbs, evaluation of the soft tissues (muscles and tendons) is of great diagnostic value.

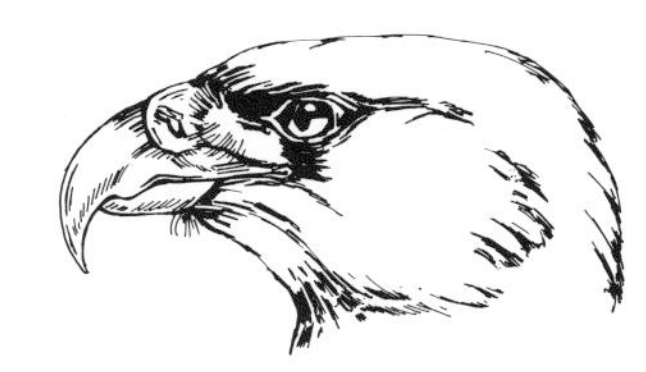

126-1

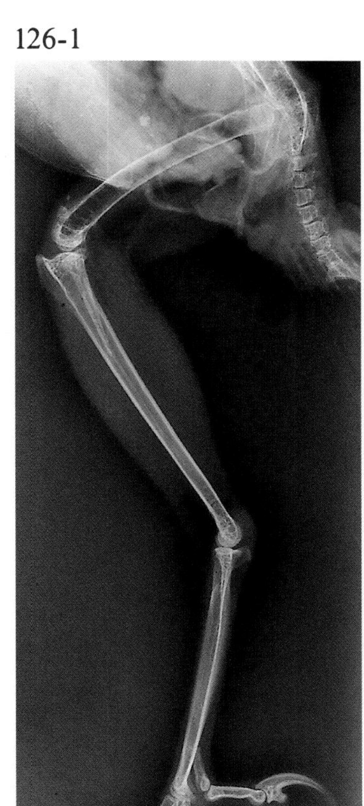

126-1 A

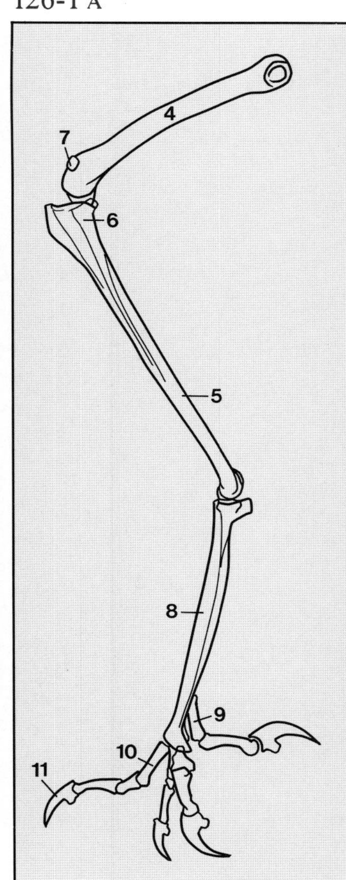

126-2

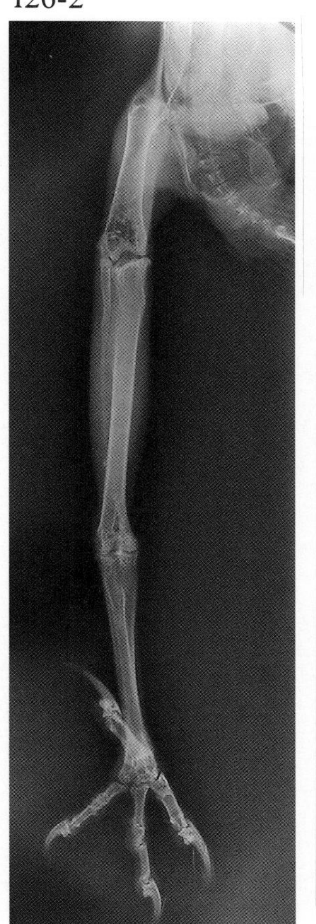

126-2 A

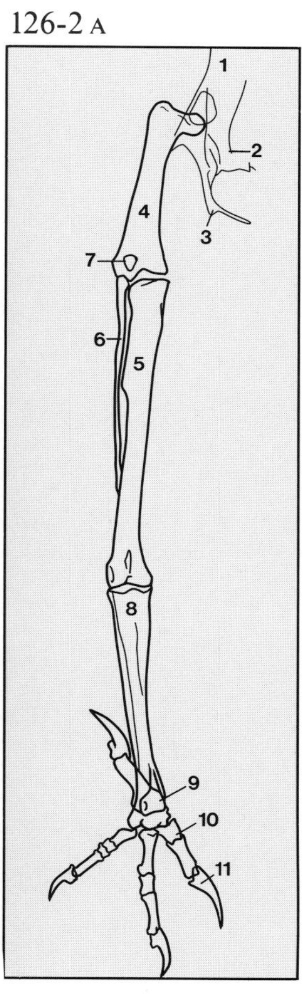

126-1/126-1A/126-2/126-2A Leg: Normal Radiographic Appearance,
mediolateral and dorsoplantar.

Common Buzzard *(Buteo buteo)*, adult.

The acetabulum is formed by the ilium (**1**), the ischium (**2**) and the pubis (**3**). The bones are difficult to distinguish on radiographs because of their fine structure. The femur (**4**) articulates in the stifle joint with the tibiotarsus (**5**) and the fibula (**6**). The patella (**7**) is well defined. Usually, the distal end of the fibula is fused with the tibiotarsus.

The strong tarsometatarsus (**8**) includes metatarsalia II, III and IV and articulates with the phalanges (**10, 11**) of the respective digits. The proximal bone of digit I corresponds to the metatarsal I (**9**).

127

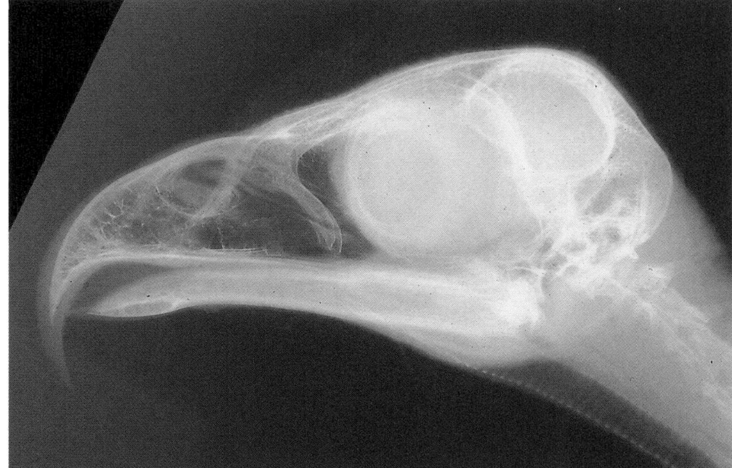

128

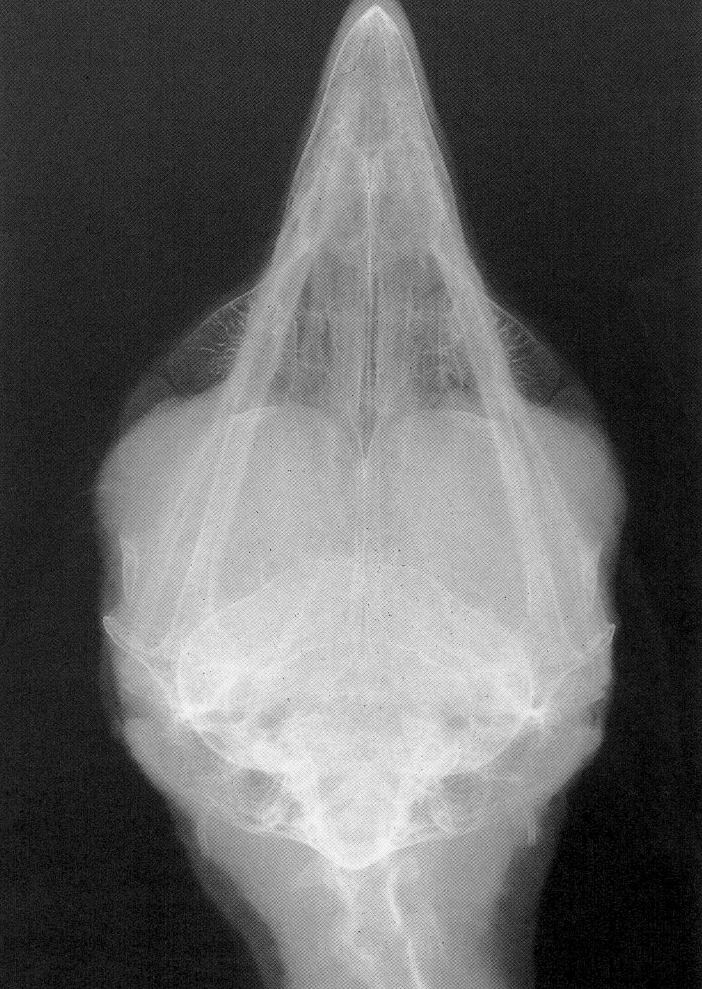

129

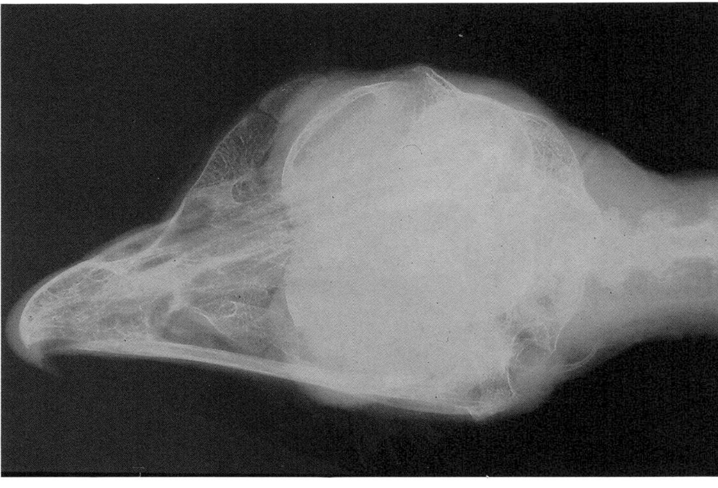

127/128/129 Skull: Normal Radiographic Appearance, ventrodorsal, lateral and oblique.

Golden Eagle *(Aquila chrysaetos)*, adult.

Several radiographic features of the skull distinguish falconiformes from the psittacines. The shape of the upper bill is unique and the nasal openings are larger, elongated, and triangular-ovoid. The nasofrontal hinge is markedly reduced in comparison with psittacines (FIG. **6-8**), although some slight moveability is maintained in most falconiformes.

Falconiformes have large, distinct prefrontal projections with a supraorbital and an orbital process. The postorbital skull is very short. The frontal bones may extend over the orbits, as with this eagle. The scleral ossicles are larger and less flat than those of the psittacines. The palatine bones of falconiformes are flat with a maximal width beneath the orbit.

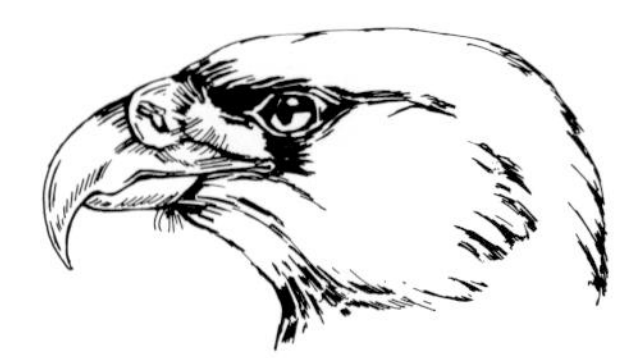

130

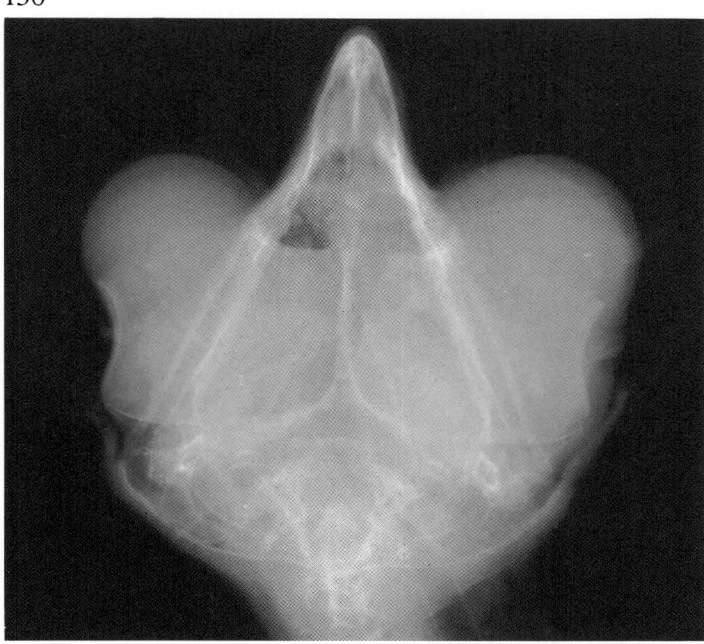

130 Trauma.

Great Horned Owl *(Bubo virginianus)*, adult.

There is an increased density in the left nasal cavity. In the left orbital region, soft tissue swelling with an increased density of the anterior portion of the globe is visible. Note the large eyes and tubular shape of the scleral ossicles characteristic of owls.

These findings indicate severe concussive trauma of the head.

131

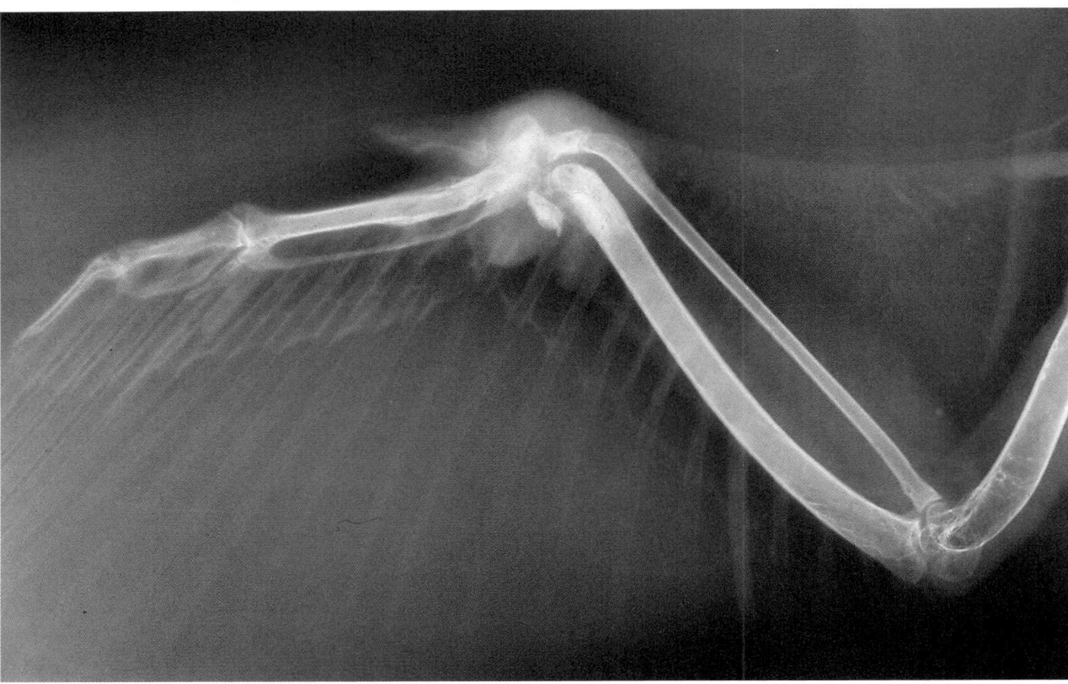

132

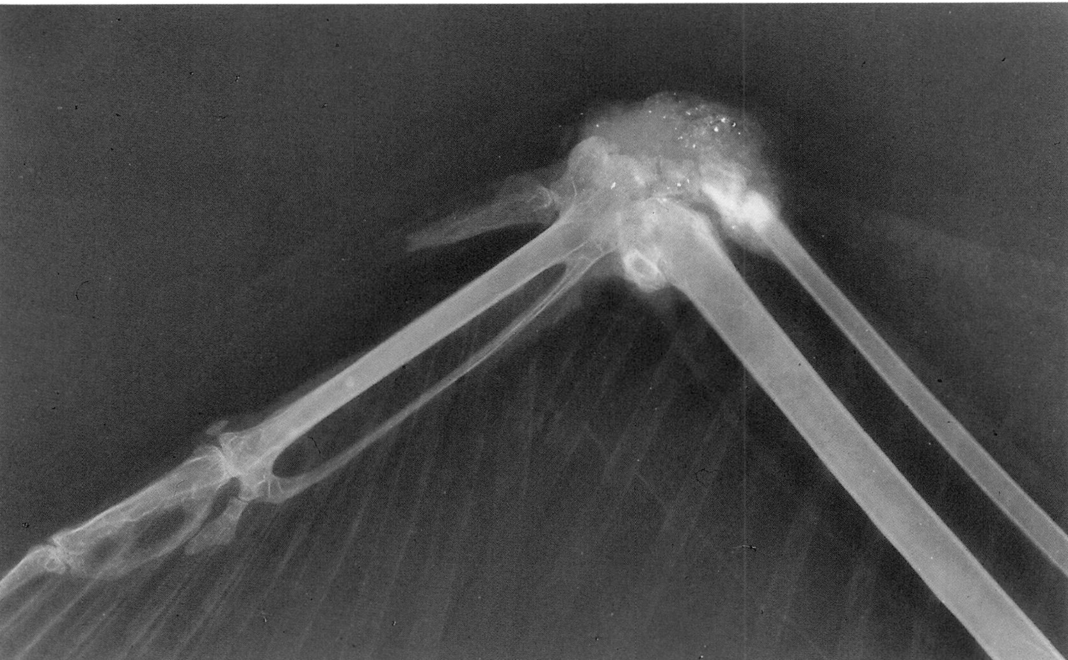

131 Infectious Arthritis.

Peregrine falcon *(Falco peregrinus)*, adult.

The area of the carpal joint is severely swollen. The carpal bones show intraarticular bone lysis and periarticular bone sclerosis. These findings are characteristic of septic arthritis. The cause of the arthritis was a mycobacterial infection.

132 Leadshot Injury.

Common Buzzard *(Buteo buteo)*, adult.

A small-sized lead pellet has penetrated the carpal joint and caused a fracture of the radius. The sclerotic changes of the bones indicate an older injury with secondary arthrosis. Some lead dust is visible within the soft tissue swelling around the joint.

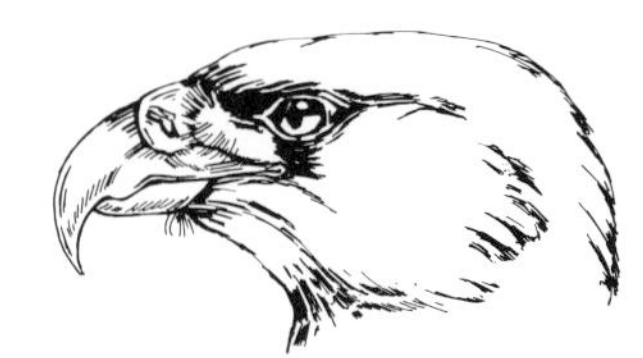

133

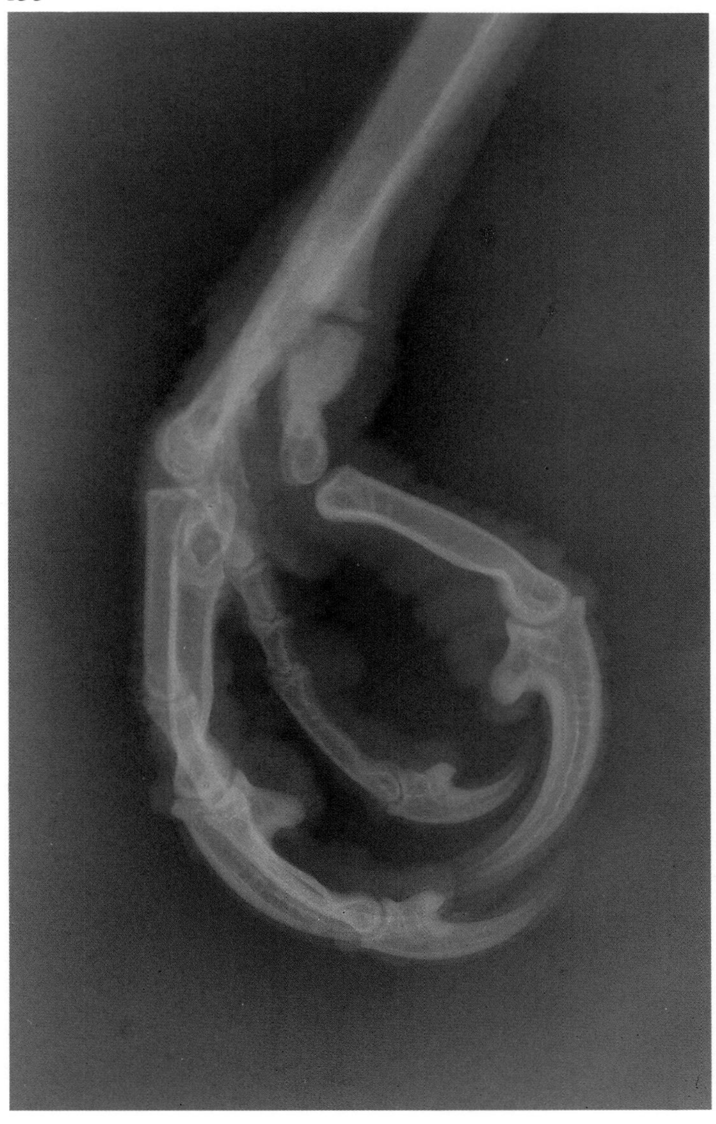

134

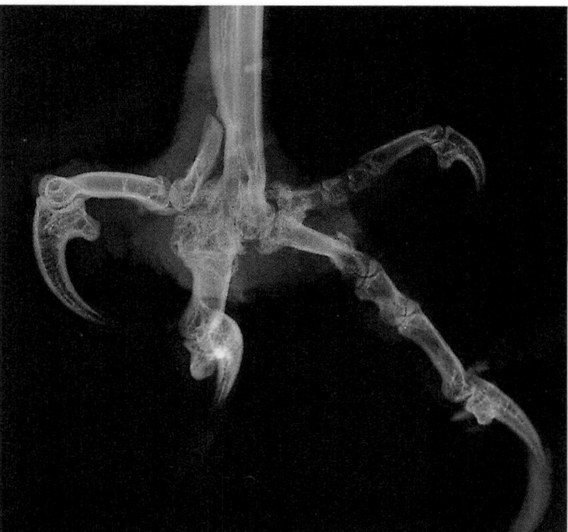

133 Arthritis.

Goshawk *(Accipiter gentilis)*, adult.

There are sclerotic bony and periosteal changes around the joint that is located between metatarsus I and tarsometatarsus. The cortex of the tarsometatarsus also has lytic changes.

134 Bumblefoot.

Spotted Eagle *(Aquila clanga)*, adult.

Lytic and sclerotic changes of all bones of the intertarsal joint justify a diagnosis of chronic infectious arthritis, in raptors called "bumblefoot". The infection is often secondary to an injury.

135

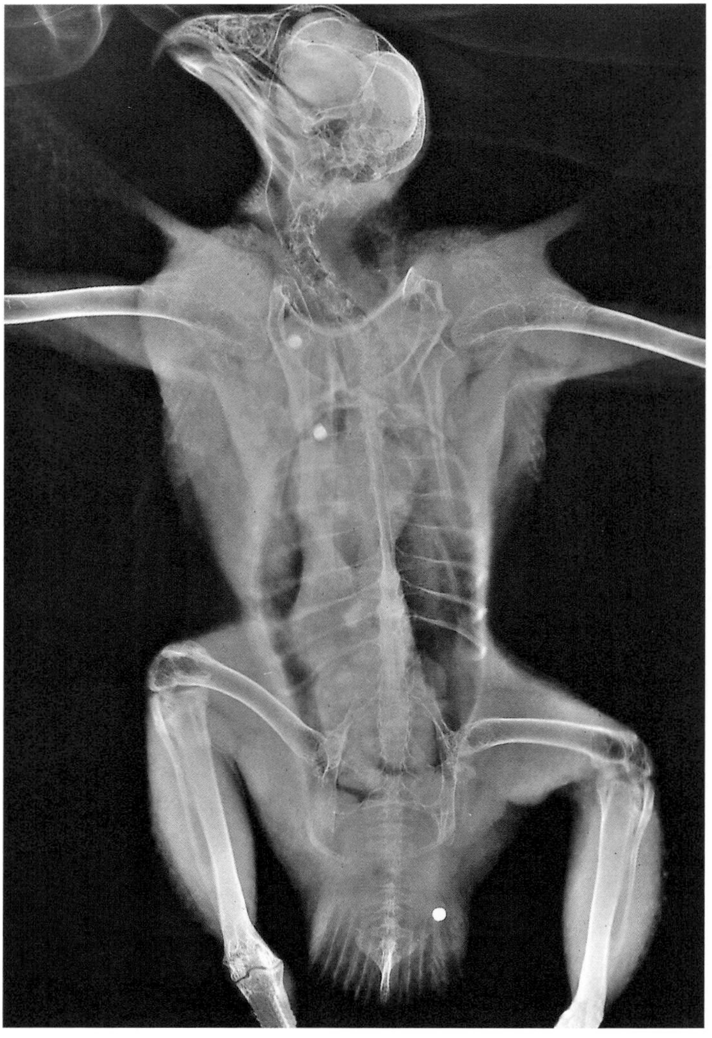

136

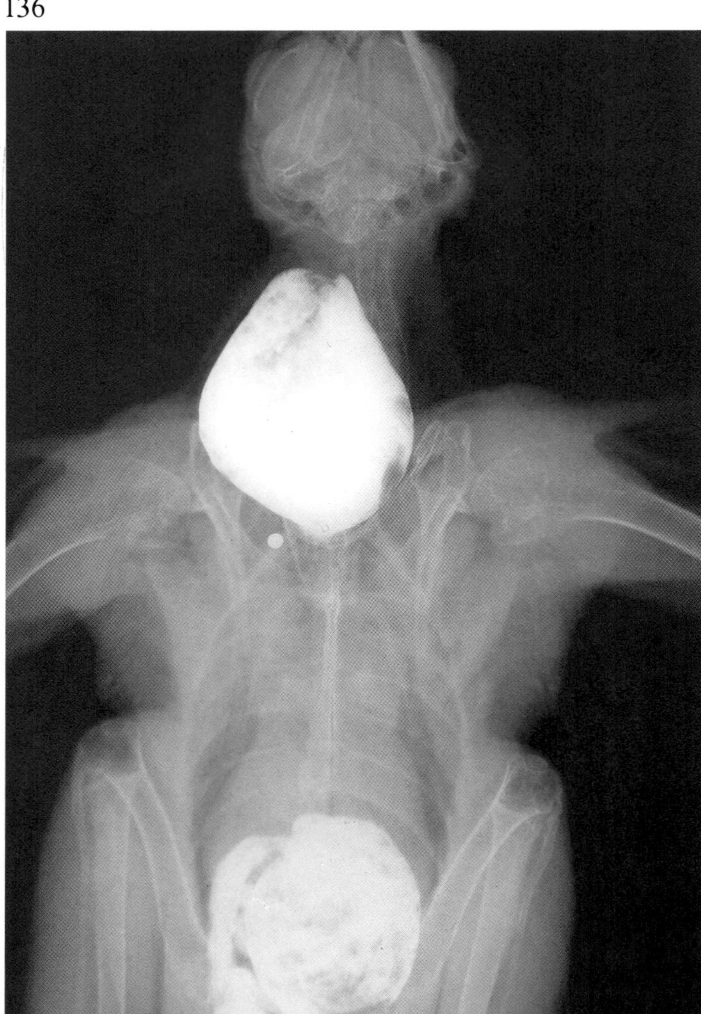

135/136 Leadshot.

Saker falcon *(Falco cherrug)*, adult.

The noncontrast radiograph shows lead pellets in the body of the falcon. The application of contrast medium (FIG. **136**) enables one to see the distance between the lead shot and the wall of the crop suggesting that the crop is undamaged.

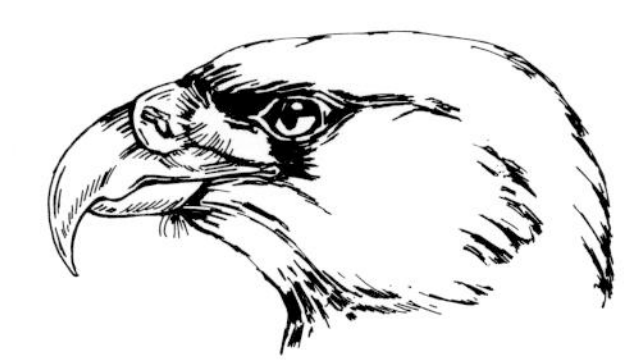

137

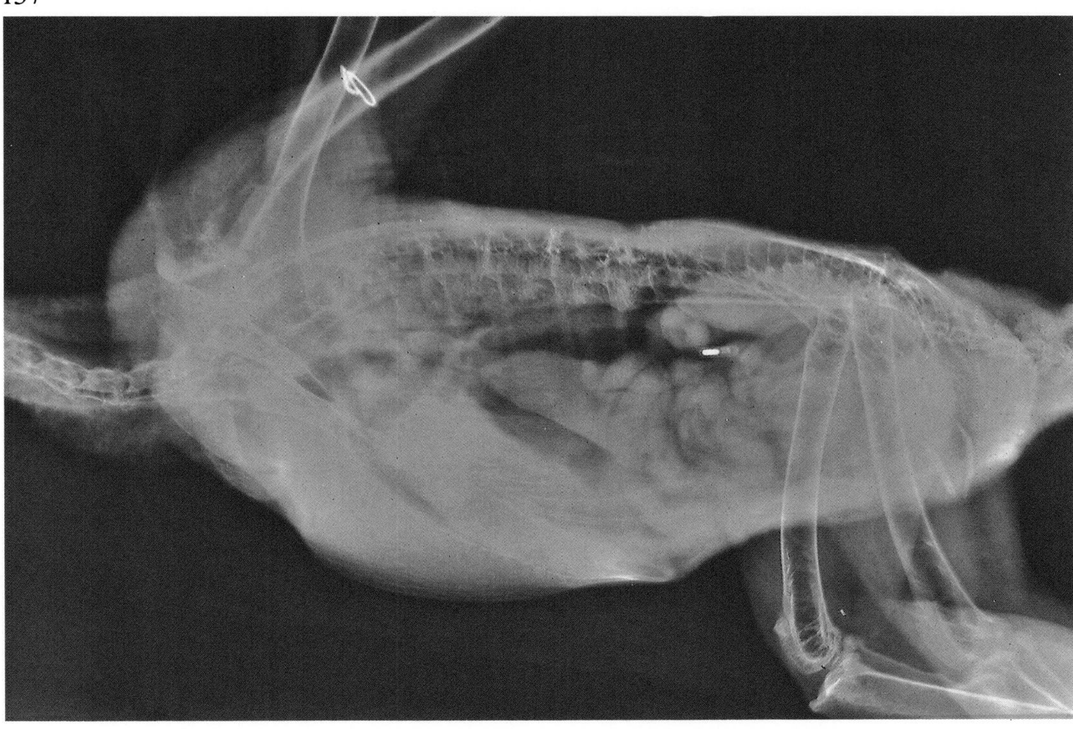

138

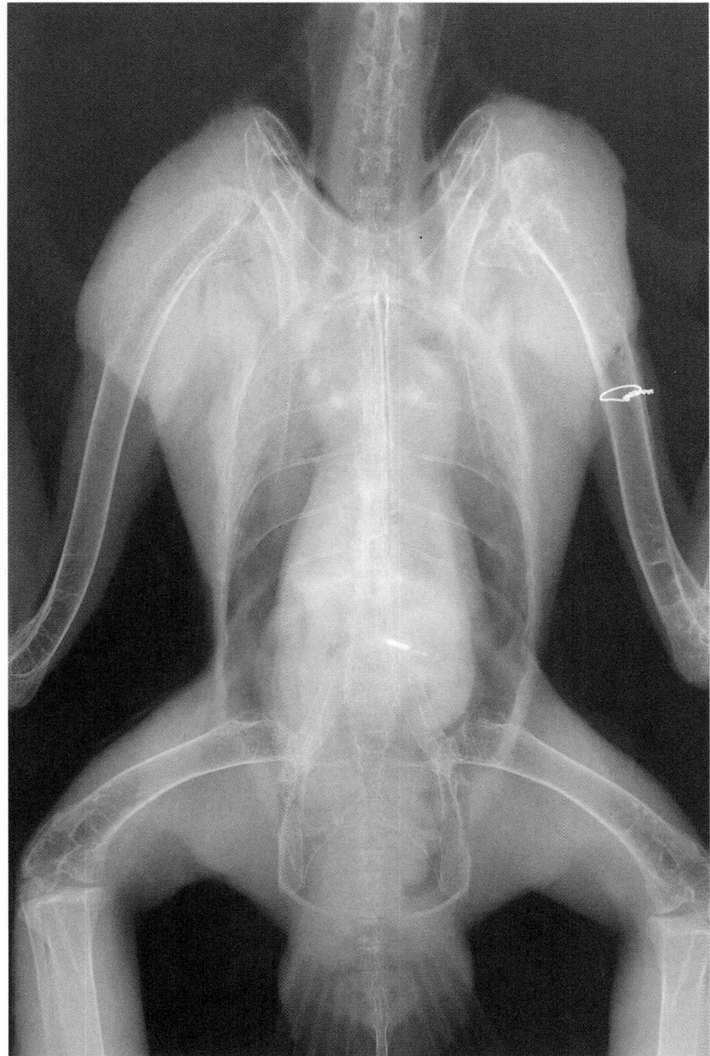

137/138 Microchip Implantation.

Common buzzard *(Buto buteo)*, adult.

A microchip for identification is implanted in the gonadal area.

Note: The cerclage-wire around the left humerus results from a fracture repair performed one year ago.

139

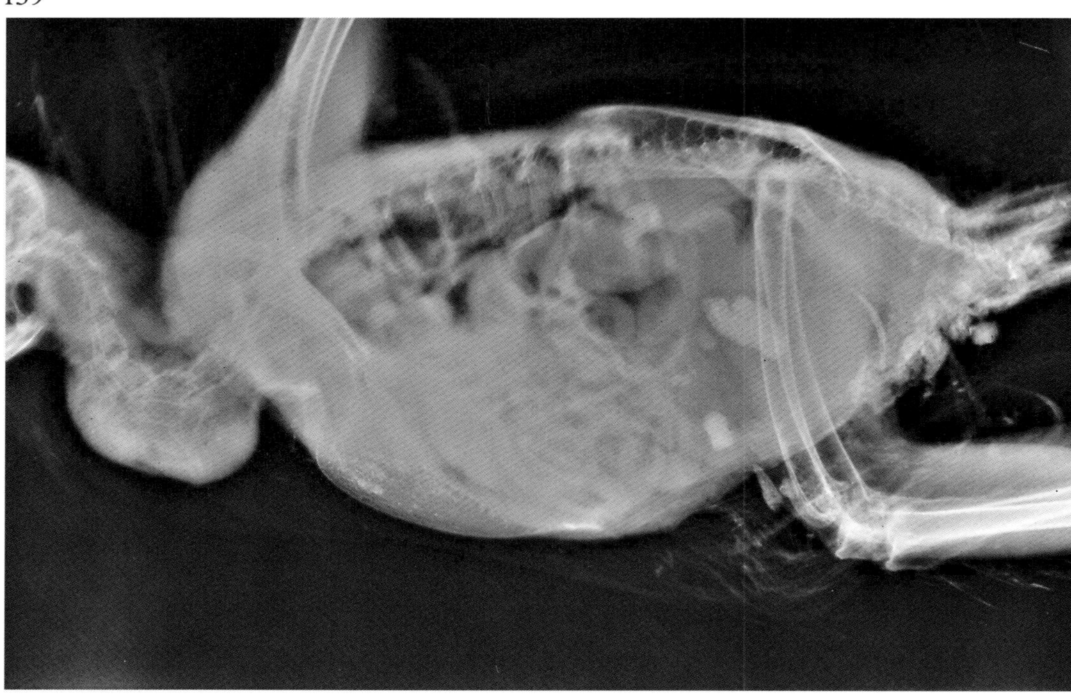

140

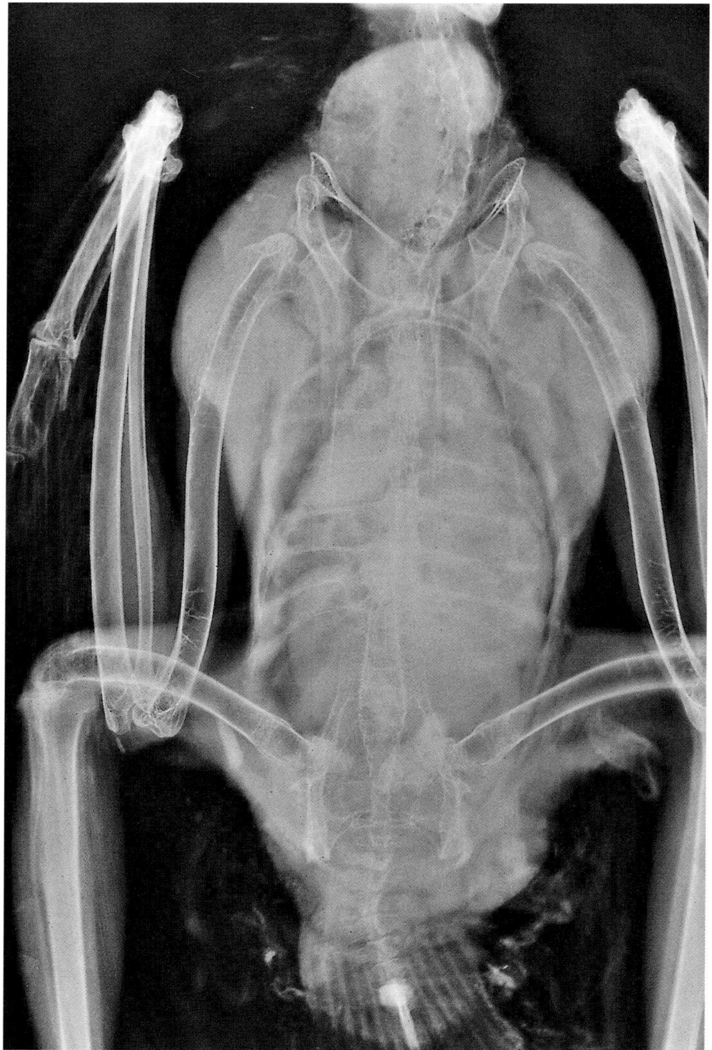

139/140 Luxation of the Thoracic Vertebral Column.

Common buzzard *(Buteo buteo)*, adult.

There is a luxation of the last two thoracic vertebrae. On the lateral radiograph, the cranial part of the synsacrum is displaced dorsally and on the ventrodorsal radiograph it is displaced to the right. Remnants of contrast medium given the day before are still present in the intestines. This indicates disturbed intestinal peristalsis and coprostasis.

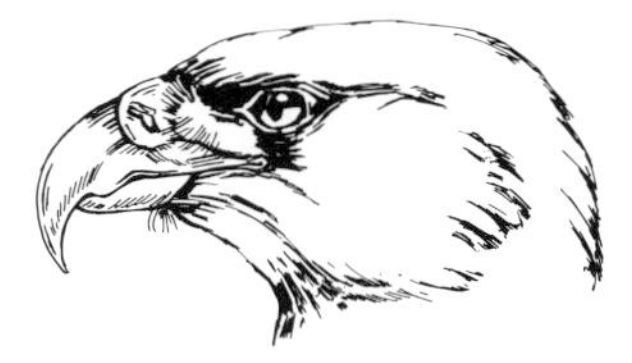

141

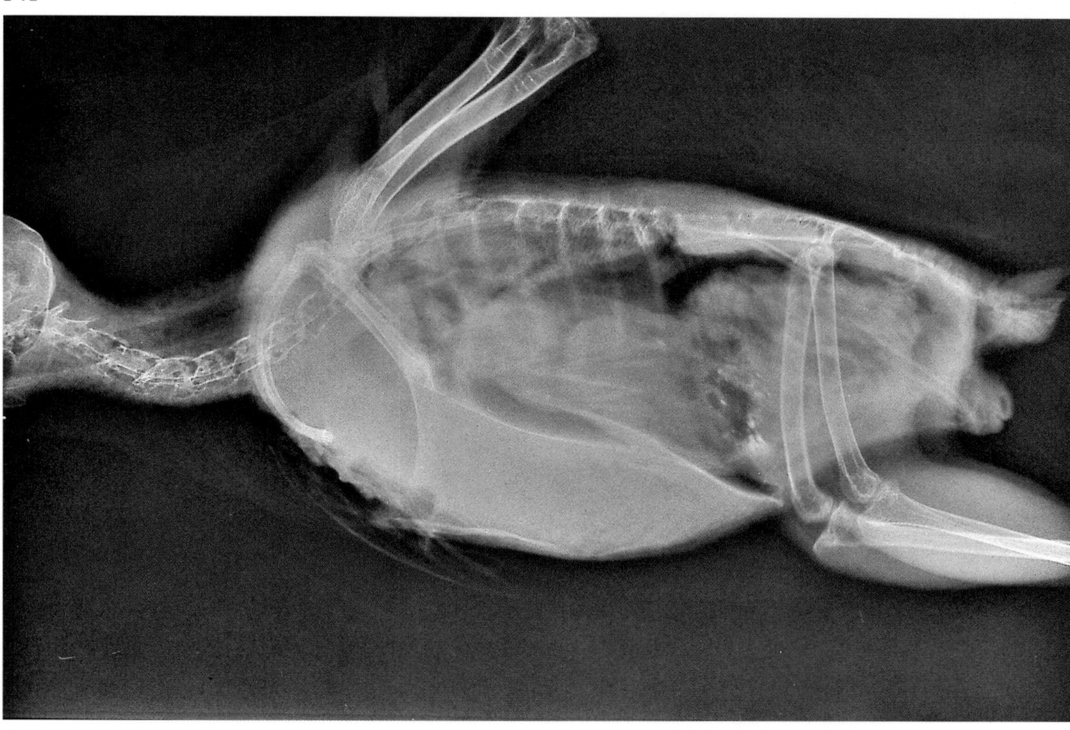

142

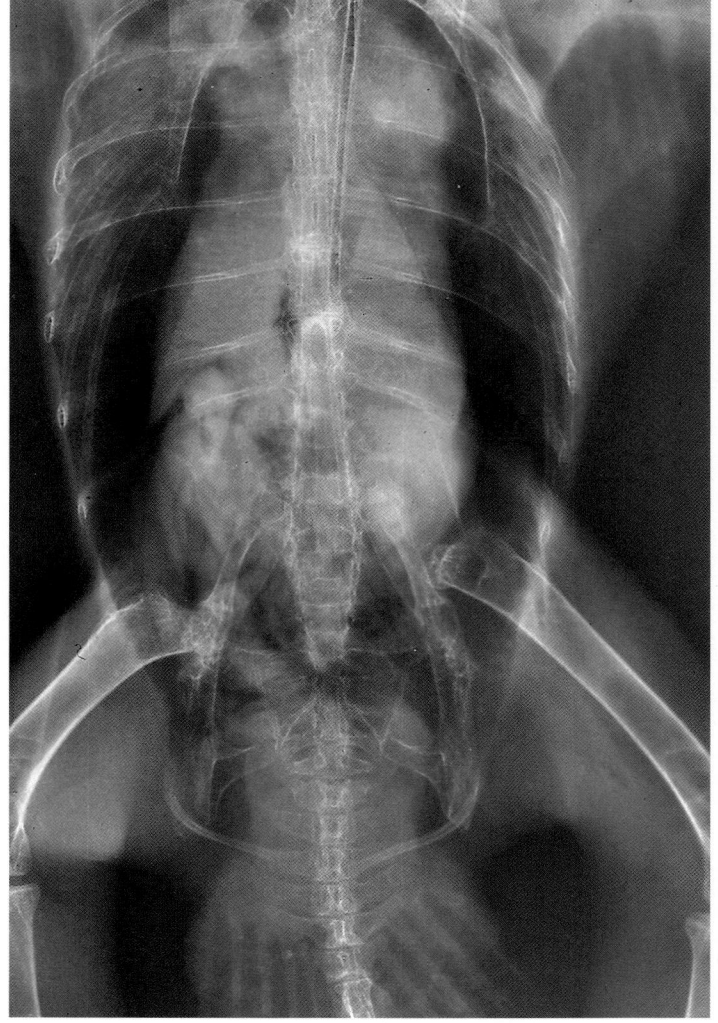

141 Injury.

Eurasian Woodcock *(Scolopax rusticola)*, adult.

The crista sterni has an abnormal outline. Soft tissue swelling is also present. These changes are often the result of a crash against an obstacle.

142 Luxation of the Hip Joint.

Common Buzzard *(Buteo buteo)*, adult.

The left hip joint is luxated. The head of the femur is displaced cranially.

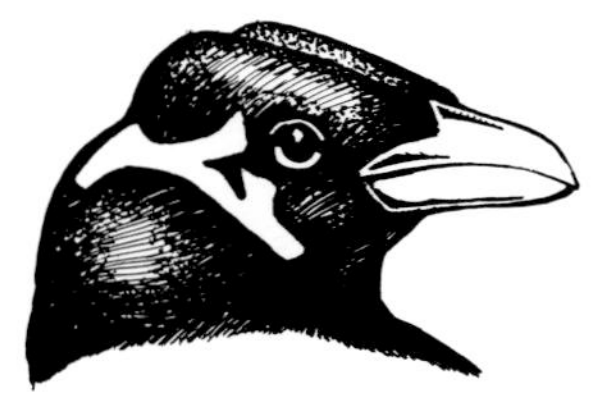

Birds: Hill-Mynah Radiographic Anatomy

143

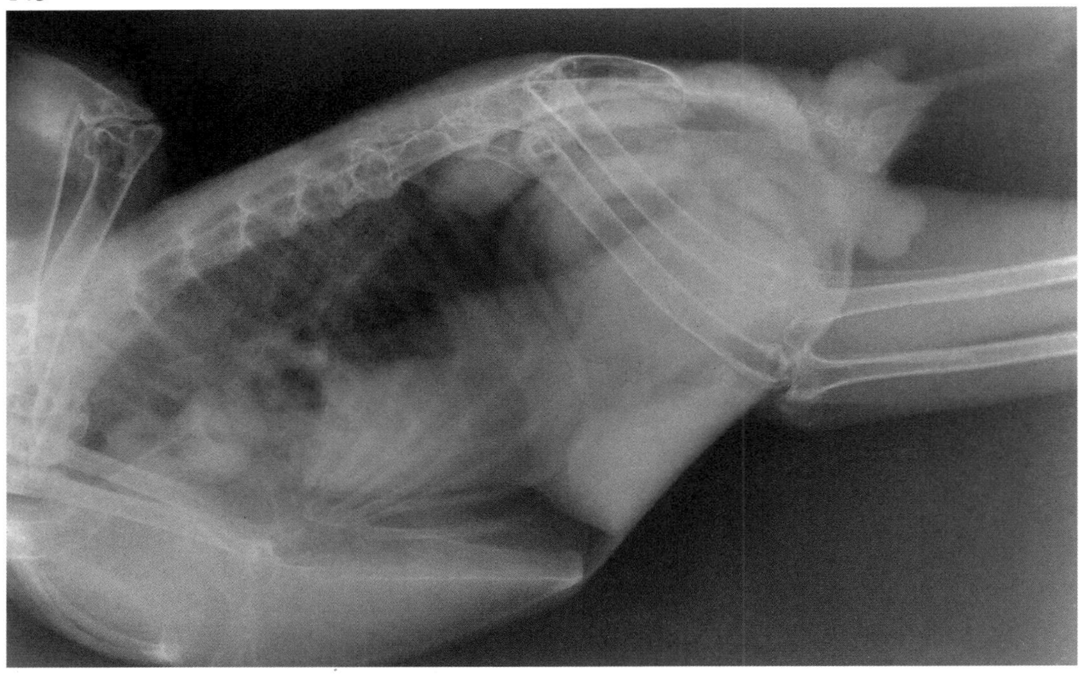

143 A

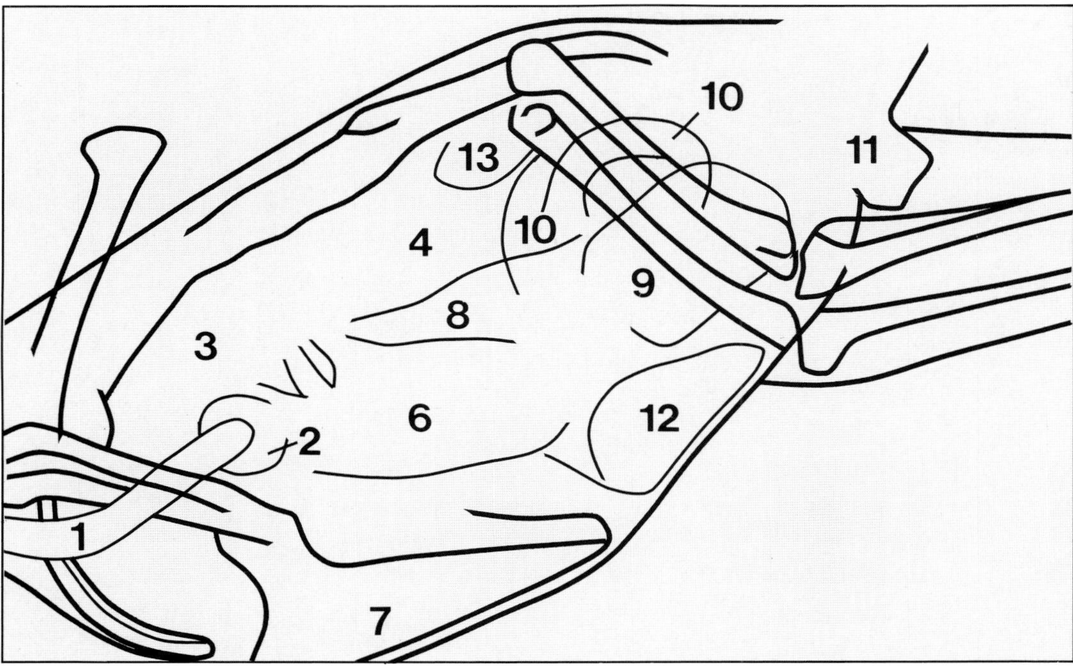

143/143A/144/144A Normal Radiographic Appearance, lateral and ventrodorsal.

Hill-Mynah *(Gracula religiosa)*, adult.

Respiratory Tract

Relative to body size, the trachea (**1**) is long and flexible. The syrinx is surrounded by a large muscle mass (**2**), which is normally found in speaking, singing and whistling birds and can easily be recognized in both views. The lungs (**3**), bronchi, and air sacs (**4**) are comparable with those of other birds. The radiolucent diverticles of the clavicular air sacs (**5**) are small because the wings are very close to the body.

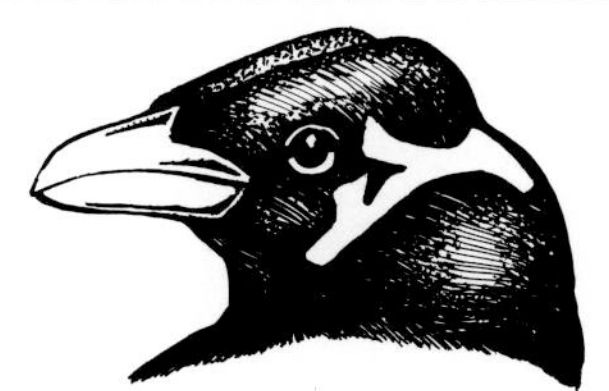

144

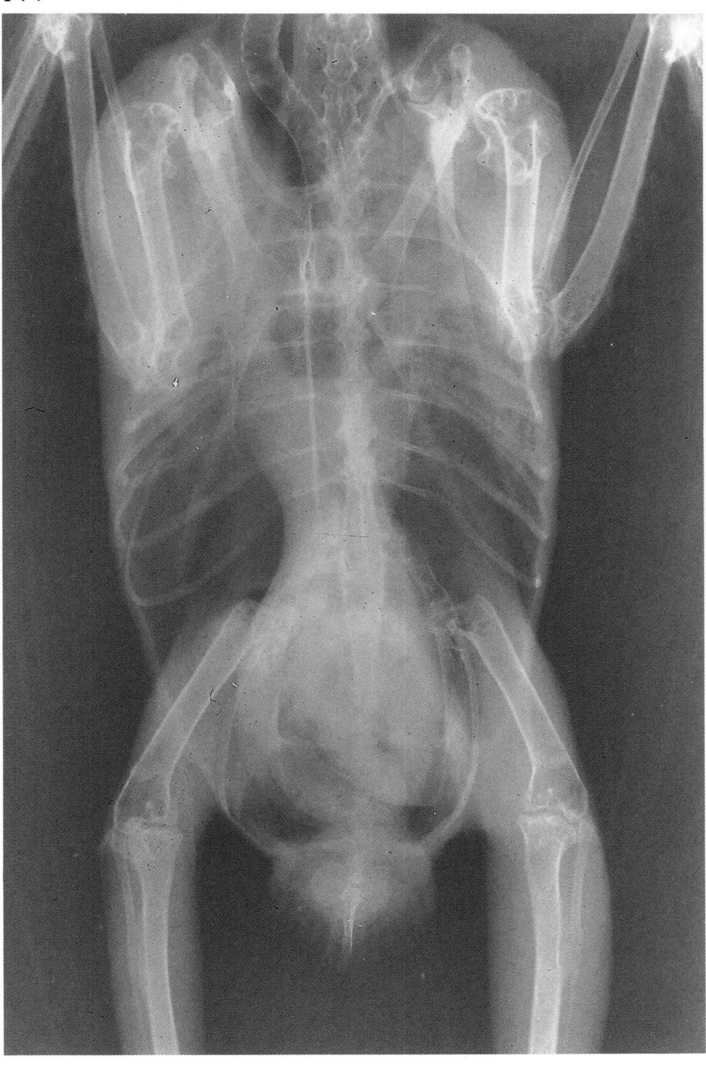

144 A

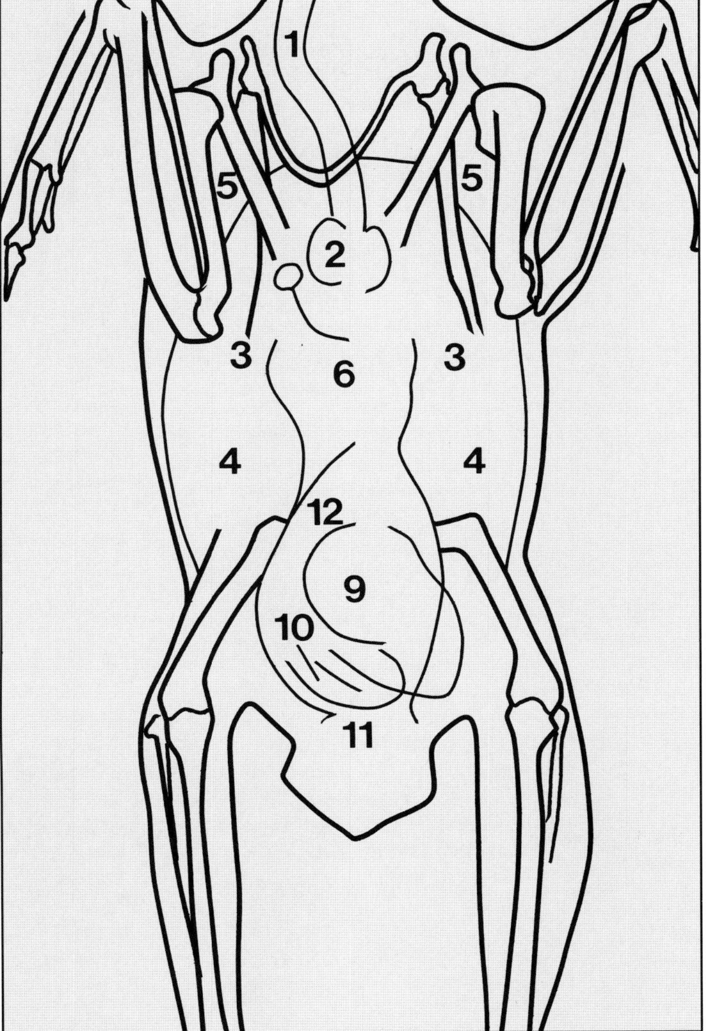

Heart and Vessels

On the lateral radiograph, the heart (**6**) of the hill-mynah is separated from the sternum (**7**) by a small distance. The large vessels are usually well visible.

Gastrointestinal Tract

Esophagus and proventriculus (**8**) are only visible on lateral radiographs. Superimposition of bony structures and of heart and liver prevents visualization on ventro-dorsal radiographs. The ventriculus (**9**) of soft food eaters is not as muscular as in seed eaters making determination difficult. Several intestinal loops (**10**) can be recognized. The shadow of the cloaca (**11**) is small.

Liver and Spleen

On the lateral radiograph, the liver (**12**) can easily be identified. Its examination is especially important in mynahs because of common occurence of hemochromatosis. The spleen is usually superimposed by the gastro-intestinal tract and cannot be recognized.

Urogenital Tract

On the lateral radiograph, the cranial lobes of the kidneys (**13**) are clearly outlined. The genital organs, especially the testes, can sometimes be seen during the breeding season.

145

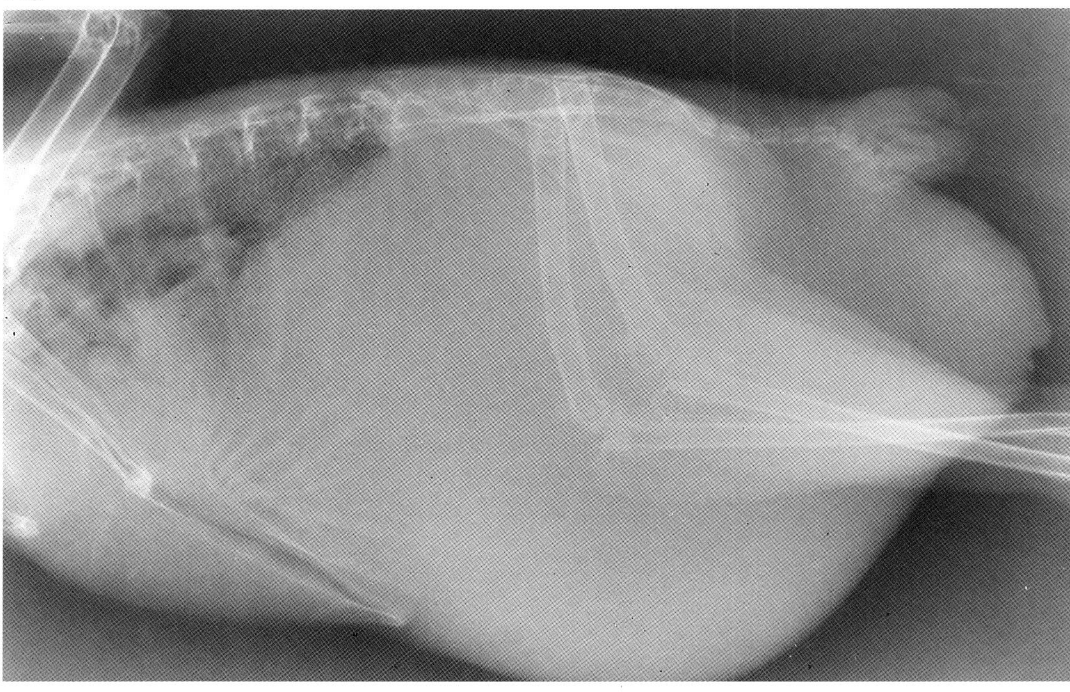

146

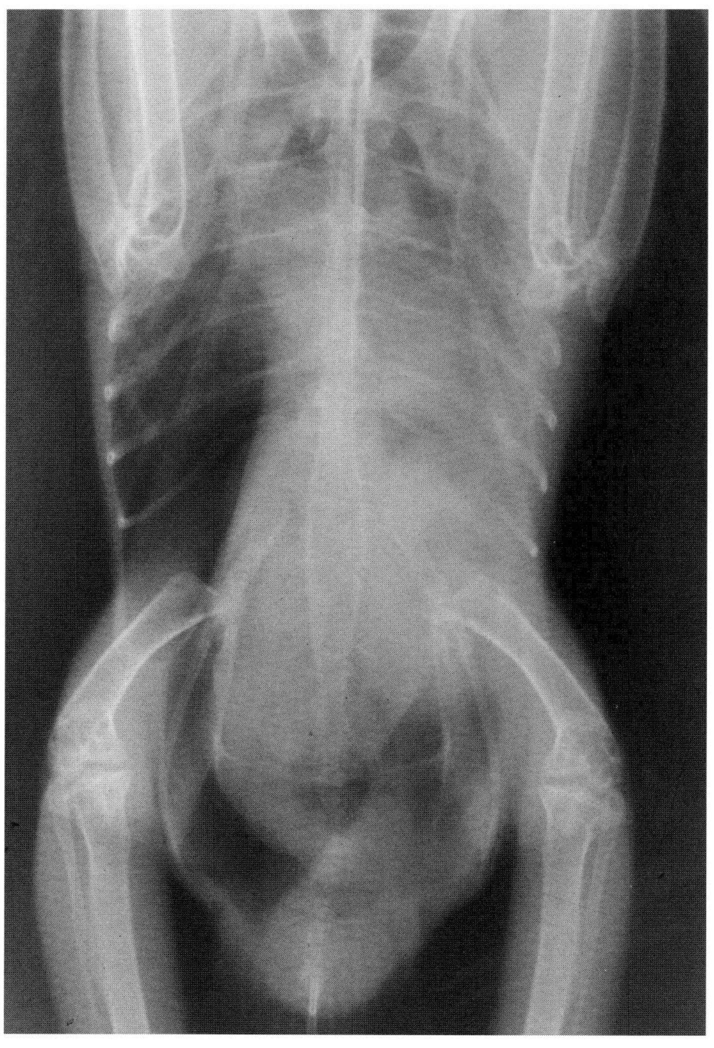

145 Ascites.

Hill-Mynah *(Gracula religiosa)*, 12 years.

The entire celomic cavity has a ground-glass appearance. The air sacs are compressed and airless. The lungs are partially compressed.

Note: Ascites is a common complication of hemochromatosis, a degenerative liver condition, being one of the most common mynah diseases.

146 Aspergillosis.

Hill-Mynah *(Gracula religiosa)*, 6 years.

The left lung and the air sacs of the left celomic cavity contain multiple mass-like densities. The contralateral air sacs are normal. On histological examination these densities proved to be aspergillomas.

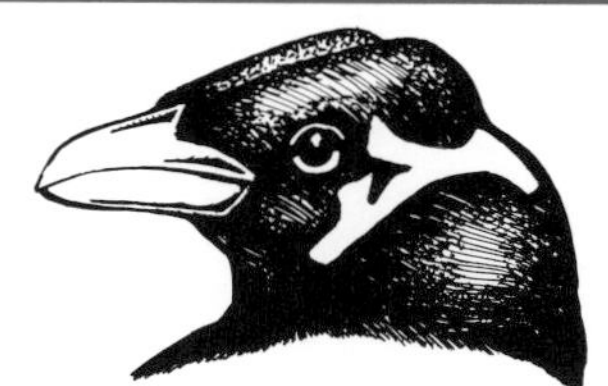

147

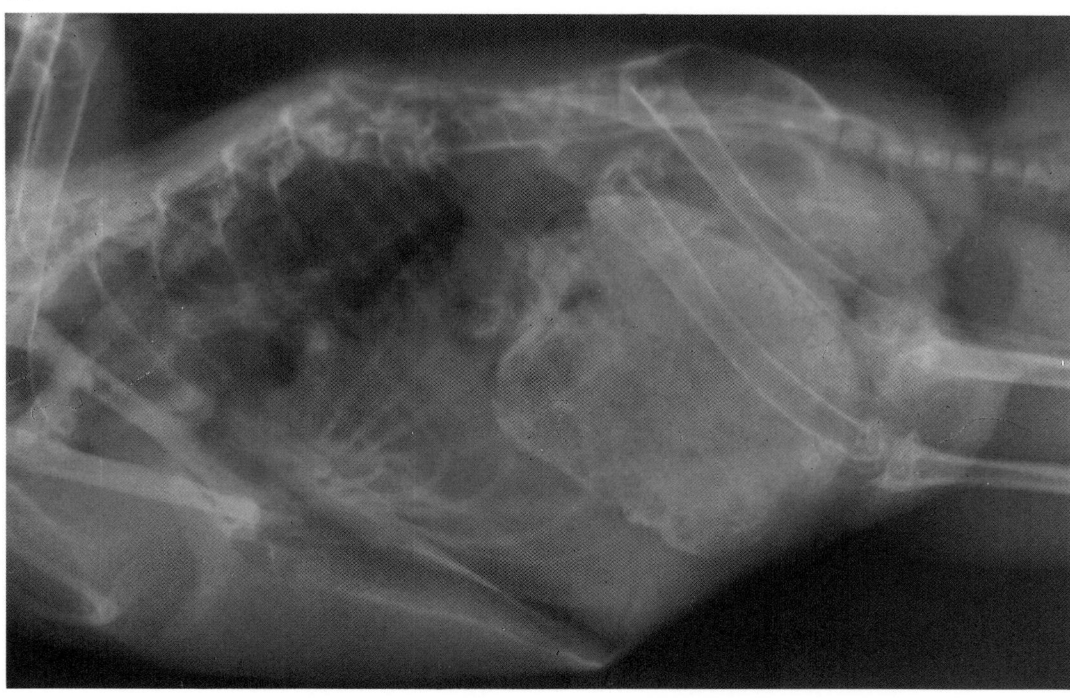

148

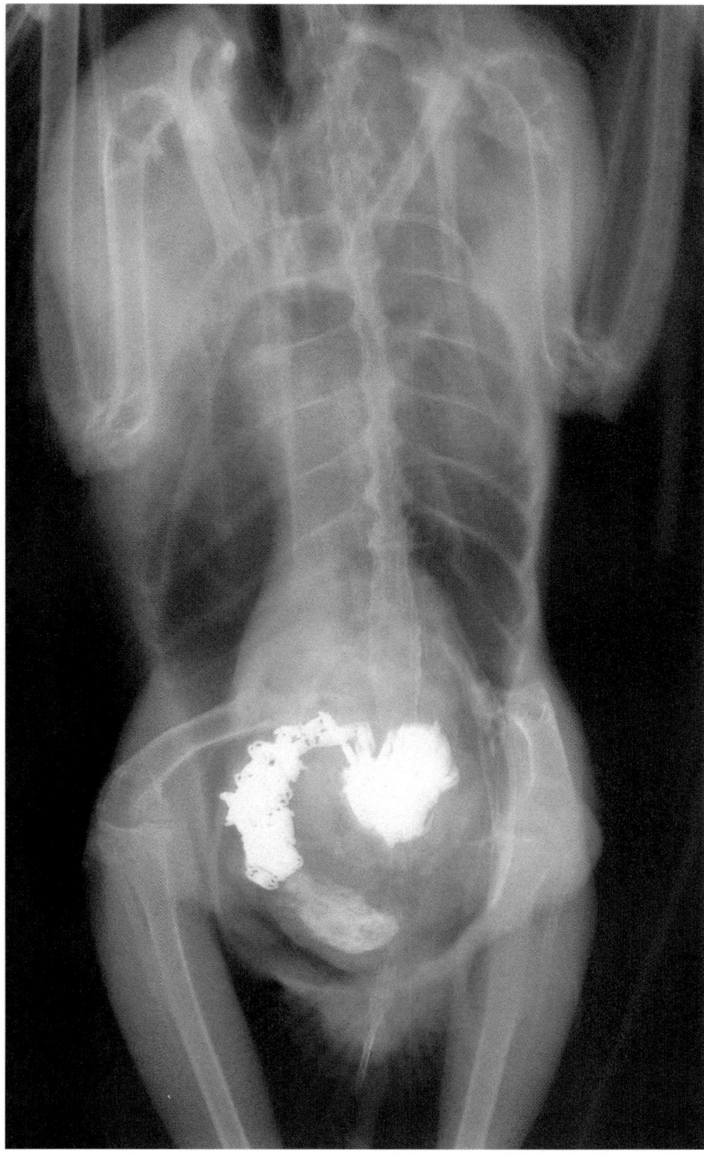

147 Foreign Body.

Hill-Mynah *(Gracula religiosa)*, adult.

In the lumen of the proventriculus and ventriculus, a large, well-defined, nonhomogeneous shadow is visible. This was a foreign body, a piece of foam rubber, that was removed orally with a forceps. An old fracture of the spine is also present.

148 Foreign Body.

Hill-Mynah *(Gracula religiosa)*, 4 years.

In the caudal celom, a foreign body is present. This was a golden necklace in the ventriculus.

Note: Hill-mynahs pick up all kinds of glittery objects and are often presented on the suspicion of having swallowed foreign bodies.

149

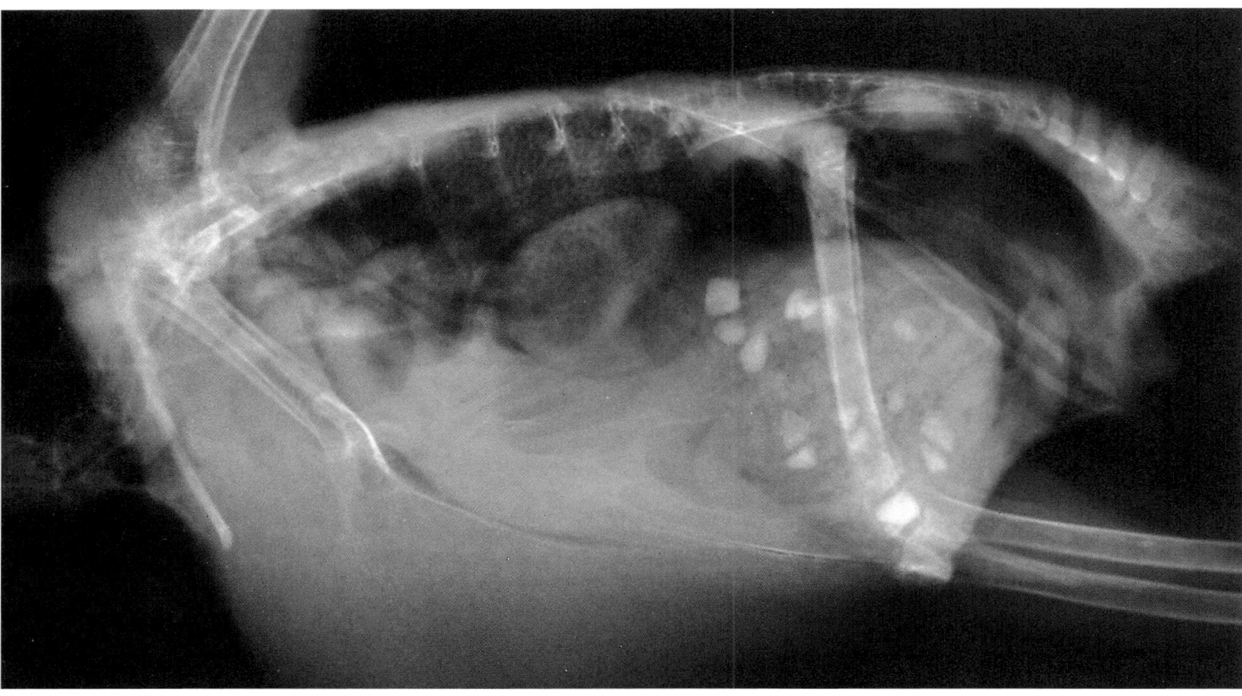

150

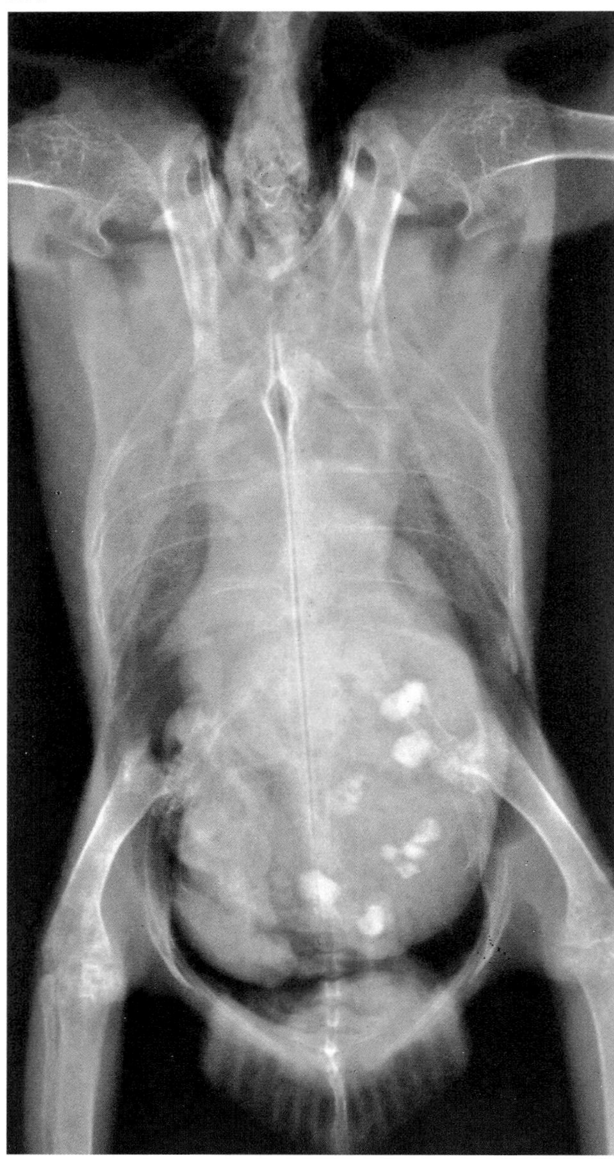

149/150 Normal Radiographic Appearance, lateral and ventrodorsal.

Domestic Pigeon *(Columba livia f. domestica)*, adult.

The trachea, lungs and bronchi are comparable with those of other birds. The gastrointestinal tract is usually very voluminous and surrounded by well-inflated air sacs. The clavicular air sacs are also well defined. The heart shadow is difficult to distinguish.

Proventriculus and ventriculus are large and food-filled. Liver, spleen and gonads are difficult to differentiate on these radiographs. The kidneys in the sublumbar area are relatively small.

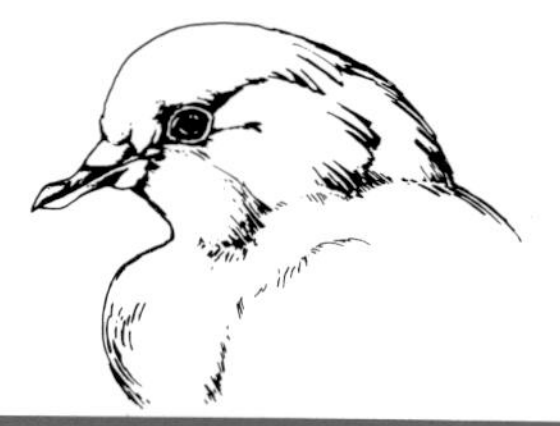

151

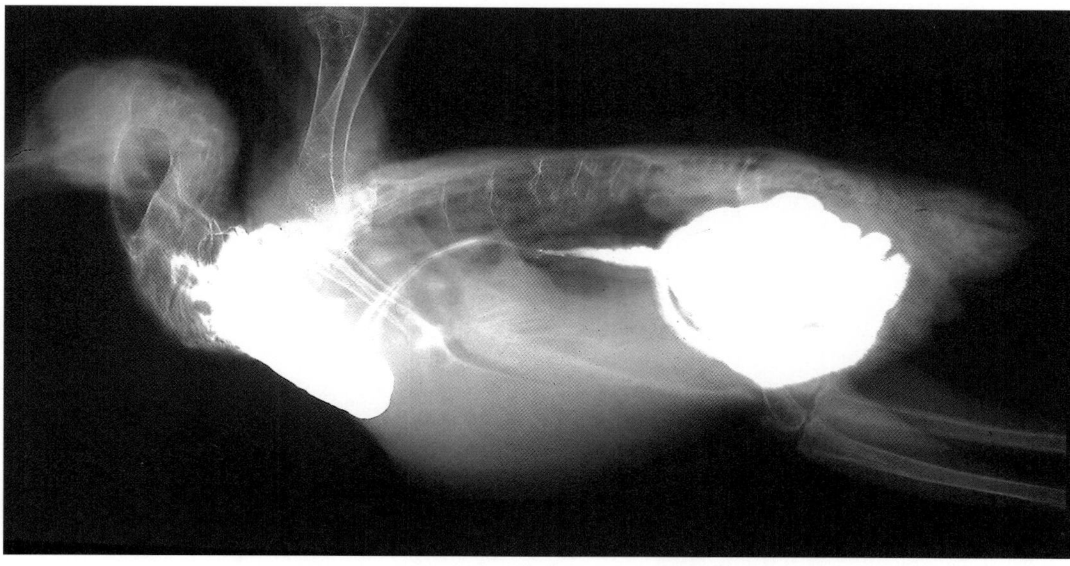

152

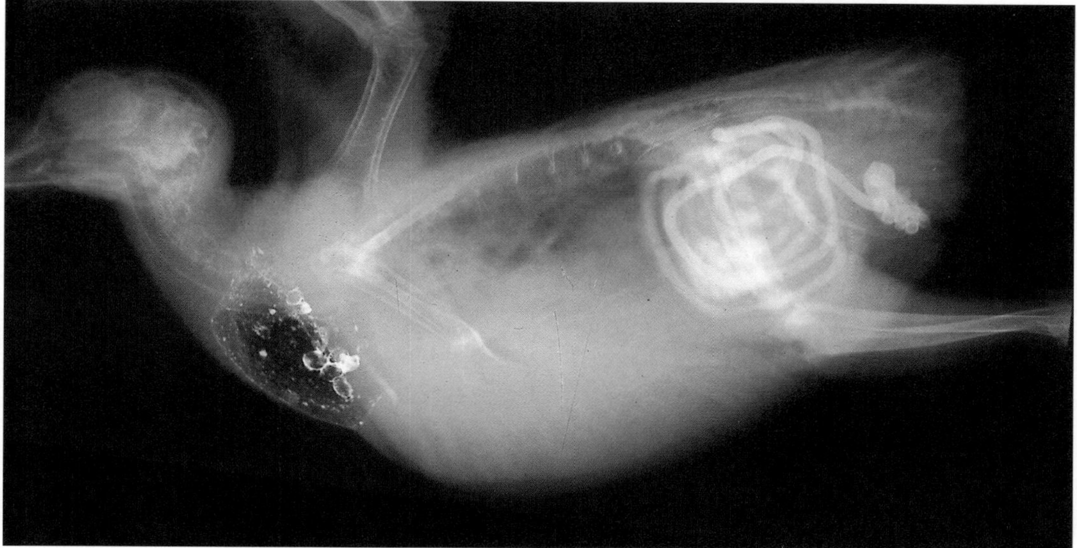

151/152 Normal Radiographic Appearance, lateral: contrast study.

Domestic Pigeon *(Columba livia f. domestica)*, adult.

Two typical pictures of the gastrointestinal passage of barium sulfate are shown. The radiographs were taken 30 and 180 min. after the administration of contrast medium.

153

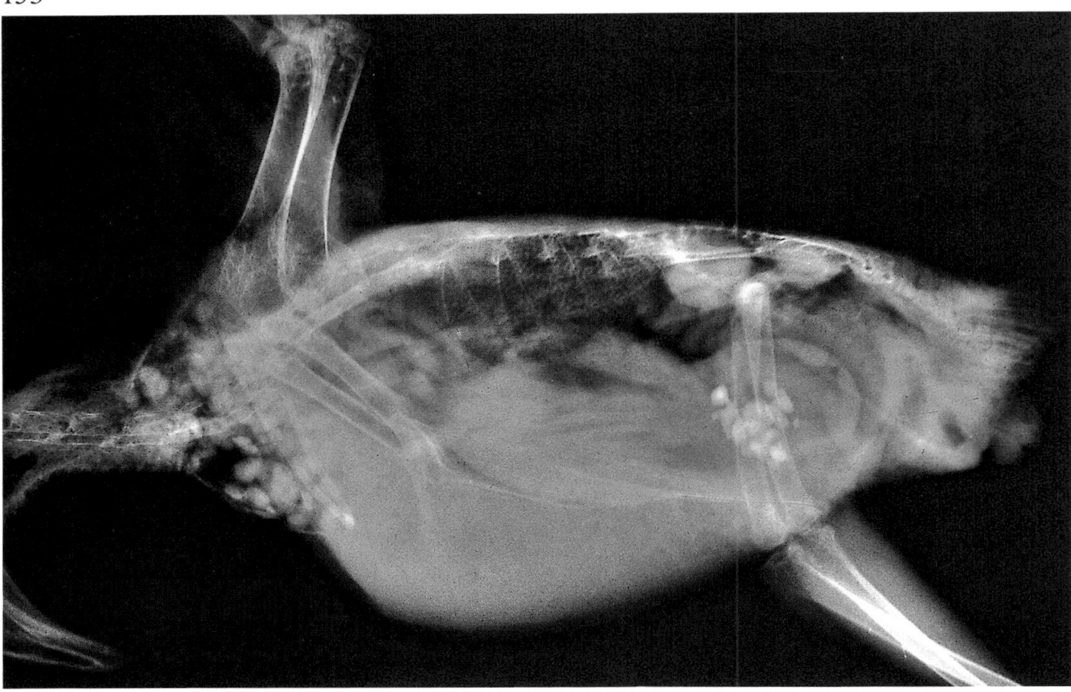

154

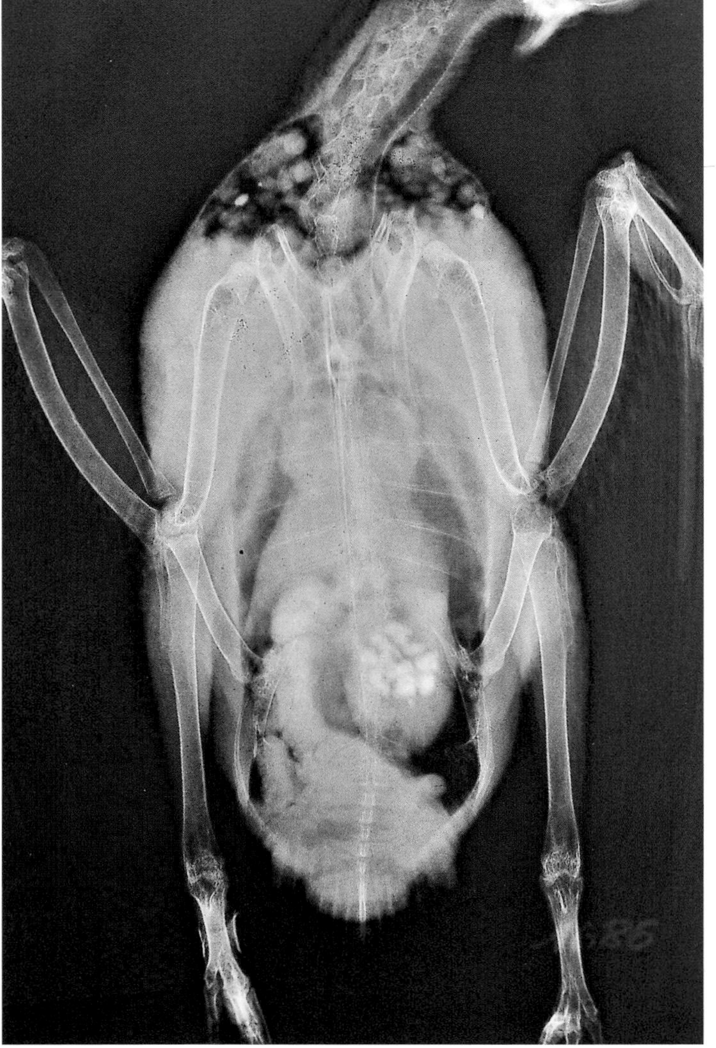

153/154 Air-filled Intestinal Loops.

Pigeon *(Columba livia f. urbana)*, adult.

The crop and gastrointestinal tract are filled with air.

An enlarged kidney can be seen, too. This pigeon ingested a pigeon regulative (a cytostatic drug) that is normally used to reduce pigeon population in towns.

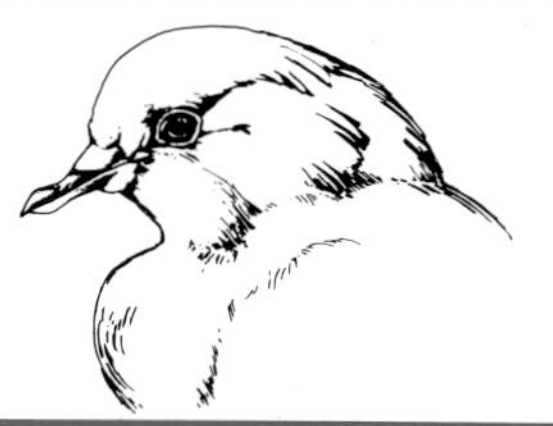

155

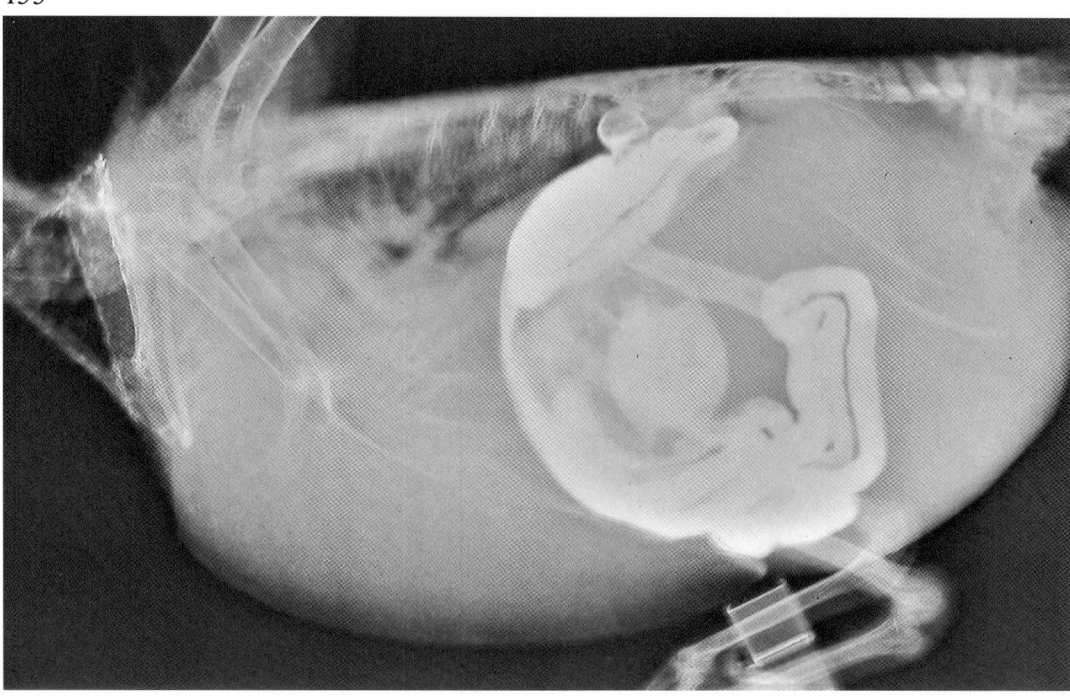

156

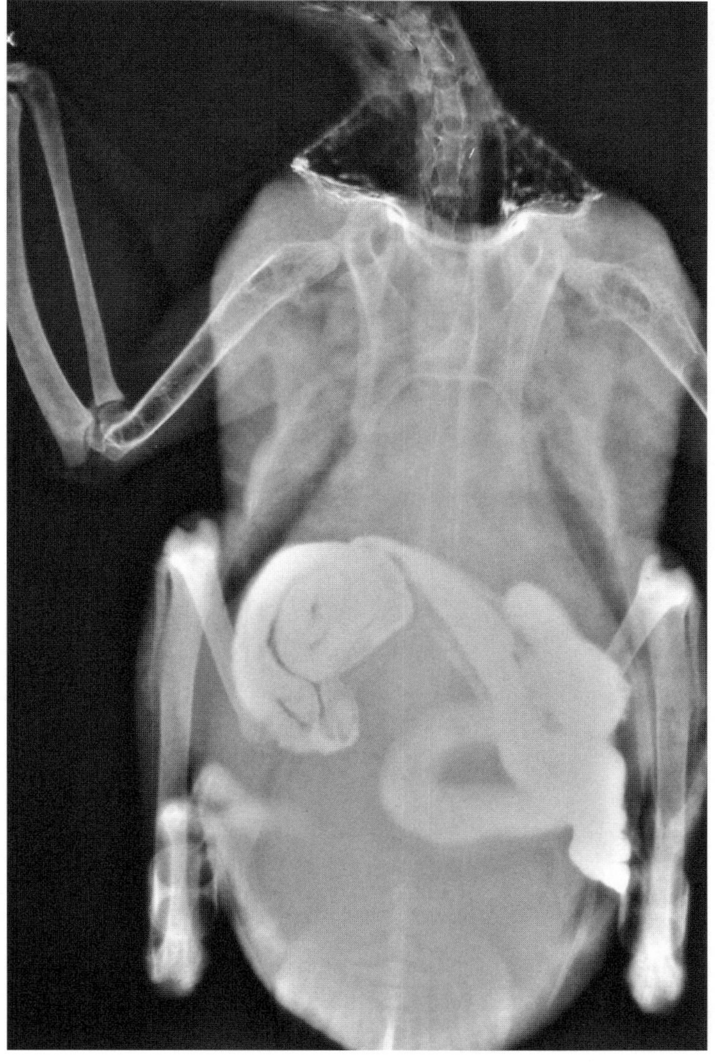

155/156 Leukosis, contrast study.

Domestic Pigeon *(Columba livia f. domestica)*, adult.

The celomic cavity is opacified by a generalized soft tissue density that prohibits organ definition. The gastrointestinal tract is dislocated cranially. Even with the use of a contrast medium, the liver, spleen and kidneys cannot be distinguished.

The liver, spleen, kidneys and gonads all showed neoplastic changes due to generalized leukosis and filled the celom.

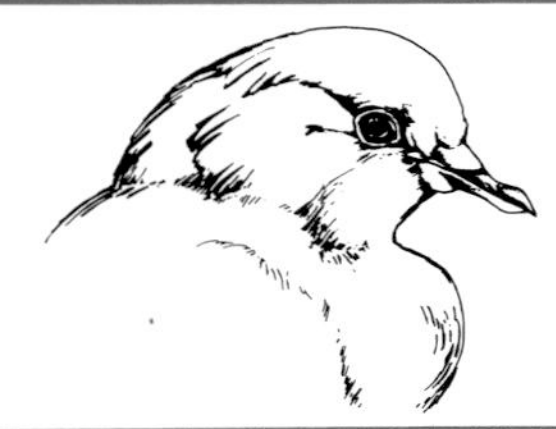

157

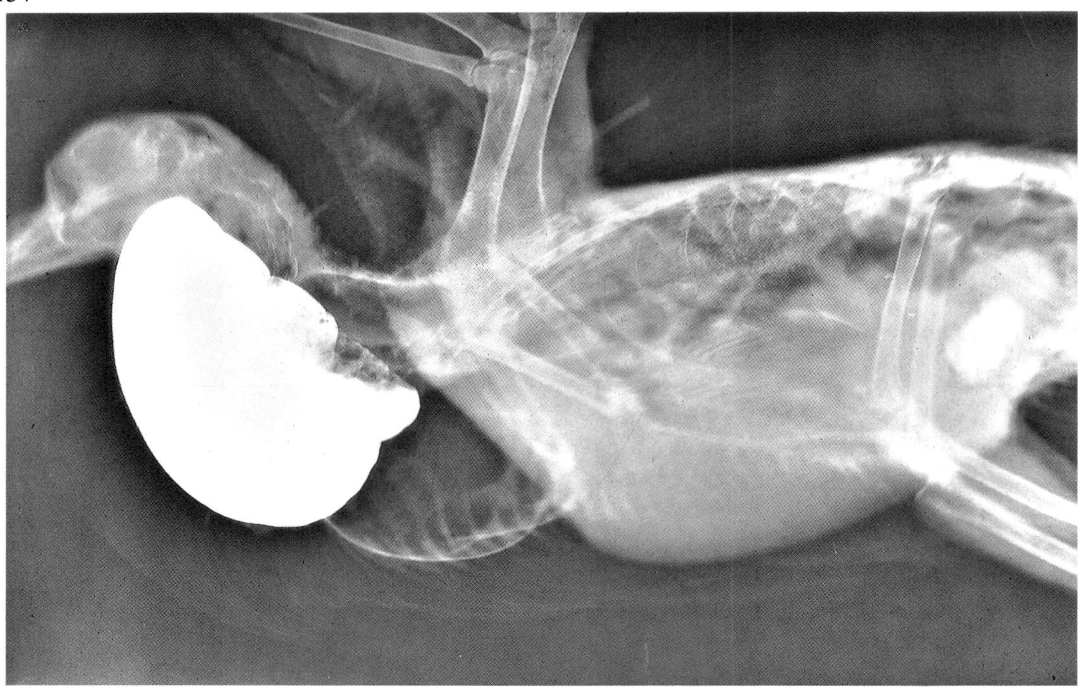

158

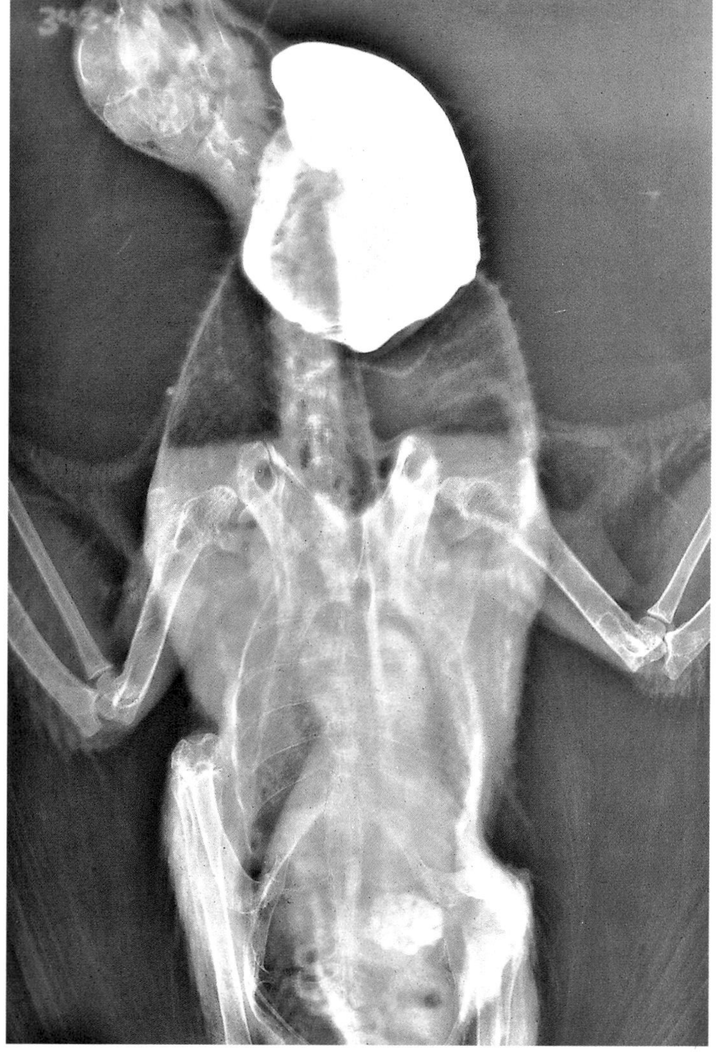

157/158 Abscess in the Crop Mucosa, contrast study.

Pigeon *(Columba livia f. domestica)*, adult.

Despite good filling of the crop with the contrast medium, there is no passage of barium sulfate into the distal esophagus. The crop seems to be dilated and inactive. These findings suggest paralysis of the crop. Postmortem examination revealed a trichomonad abscess in the wall of the crop. The abscess was not visible on the radiographs.

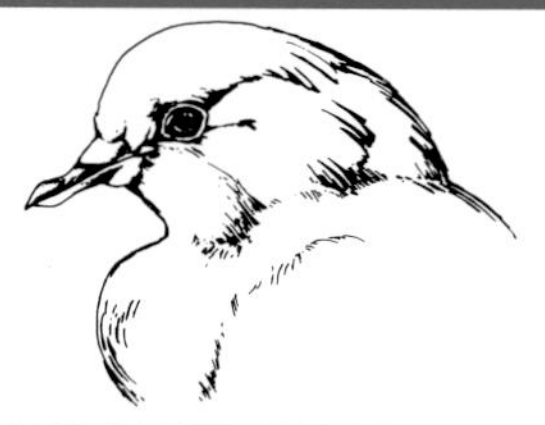

159

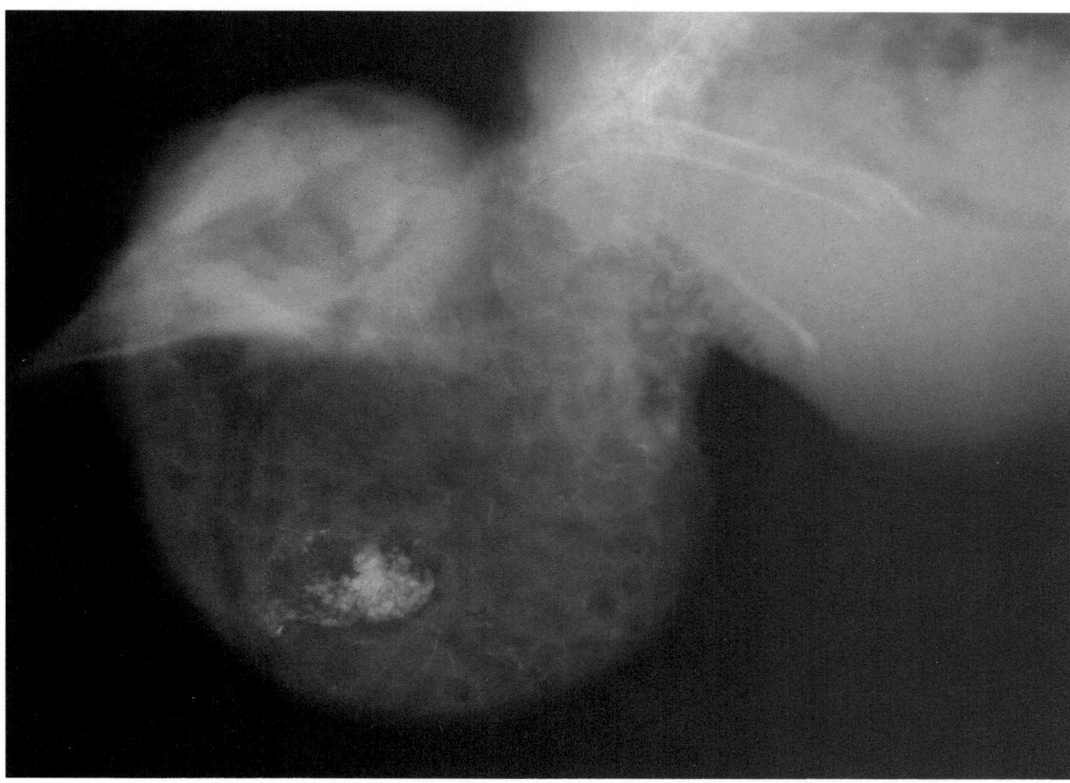

159 Abscess and Ulceration of the Crop Mucosa, contrast study.

Pigeon *(Columba livia f. domestica)*, adult.

Remnants of contrast medium are present in the crop that is filled with food. The residual barium has a focal location and seems to adhere to the wall.

Postmortem examination revealed a cherry-sized trichomonad abscess with ulcerations in the wall of the crop.

160

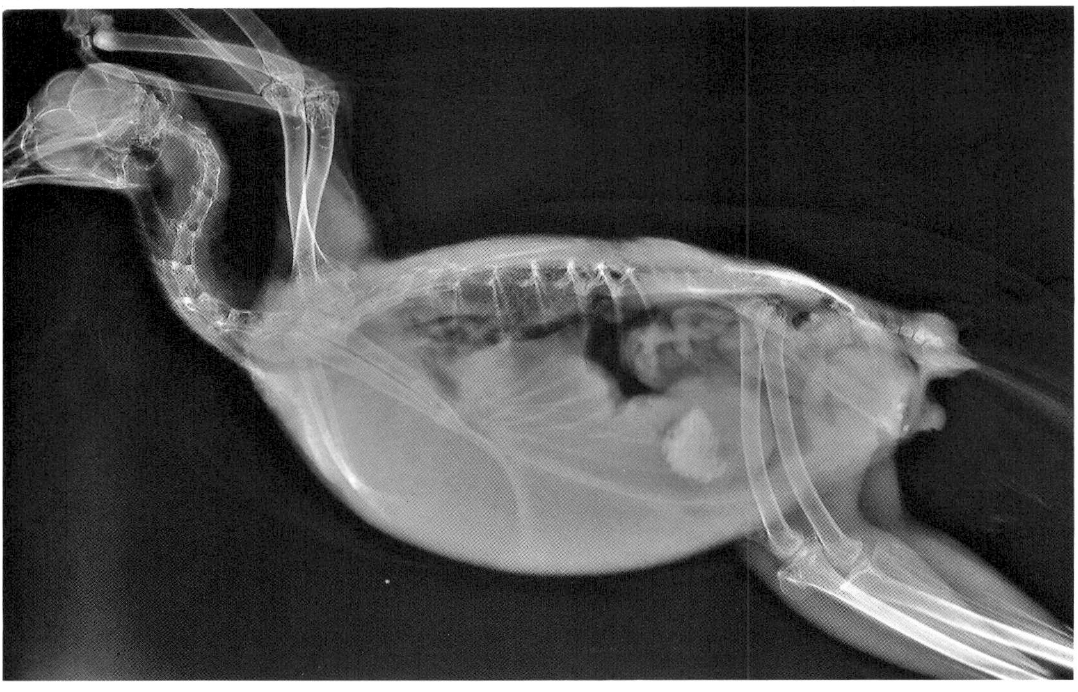

161

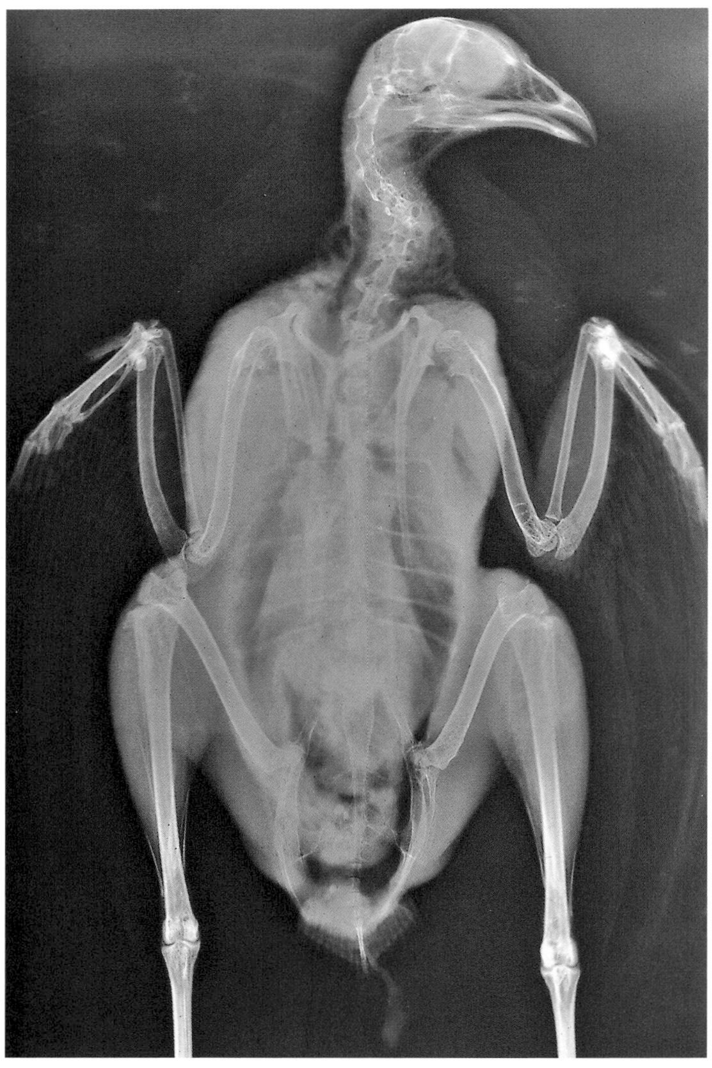

160/161 Normal Radiographic Appearance, lateral and ventrodorsal.

Partridge *(Perdix perdix)*, adult.

The far caudal extension of the sternum and the scapulae is typical for Phasianidae.

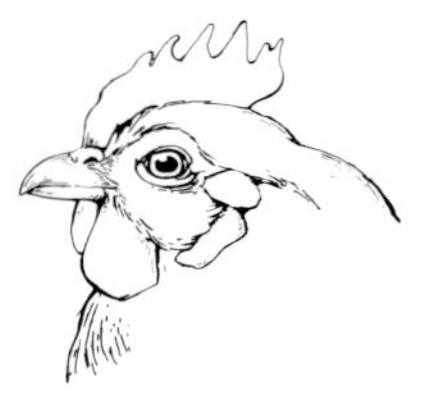

162

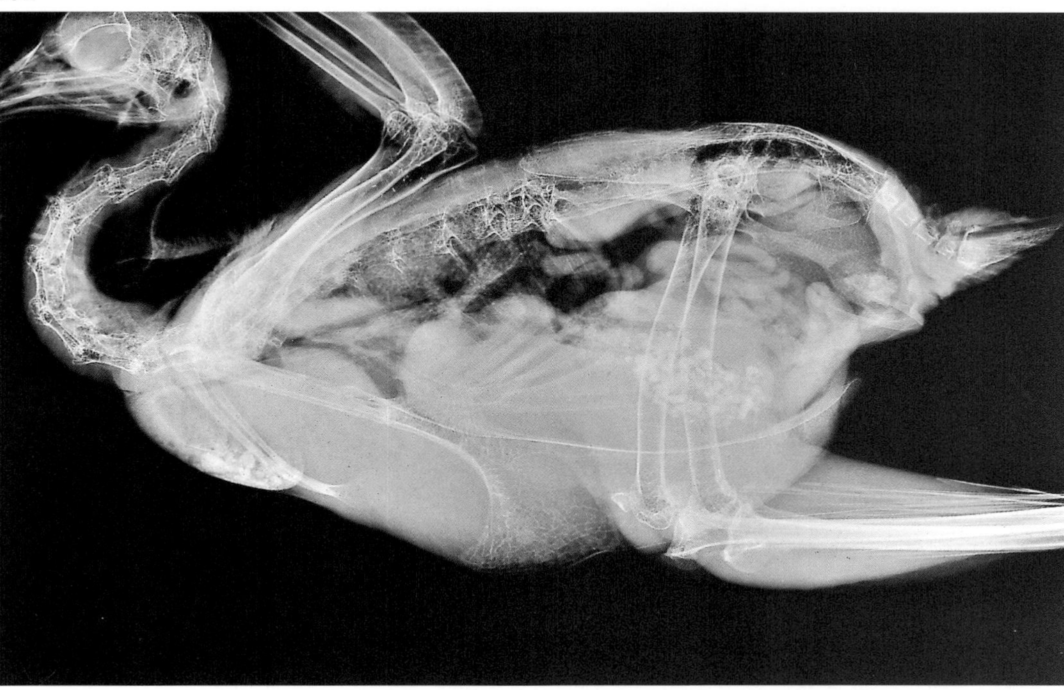

163

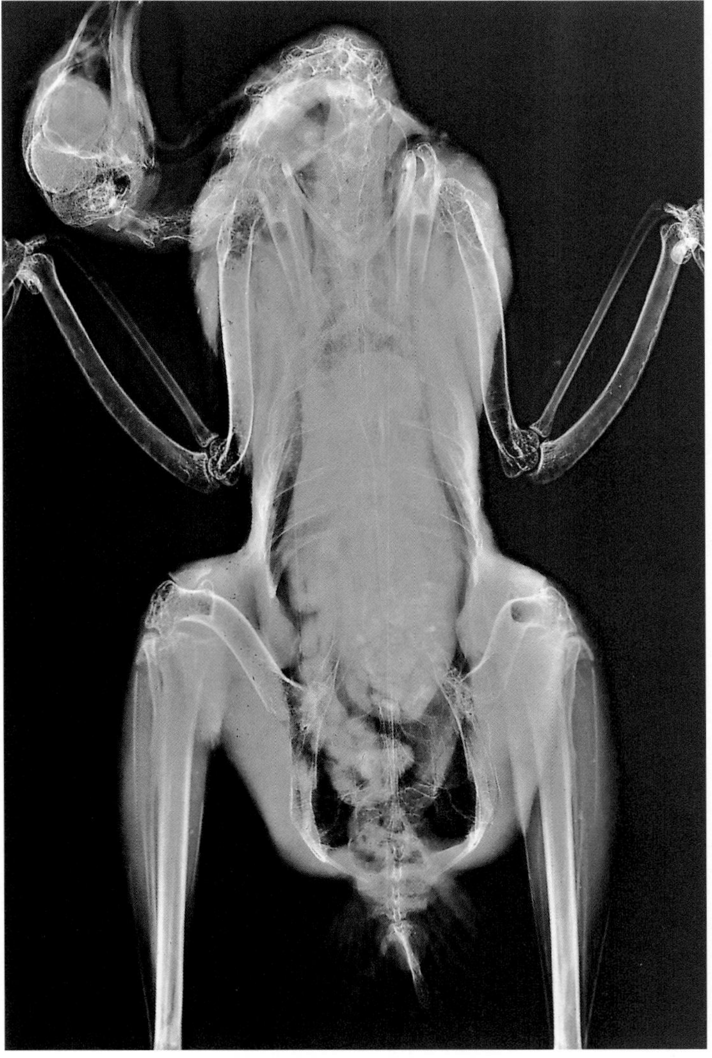

162/163 Mycotic Infection.

Sclater's Monal *(Lophophorus slateri)*, adult.

The soft tissue densities in the lung and air sacs are caused by mycotic granulomas.

Note: With the exception of the lungs and air sacs, this radiograph illustrates the normal radiographic anatomy of a fasan.

164

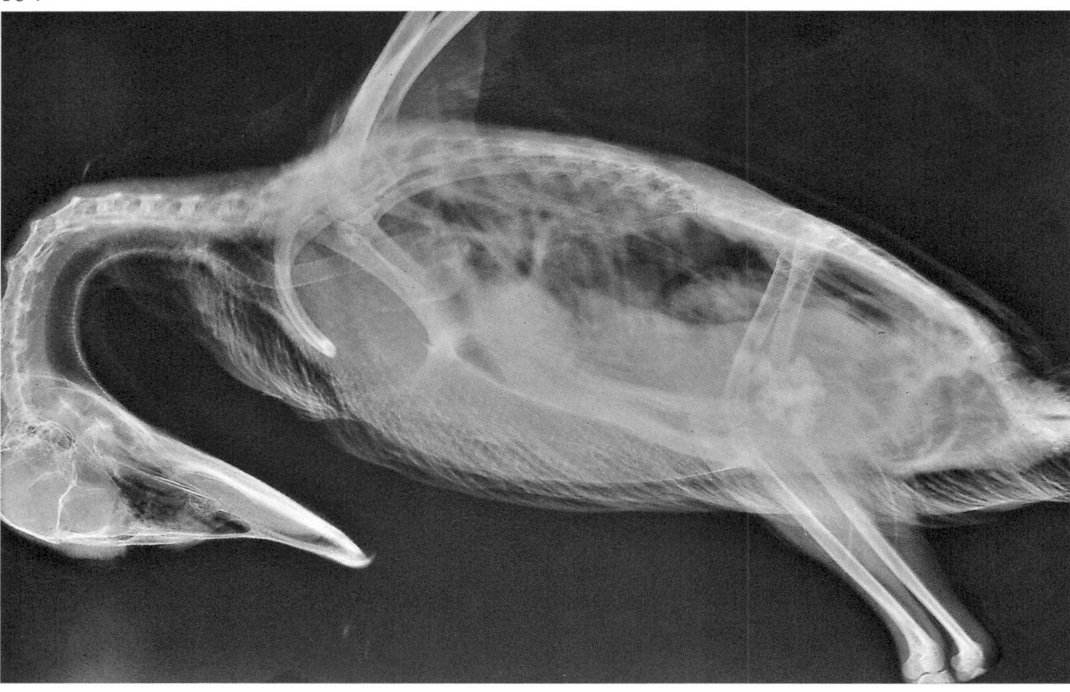

165

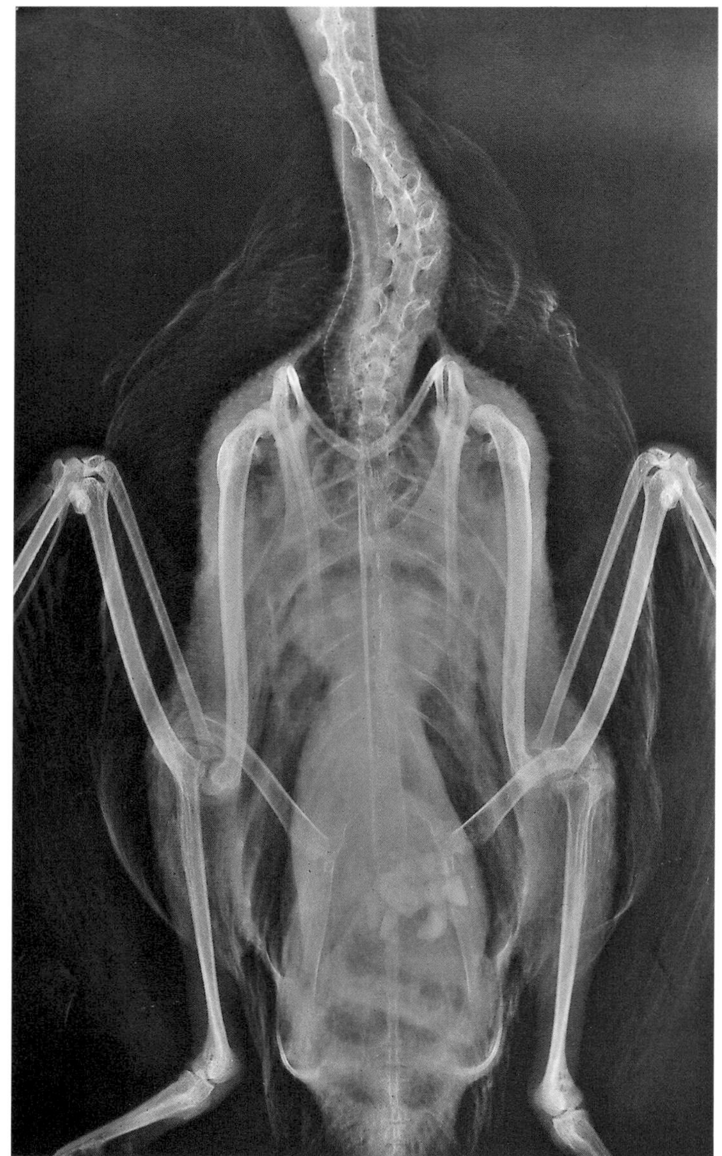

164/165 Normal Radiographic Appearance, lateral and ventrodorsal.

Tufted duck *(Aythya fuligula)*, adult, male.

Notice the bulla at the caudal end of the trachea, typical for male ducks.

The other anatomical structures are comparable with other birds.

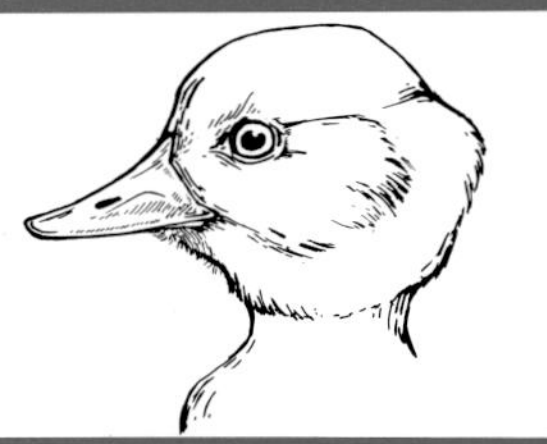

166

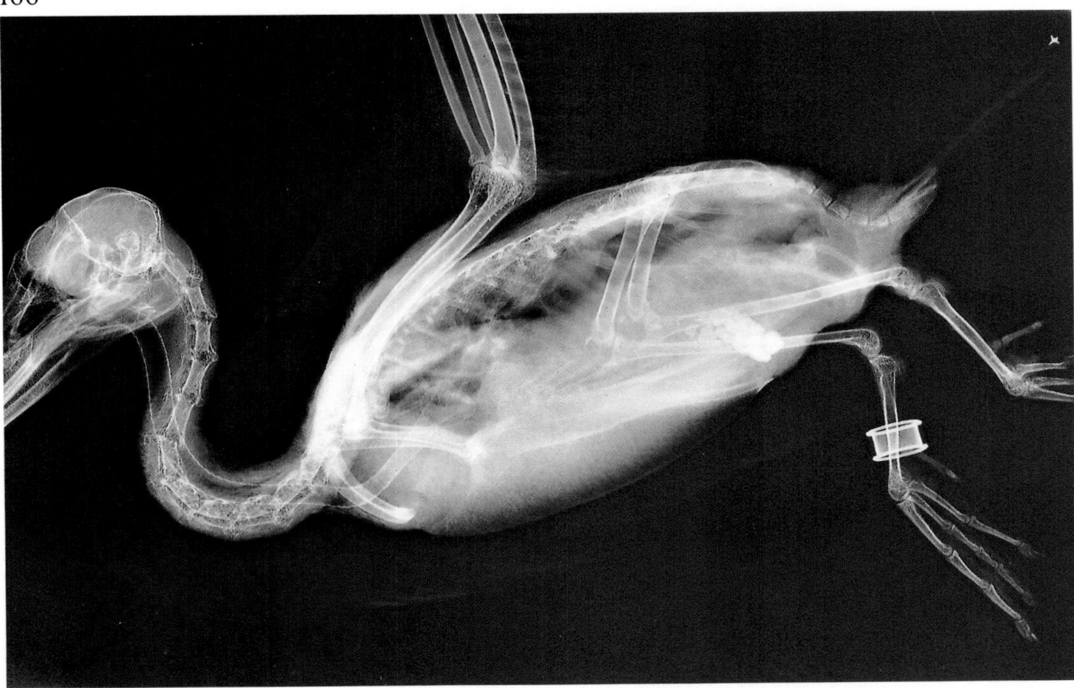

167

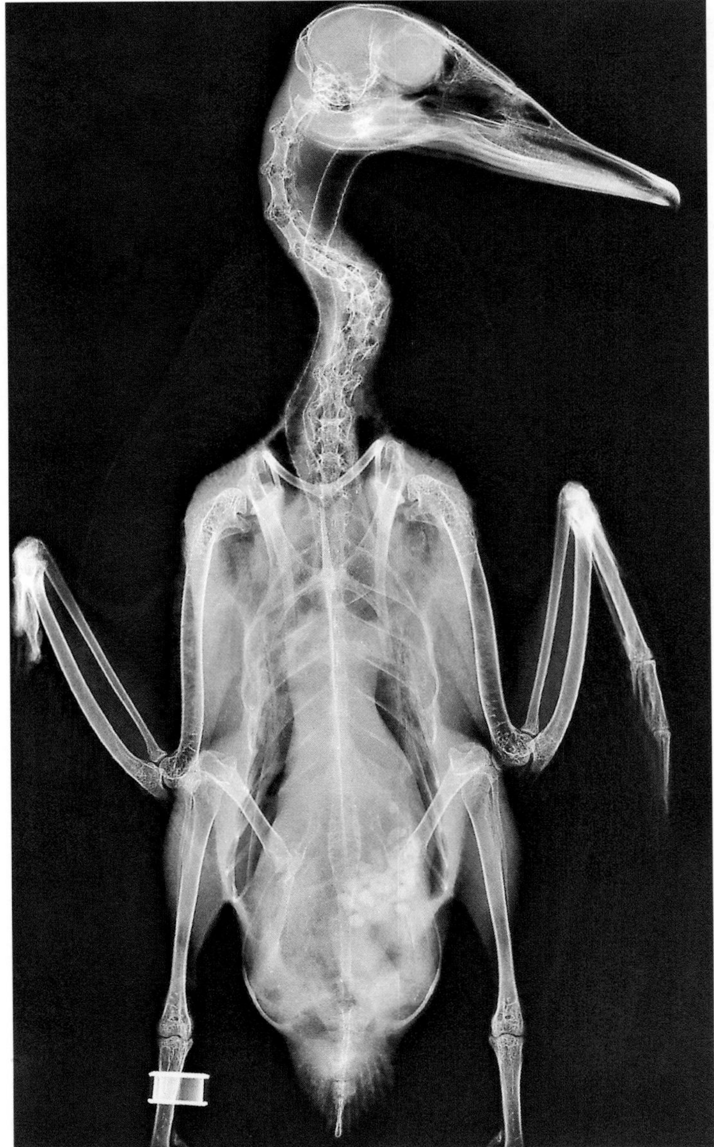

166/167 Normal Radiographic Appearance, lateral and ventrodorsal.

Ringed teal *(Callonetta leucophrys)*, adult, male.

As in the tufted duck, the male shows the typical bulla.

168

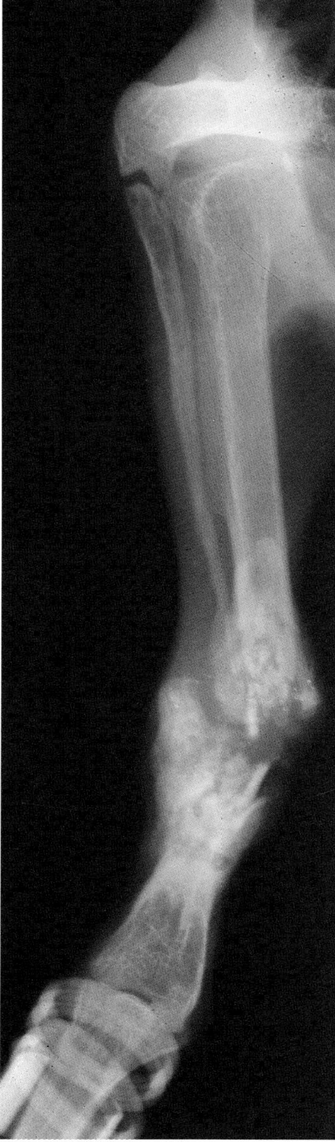

169

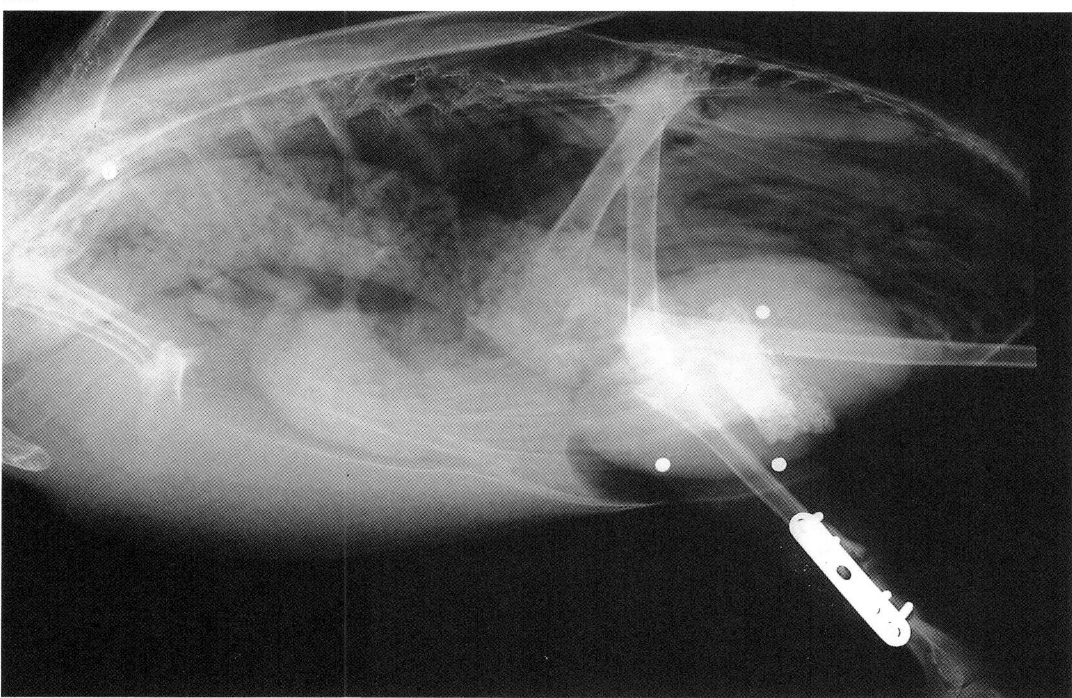

168/169 Bullet Injury and Osteosynthesis.

Greylag Goose *(Anser anser)*, adult.

The distal tibiotarsus has been crushed by a high-velocity bullet. Fine lead dust is present at the fracture site. Additionally, a lead pellet can be recognized in the area of the stifle joint.

FIG. **169** shows the tibiotarsus after osteosynthesis with a bone plate.

Note: The grain-filled caudal esophagus is a typical finding after starvation.

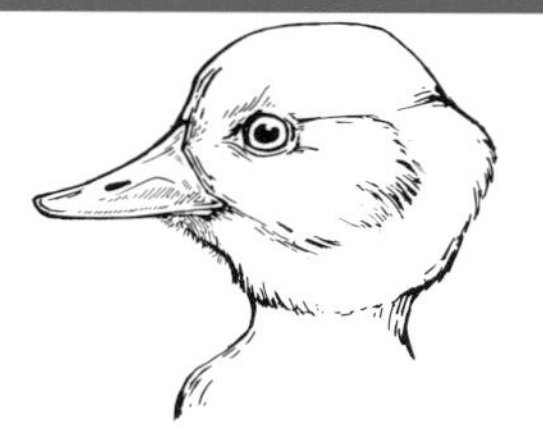

170

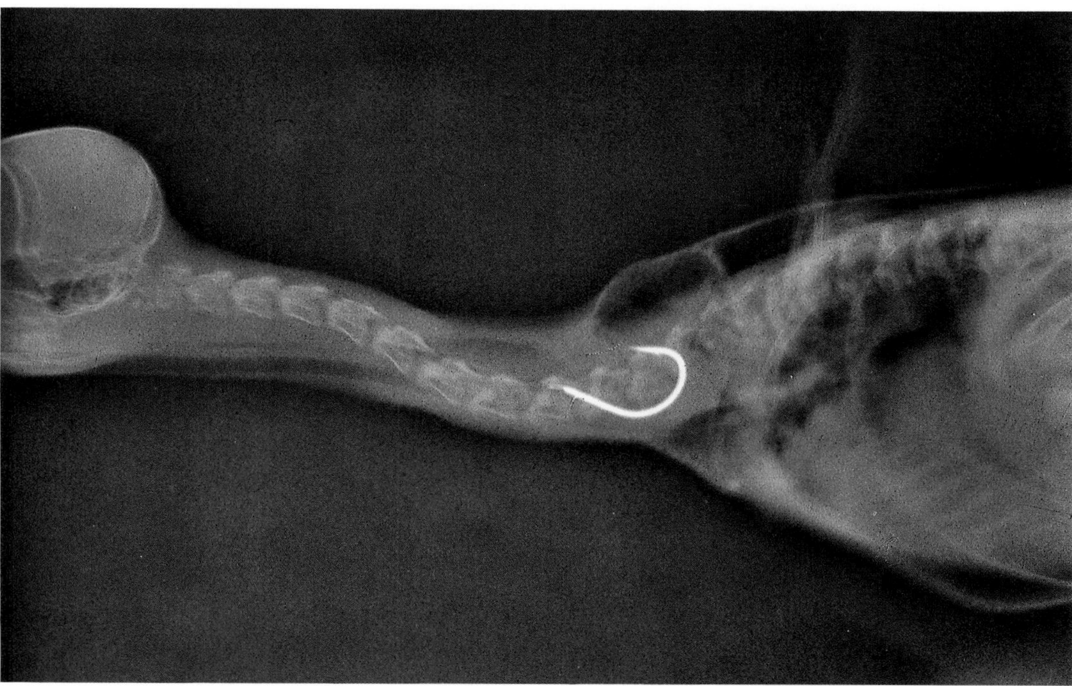

171

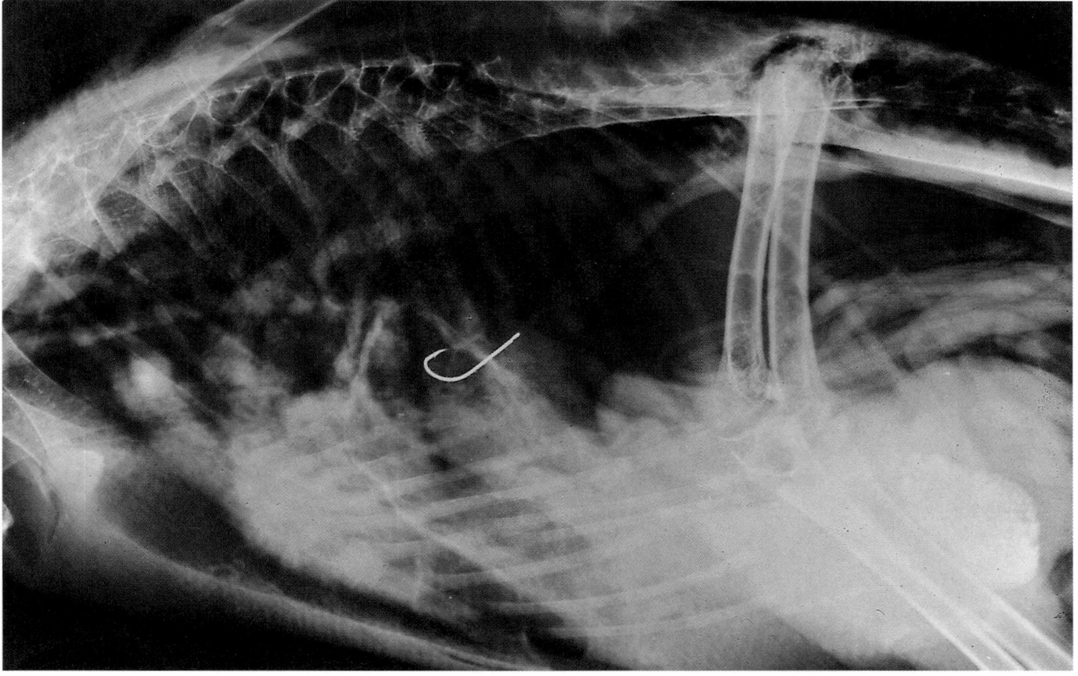

170 Fish-hook.

Mallard *(Anas platyrhynchos)*, juvenile.

There is a fish-hook in the area of the crop, probably stuck in the wall of the crop.

171 Fish-hook.

Mute swan *(Cygnus olor)*, adult.

A fish-hook is present in the distal esophagus.

172

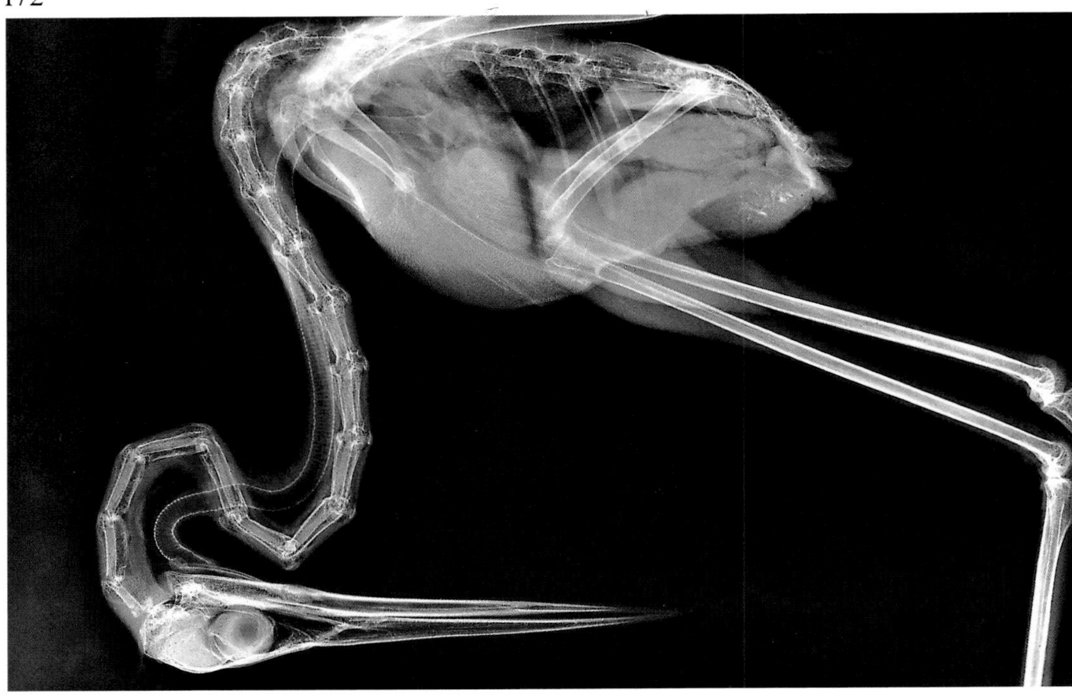

173

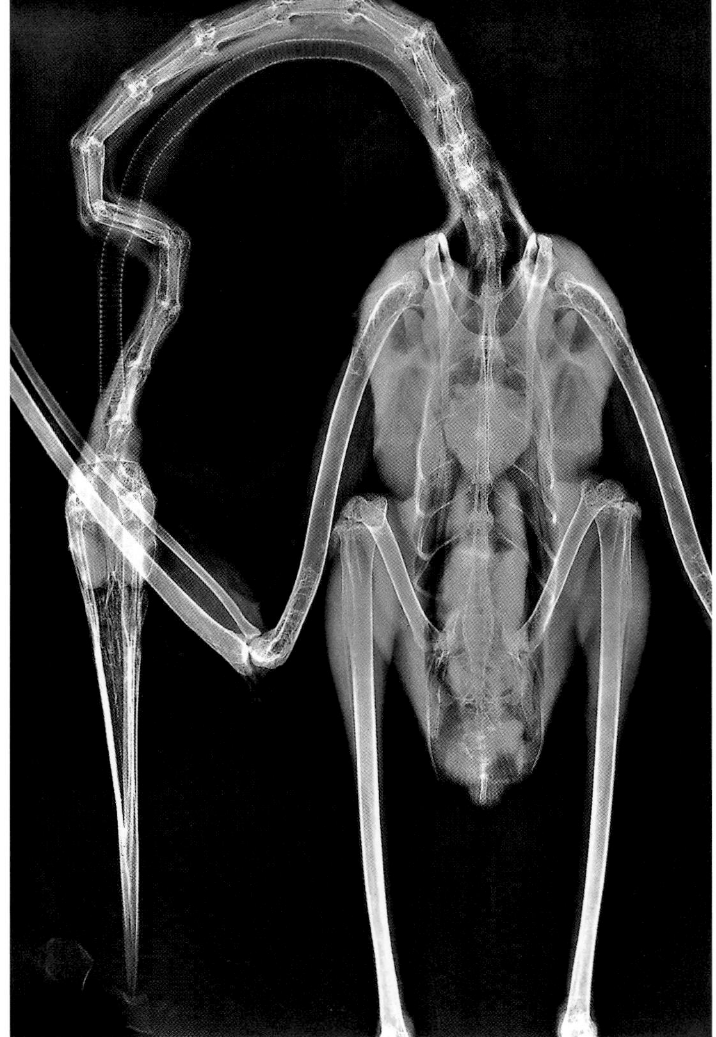

172/173 Trachea: Normal Radiographic Appearance, lateral and ventrodorsal.

Little Egret *(Egretta garzetta)*, adult.

The trachea and its unusual course to the syrinx is well outlined.

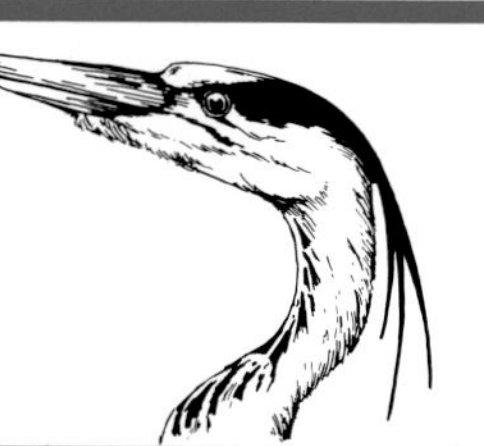

174

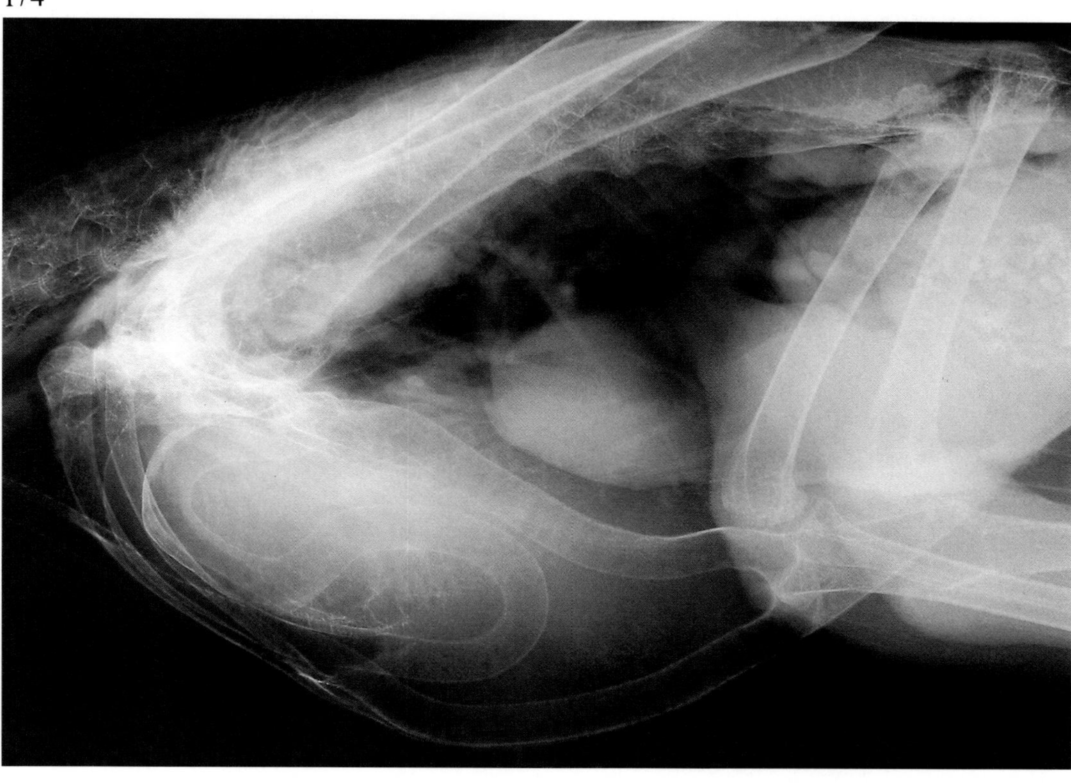

174 A

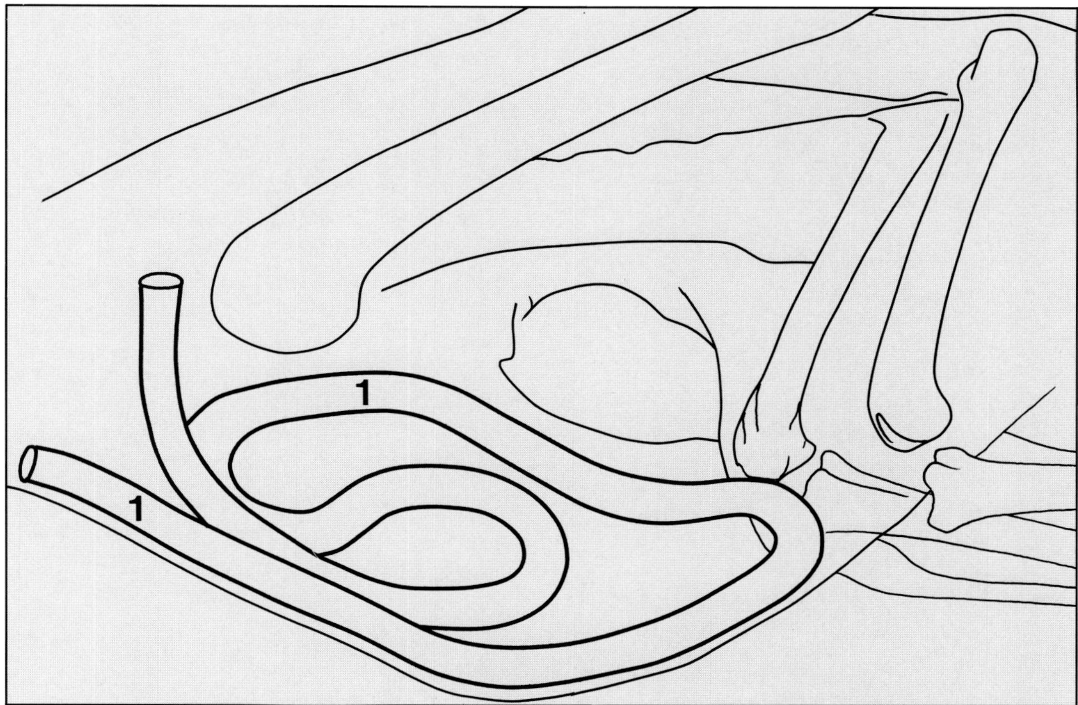

174/174A Course of the Trachea:
Normal Radiographic Appearance, lateral.

Crane *(Grus grus)*, adult.

The very long trachea (**1**) has a folded appearance. A schematic drawing is included.

175

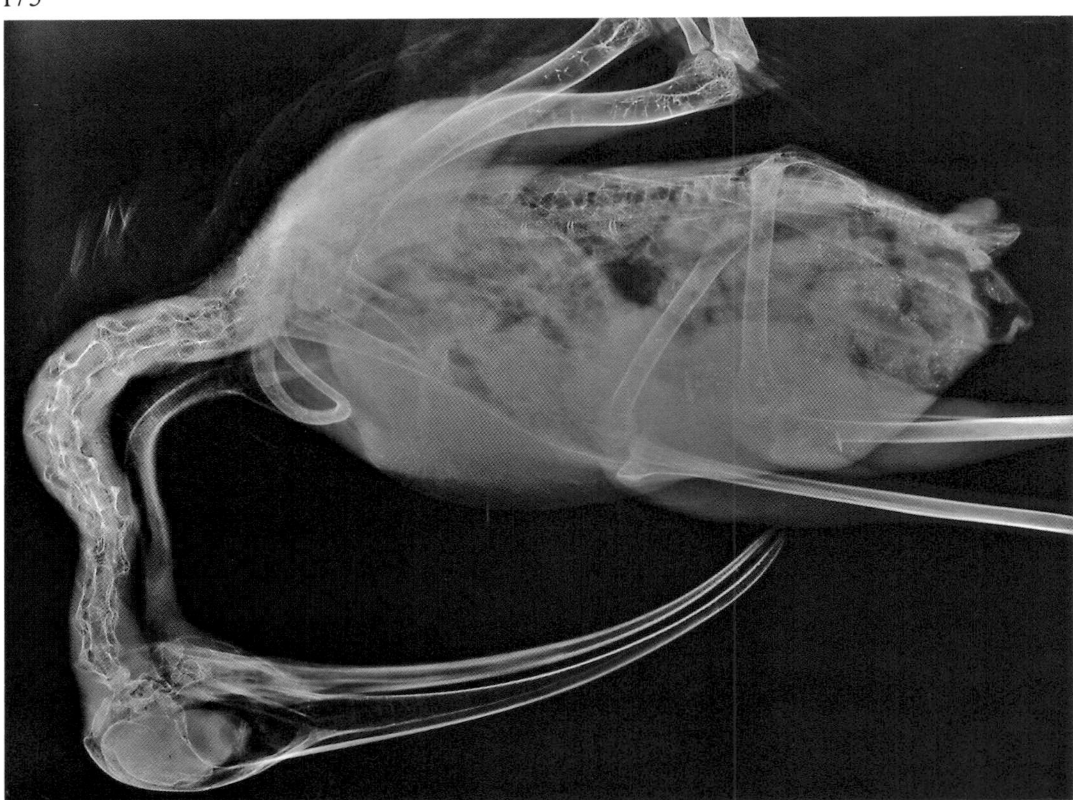

176

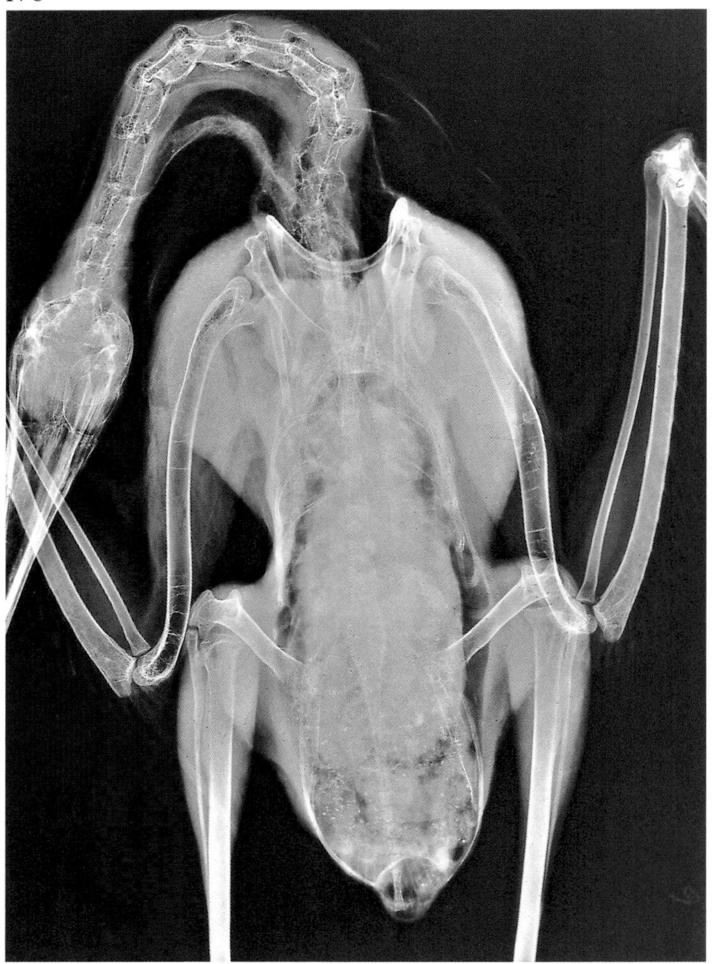

175/176 Visceral Gout.

Indian black-necked ibis *(Threskiornis melanocephalus),* adult.

The internal organs appear abnormally radiodense due to the presence of urate deposits on the serosal surfaces. In addition to the visceral gout, the trachea is partially filled with exudate.

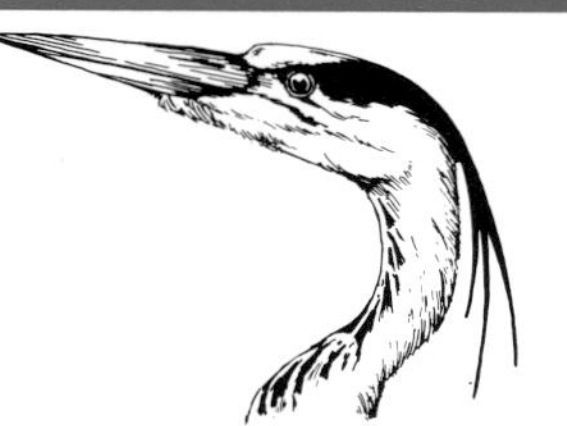

177

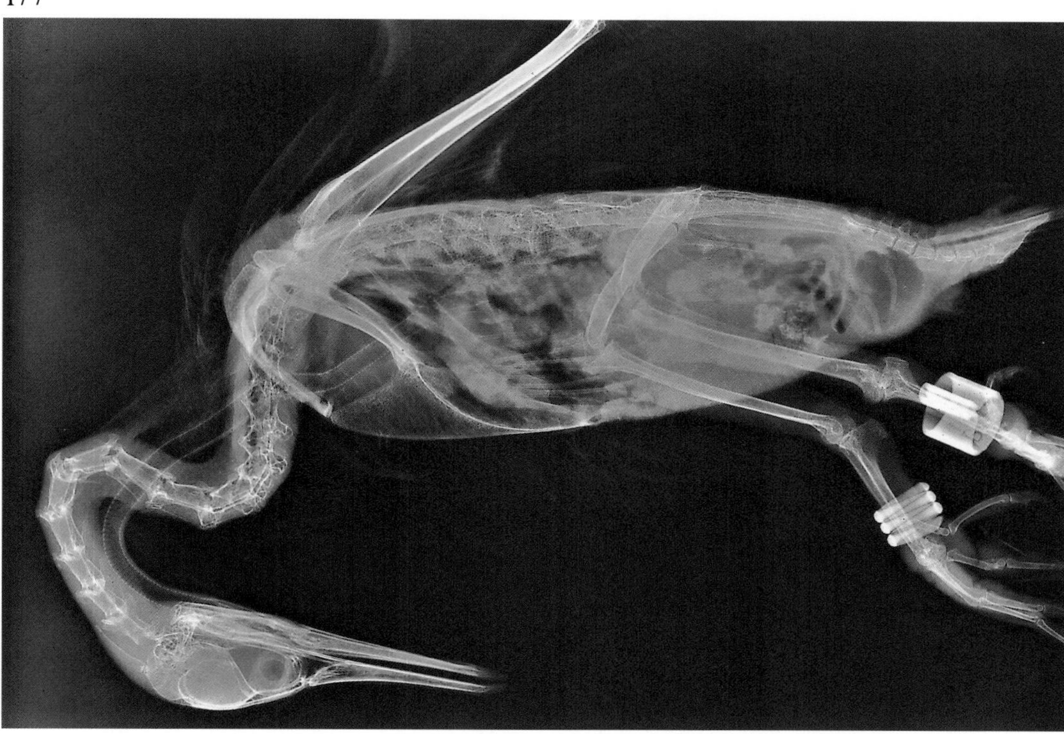

178

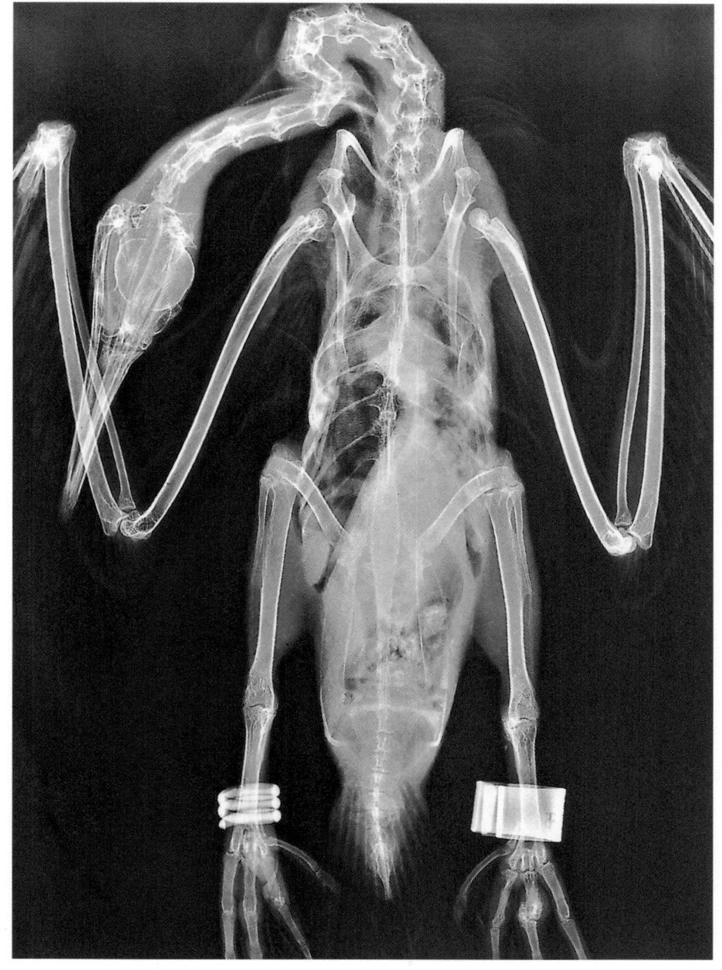

177/178 Aspergillosis.

Pygmy cormorant *(Microcarbo pygmeus)*, adult.

In the pygmy cormorant, the strongly developed shoulder girdle keeps a relatively small sternum in place.

The densities in the lungs and left thoracic air sacs were due to fungal granulomas *(Aspergillus sp.)*.

Contents

Reptiles and Amphibians

Radiographic Technique:
Tortoises and Turtles 176
Lizards 178
Snakes 178
Amphibians 179

Tortoises and Turtles:
Radiographic Anatomy
Internal Organs and Skeleton 180
Contrast Radiography of the Alimentary Tract 184
Radiographic Abnormalities
Skeleton 188
Lungs 190
Gastrointestinal Tract 191
Urogenital Tract 194

Lizards:
Radiographic Anatomy
Internal Organs and Skeleton 196
Contrast Radiography of the Alimentary Tract 199
Radiographic Abnormalities
Skeleton 200
Gastrointestinal Tract 204
Urogenital Tract 206
Miscellaneous 208

Snakes:
Radiographic Anatomy
Internal Organs and Skeleton 210
Contrast Radiography of the Alimentary Tract 213
Radiographic Abnormalities
Skeleton 216
Gastrointestinal Tract 218
Urogenital Tract 220

Amphibians:
Radiographic Anatomy 222
Radiographic Abnormalities 224

A

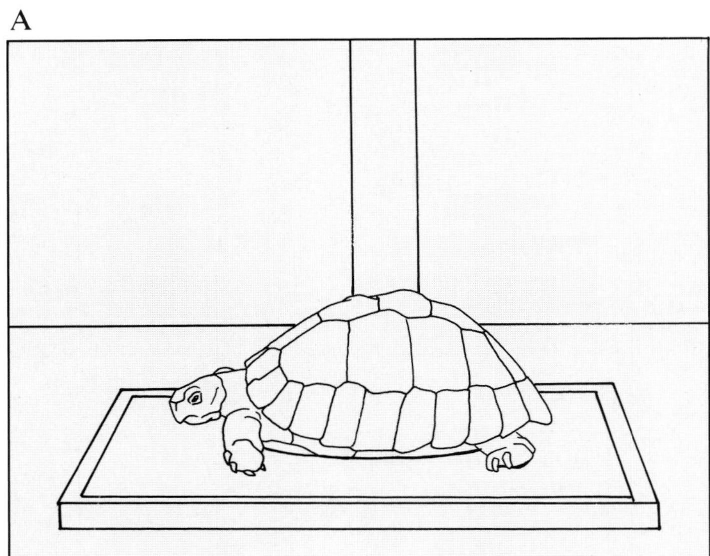

B

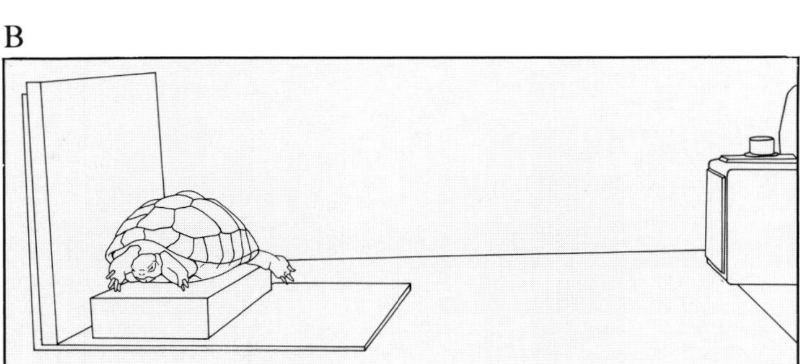

C

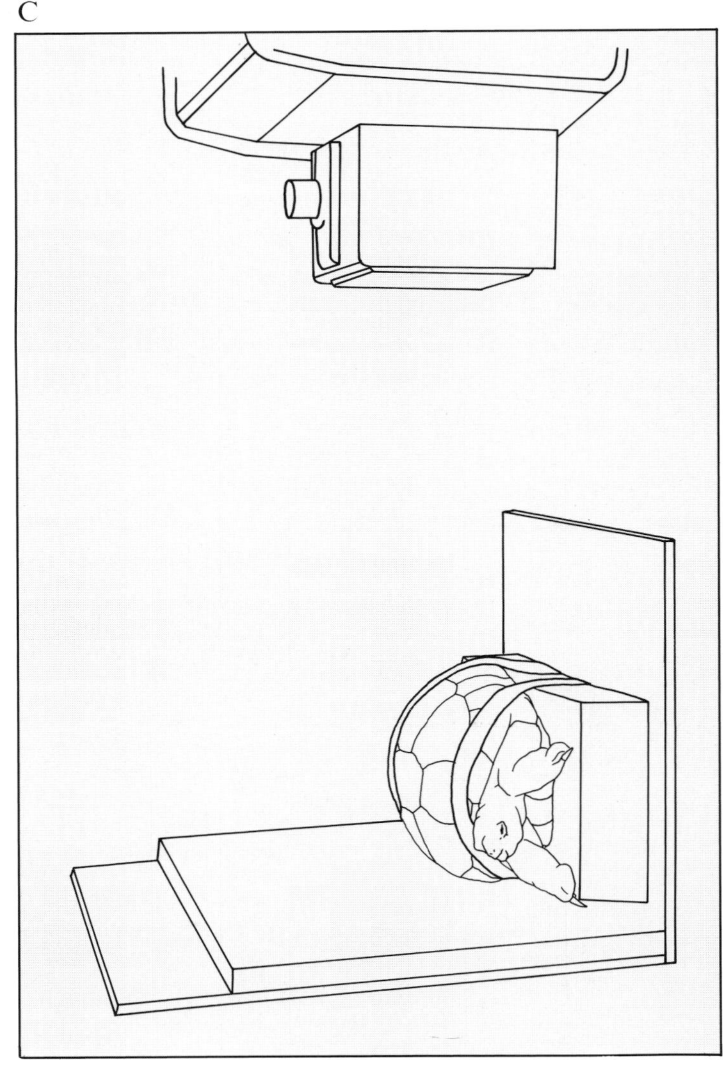

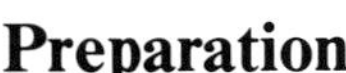

Preparation

Due to their special anatomy radiographic examination of chelonians is difficult. The shell of the chelonians complicates radiographic examination of the celomic organs. It is possible, however, to partially avoid this difficulty by special positioning of the tortoise.

Under normal circumstances, the chelonians are calm and slow. Most of the time, it is possible to examine these animals radiographically without sedation. In order to prepare the chelonian for radiography, it is turned onto its back. Just before the radiograph is made, the animal should be turned back into normal position. The chelonian needs a short period for reorientation. The head and the limbs extend from underneath the shell. This is the moment to make the radiograph. Sometimes it is possible to restrain a restless tortoise is by using adhesive tape or to put the animal into a plastic or paper box so that its motion is reduced. It is important to remember that some tortoises may bite. If it is necessary to sedate the animal, this can be done using ketamine hydrochloride. The dosage is 25-80 mg/kg bw.

Positioning

The radiographic investigation is performed in three projections: dorsoventral, laterolateral and craniocaudal.

a. dorsoventral (FIG. **A**)

Vertical X-ray beam with tortoise in prone position. The tortoise is laid down on the radiographic cassette. To determine the appropriate exposure data, the diameter at the thickest portion of the body (shell) should be measured and the two sides should be marked with letters ("L"/"R").

b. laterolateral

1. Horizontal X-ray beam with tortoise in normal position. The animal is put on top of a sponge. The X-ray beam should be directed parallel to the sponge. The cassette is positioned vertically in close contact with the carapace (FIG. **B**).

2. Vertical X-ray beam with tortoise fixed on its side. If for technical reasons the X-ray tube cannot be turned in horizontal position, the tortoise may be fixed on a rack. The rack (right-side position) should be positioned in such a way that the central X-ray beam penetrates the body laterolaterally. The lower edge of the shell should

D

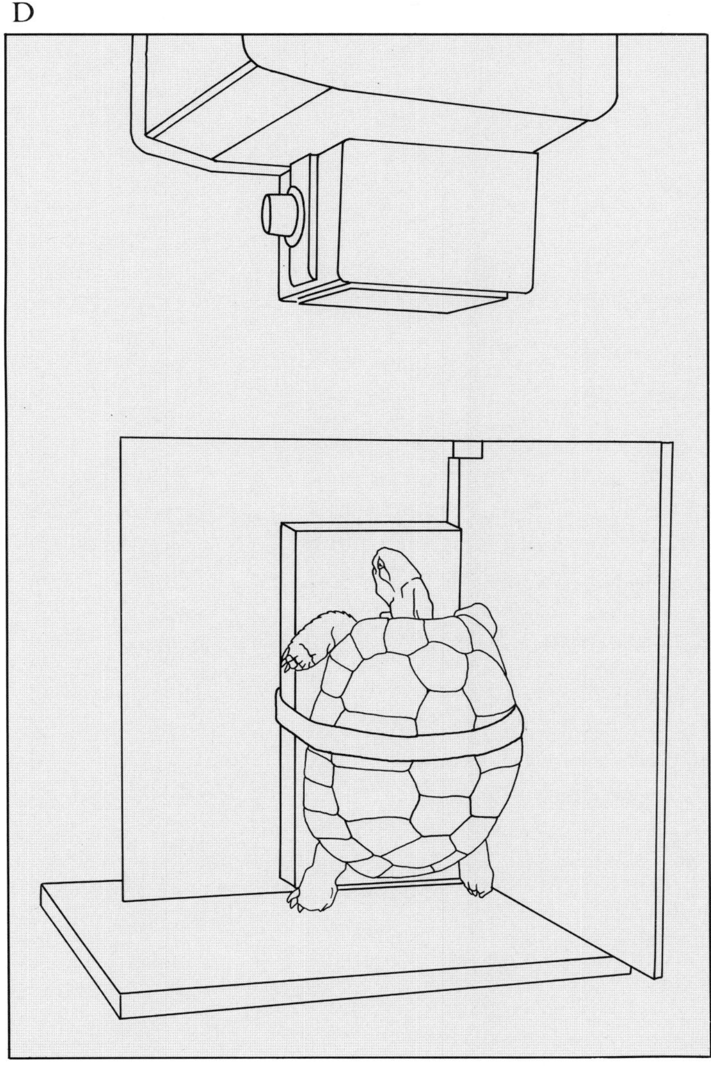

rest on the X-ray cassette (FIG. **C**). The X-ray beam is directed at the centre of the carapace.

c. craniocaudal

1. Horizontal X-ray beam with tortoise in prone position. The animal is immobilized on a radiolucent sponge. The X-rays should pass through the body from head to tail. The cassette should be placed vertically and behind the animal. As soon as the limbs of the animal come out from underneath the shell, the radiograph should be made.

2. Vertical X-ray beam with tortoise fixed upright (FIG. **D**). It is helpful to place the animal on a rack which is positioned vertically and parallel to the X-ray beam. The centre of the beam should be directed at the head. Don't forget to mark the position ("L"/"R"). The length of the body is measured from head to tail.

Radiographic Contrast Studies

The use of barium sulfate is recommended for outlining details of the stomach and intestines of chelonians. The dosage is 20 cc/kg bodyweight. To obtain detailed visualization of the gastric mucosal surface a combination of barium and air can be administered into the stomach using a stomach tube. The double-contrast radiographs obtained by this method may be excellent and can be very helpful in interpretation of gastric abnormalities. Intestinal studies are more difficult, because the passage of barium sulfate in chelonians can be very slow. In tortoises, the passage time may be 24-40 days, in turtles it can be shorter.

Another important point is that the passage time changes with the environmental temperature (poikilothermy), with times of high activities (spring, autumn) and during digestion of food. With gastrointestinal disease the passage time may be very fast (diagnostic criterion).

E

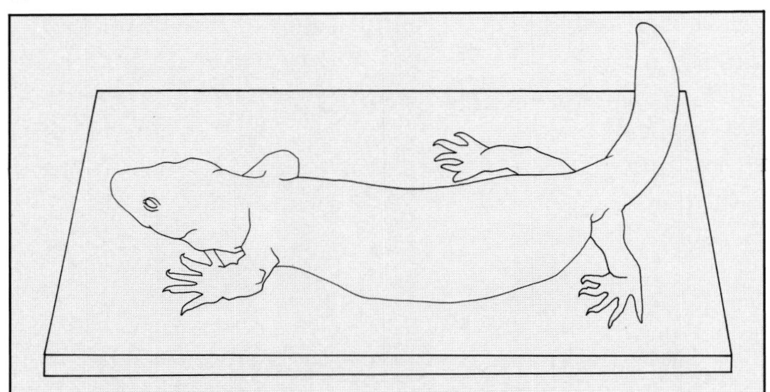

F

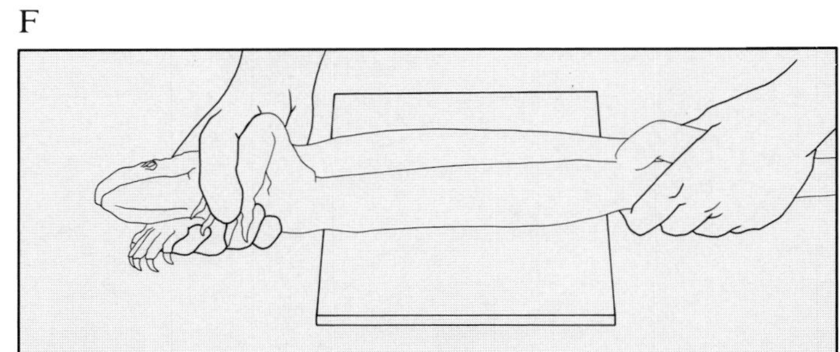

Lizards

Preparation

Radiographic examination of lizards is sometimes difficult because handling of the animals is sometimes difficult. Monitors, geckos, and flat lizards normally have to be sedated while most larger skinks, green iguanas and agamids can be fixed manually.

In this active, restless species, a sedative such as ketamine hydrochloride provides very good results. The dosage is 20-50 mg/kg bodyweight. Sometimes, it is sufficient to cover the animals with both hands and withdraw them just before the exposure is made. Very calm animals can be taped on the X-ray cassette. Removing of the tape should be done carefully in order not to damage the scales. Aggressive lizards and crocodiles should be X-rayed with the snout tied. In some species, the tail has to be fixed too. This should not be done with lizards that are capable of autotomy.

Positioning

For best results, a radiographic examination of lizards must include at least two views, a dorsoventral and a laterolateral view.

a) dorsoventral, vertical X-ray beam with animal in prone position (FIG. **E**)

The animal is placed directly onto the cassette. The body must be stretched and the limbs extended. Don't forget to mark "right" and "left" on the cassette. This position provides a good full-body view and is useful for examination of the skeletal system, the gastrointestinal tract, and the lungs.

b) laterolateral

1. Horizontal X-ray beam with animal in prone position.

The animal can be fixed with tapes. The cassette is placed vertically alongside the animal and parallel to the vertebral column. The X-ray beam is directed horizontally at a perpendicular angle to the vertebral column.

2. Vertical X-ray beam with lizard lying on its side (FIG. **F**).

Many lizard species can be fixed in a lateral position by a firm grip relaxing after a few seconds. When not successful, sedation is necessary. In lateral position, the vertebral column, cardiovascular system, lungs and urogenital system can be evaluated.

Radiographic Contrast Studies

For contrast examination of the gastrointestinal tract, the dosage of barium sulfate is up to 50 ml/kg bodyweight. The passage time in active carnivorous lizards such as monitors is short, being 3 to 6 days. In herbivorous lizards such as the green iguanas with considerable quantities of plant material in the voluminous and partially septated digestive tract, the passage time can be 15 to 30 days. In addition, passage time also depends on temperature and activity (e.g., aestivation, hibernation).

In lizards with a low oral water uptake and long passage time (e.g. larger skinks), the barium sulfate suspension can become dehydrated in the digestive tract and can cause constipation. To avoid this, 5 percent iodinized contrast medium is added to the barium sulfate suspension and sufficient water is administered to the lizards.

Snakes

Preparation

Because of their special anatomy, snakes are difficult to radiograph. Localization of the organs might be a problem. Especially in the lateral position, it is necessary to radiograph snakes segment by segment.

Small non-poisonous snakes can be placed directly upon the cassette. If they are active and try to escape, it is possible to use a plastic box without a bottom and top (FIG. **G**). In very restless and especially in poisonous species, sedation is required. Ketamine hydrochloride, with a dosage of 25-75 mg/kg bodyweight, is used for sedation. Another solution is the use of a X-ray permeable plastic tube. Most snakes will crawl into these tubes immediately. After closing the open ends, the snake can be radiographed lengthwise inside the tube.

Reptiles: Snakes/Amphibians Radiographic Technique

G

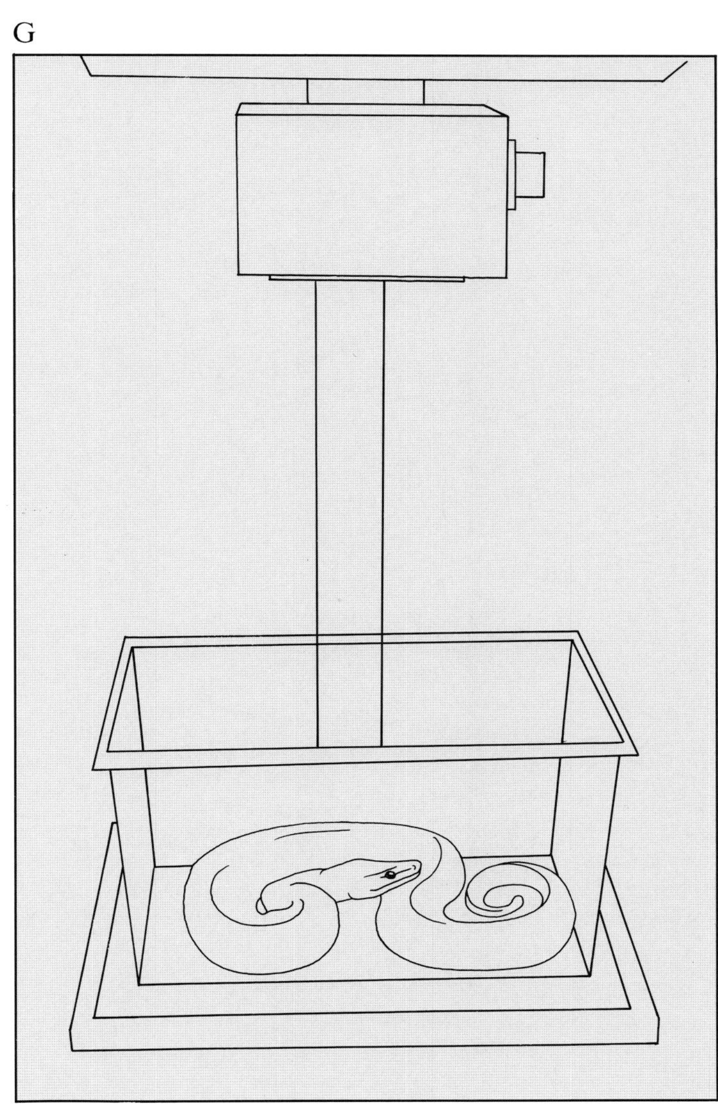

H

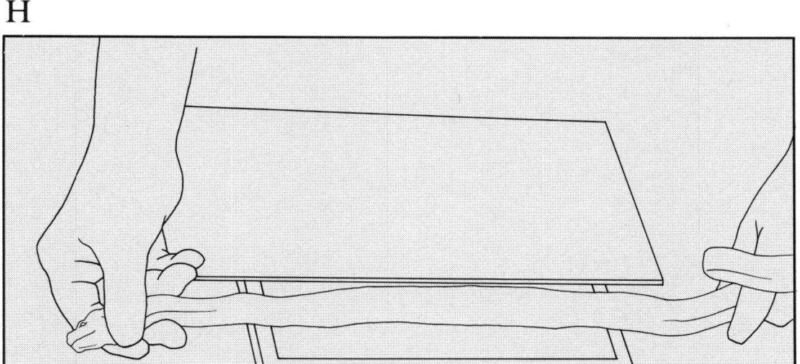

Positioning

a) dorsoventral (FIG. **G**)

The animal is usually left coiled up in a physiological orientation or fixed in an extended position in a plastic tube. In this way, a complete body survey can be made in order to investigate the digestive system. For the lungs, the first two-thirds of the body are radiographed. It is useful to mark "L" and "R", and even use leaded numbers positioned at regular distances along the vertebral column in order to be able to localize changes on the radiograph and arrange the radiographs in the right order.

b) laterolateral (FIG. **H**)

In longer snakes, it is necessary to radiograph the animal in segments, or concentrate upon a certain segment of the body. In most cases, it is possible to fix the animal manually. In animals in plastic tubes, it is necessary to rotate the tube until the snake is positioned on its side.

Radiographic Contrast Studies

To investigate the digestive system a barium sulfate suspension is administered through a stomach tube. The passage can be accelerated if the body is held vertically, head upright, and the belly is massaged gently from neck to cloaca. With this method, it is possible to achieve complete passage of barium sulfate within one hour. Otherwise, the passage time depends on the same circumstances as in other reptiles and might take even longer if a snake refuses to eat.

Localization of Internal Organs

The orientation and localization of anatomical structures and abnormalities on segmental radiographs is difficult. JACKSON and COOPER (1979) published a schedule which allows an easier coordination of radiographs. The computation is performed as follows: length from nose to anatomical structure or pathological change divided by total length from nose to cloaca multiplied by 100 equals x percent. The following table has been worked out in boas and pythons and may differ in other groups.

Table

Orientation of the Organs of Python and Boa

Organ	% total length
Heart	22— 33 %
Lung*	33— 45 %
Airsac	45— 64 %
Liver	38— 56 %
Stomach	46— 67 %
Small intestine	68— 81 %
Cranial kidney (right)	67— 69 %
Caudal kidney (left)	74— 82 %
Large intestine	81—100 %

* Pythons and boas possess both lungs (the left one is smaller), most other species only have a right lung.

Amphibians

For amphibians, the same adapted radiographic techniques as in other exotic pets are suitable.

Methoxyflurane inhalation is preferred for sedation or anaesthesia. One can also use Ketamine applicated into the dorsal lymph sac or a dipping in MS 222.

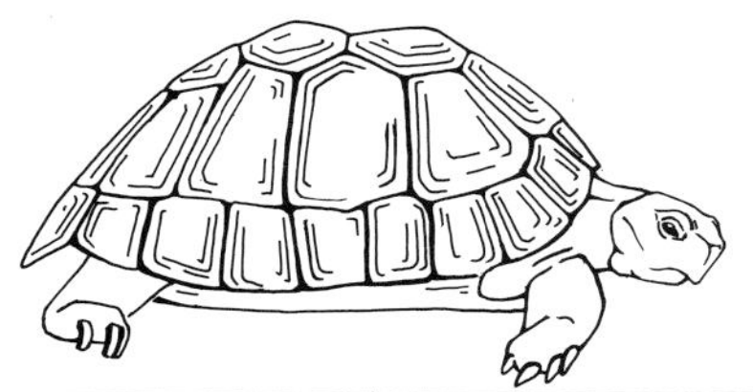

Reptiles: Tortoises and Turtles

Radiographic Anatomy
Internal Organs
and Skeleton

1

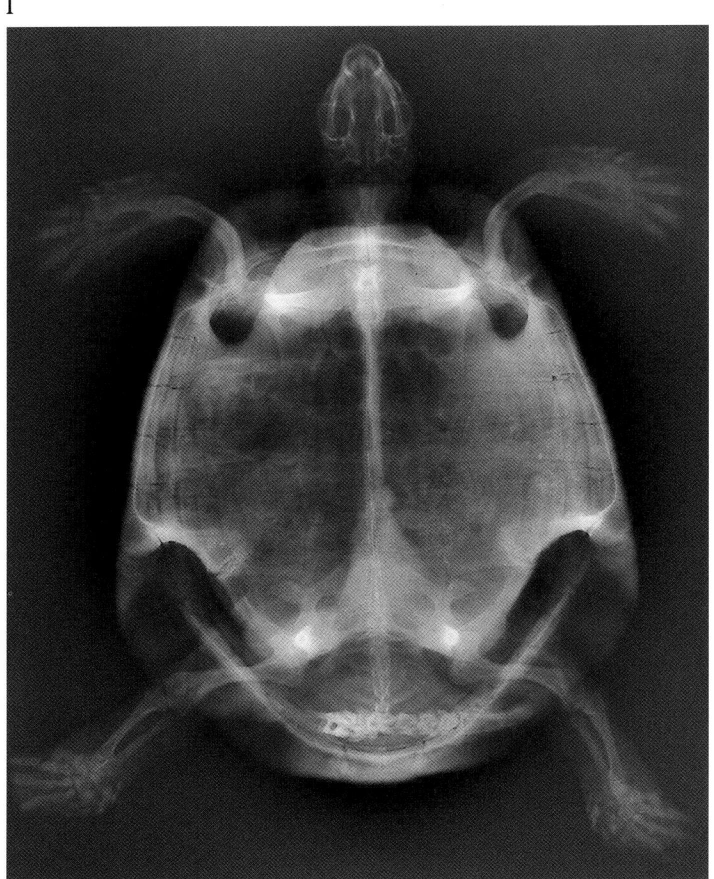

1 A

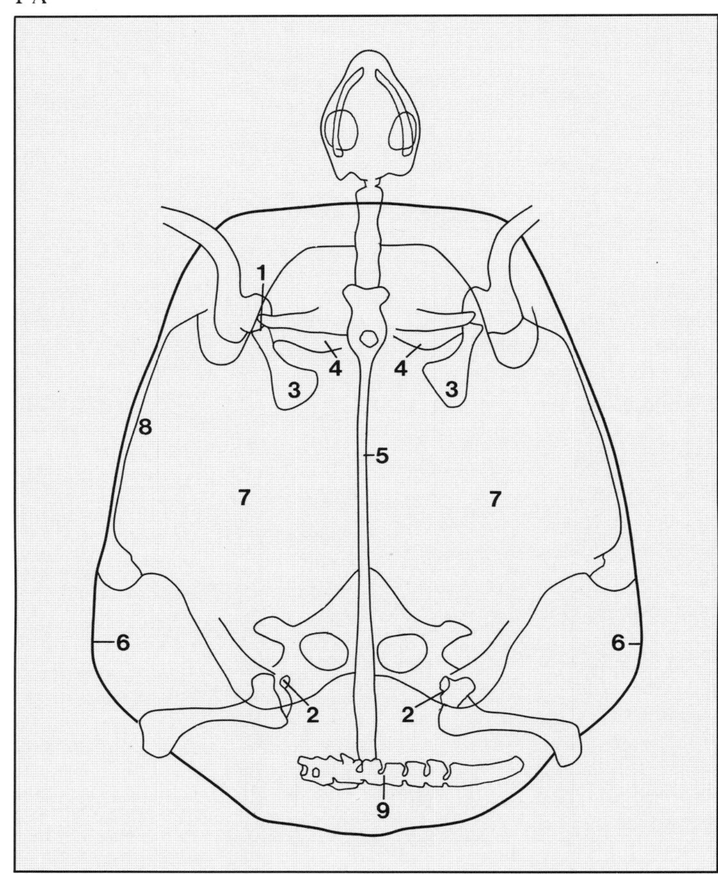

1/1A Normal Radiographic Appearance, dorsoventral.

Hermann's Tortoise *(Testudo hermanni)*, male.

The sutures between the bony plates, one median line (neuralia) and two lateral lines (pleuralia), are visible. The bony plates do not correspond with the keratinized shields. On the dorsoventral radiograph, the internal organs can be evaluated rarely because of the superimposition of the bony carapace and plastron.

In female animals, a transverse line of connective tissue from knee to knee can be seen. This tissue allows the caudal part of the plastron a certain degree of moveability when eggs are laid (see FIG. **6**).

The shoulder joint (**1**) and hip joint (**2**) are visible. Coracoid (**3**) and scapula (**4**) can be differentiated. The reduced, fused vertebral column (**5**) can be seen as a median stripe. The dorsal shell (carapace) (**6**) and ventral shell (plastron) (**7**) are fused by a bony bridge (**8**) that extends from the knee to the shoulder sinus. The coccygeal vertebrae (**9**) inside the flexed tail are visible in the cloacal area.

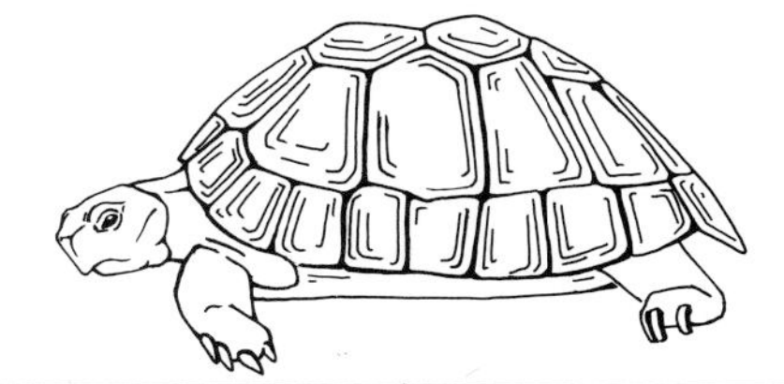

2

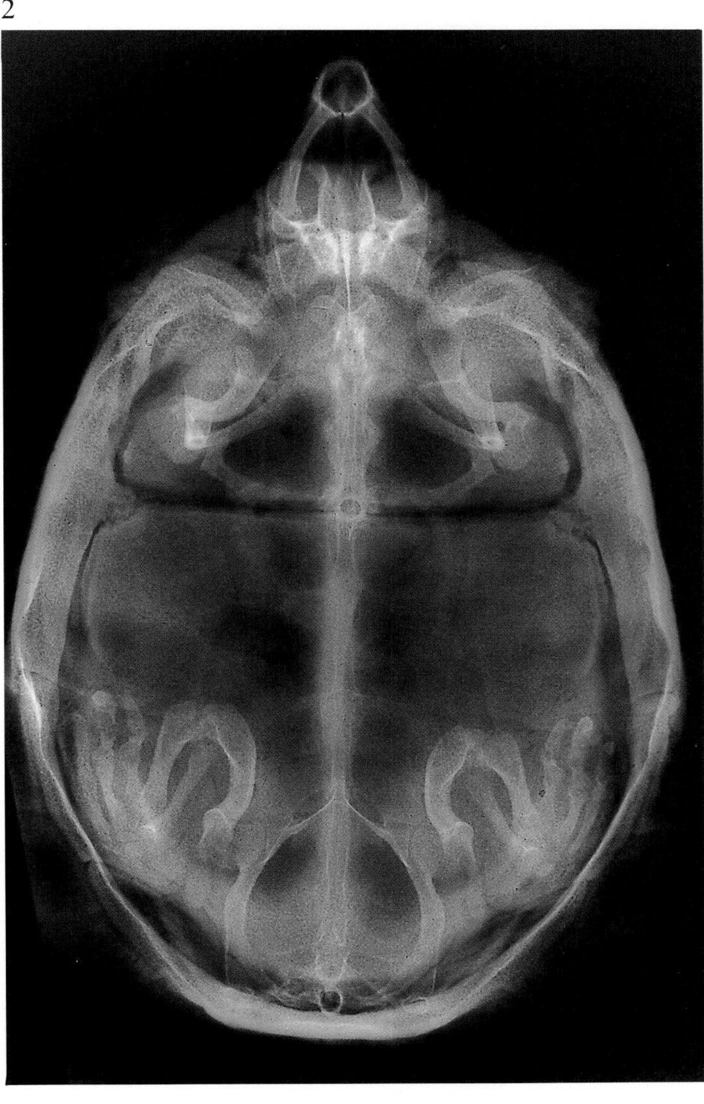

2 Normal Radiographic Appearance, dorsoventral.

Box turtle *(Terrapene carolina).*

In the box turtle as in many other species, we find a transverse hinge in the plastron. The cranial and the caudal part of the plastron can move dorsally around this hinge, enabling the turtle to close the shell tightly after withdrawal of head and limbs (Box Turtle).

3

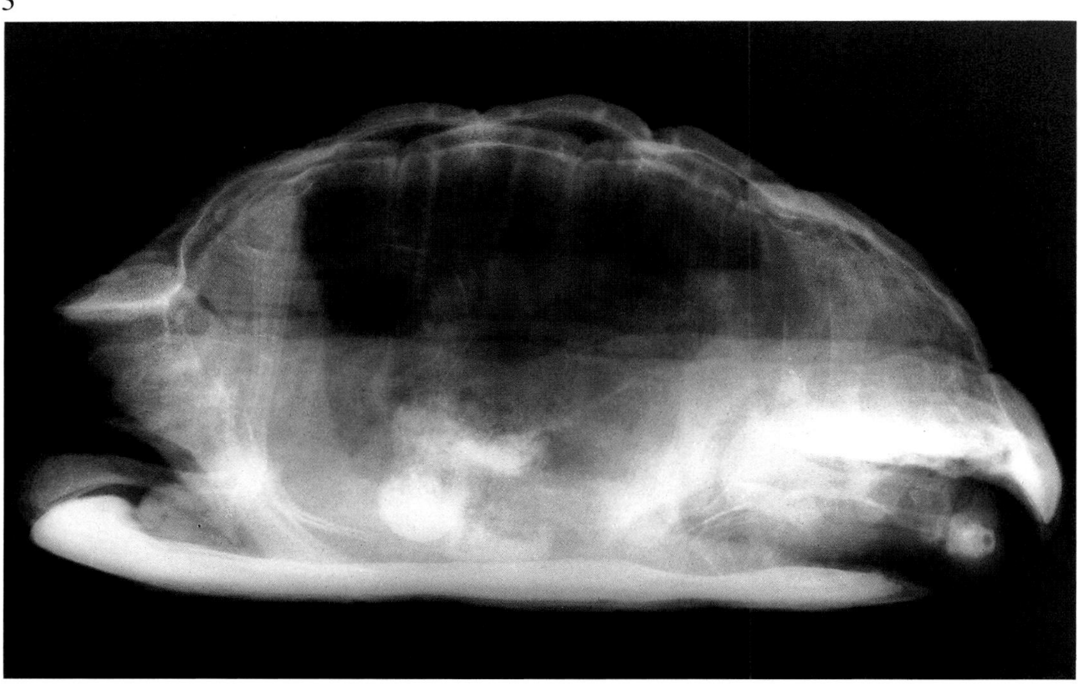

3A

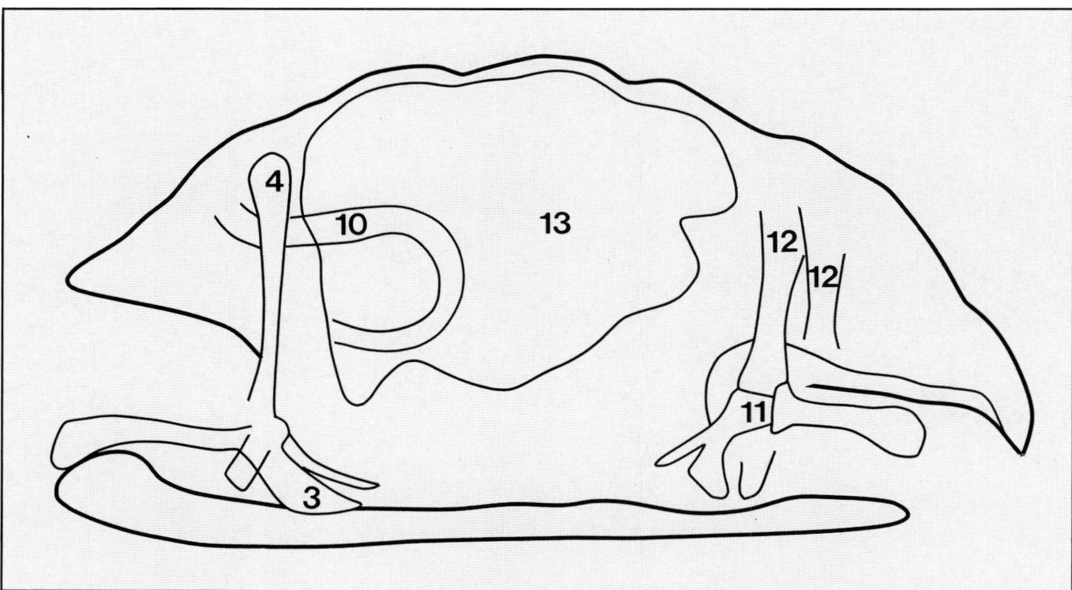

3/3A Normal Radiographic Appearance, lateral.

Hermann's Tortoise *(Testudo hermanni)*, male.

In cryptodire turtles, which include all species except the sidenecks (pleurodires), the S-like curvature of the cervical spine (**10**) is visible. The coracoid (**3**) and the scapula (**4**) connect the plastron and carapace cranially, the os pubis (**11**) and the os ilium (**12**) caudally. The shadows of both lungs (**13**) are clearly visible. Stomach, intestines, liver, heart, and spleen cannot be identified separately.

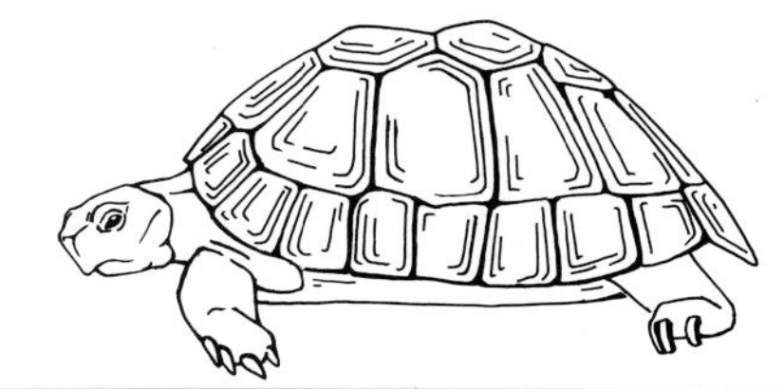

4

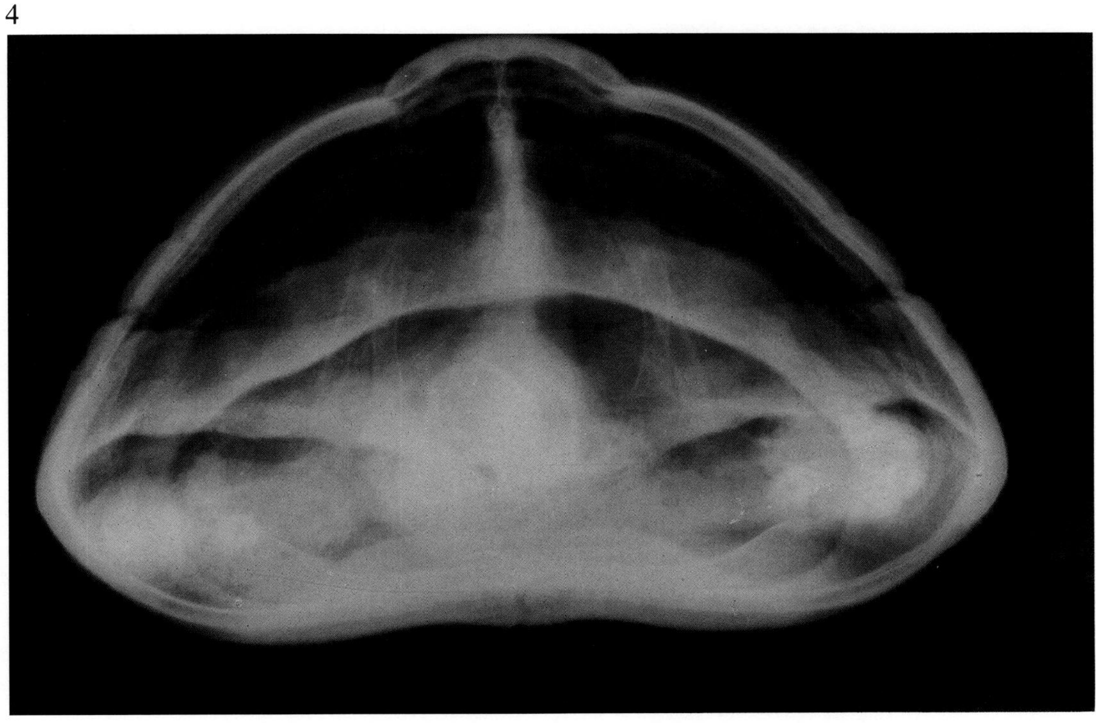

4A

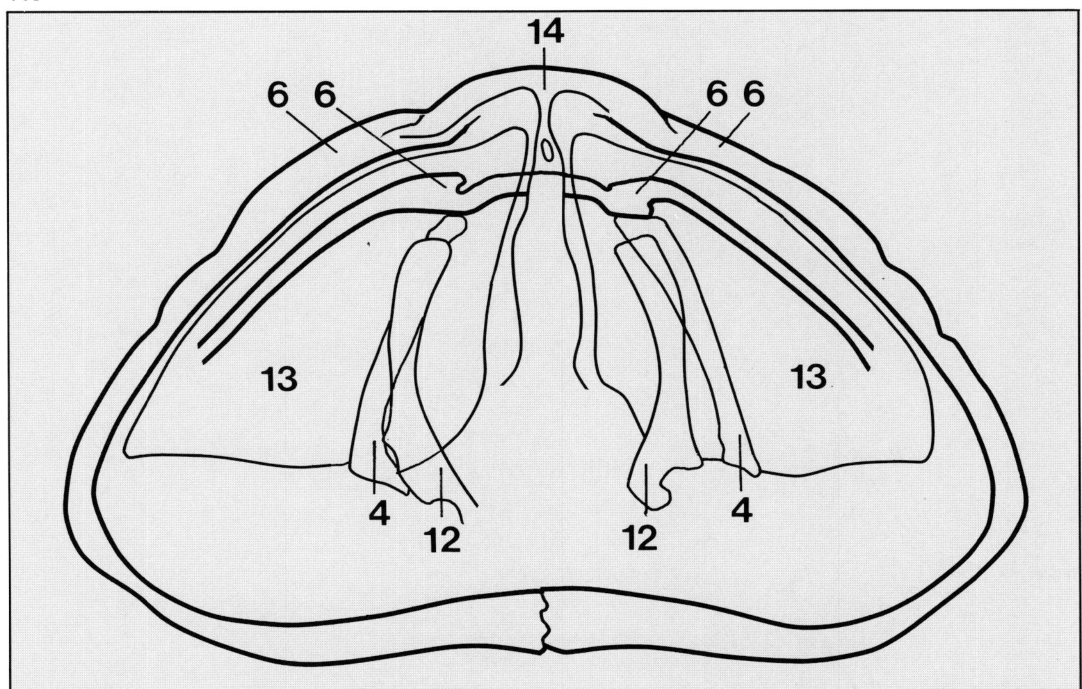

4/4A Normal Radiographic Appearance, craniocaudal.

Hermann's Tortoise *(Testudo hermanni)*, male.

The craniocaudal view is especially useful to evaluate both lungs and to compare both sides of the lungs (**13**). Superimposed on the lungshadows, parts of the carapace (**6**), vertebral column (**14**), scapula (**4**) and ilium (**12**) are visible.

5

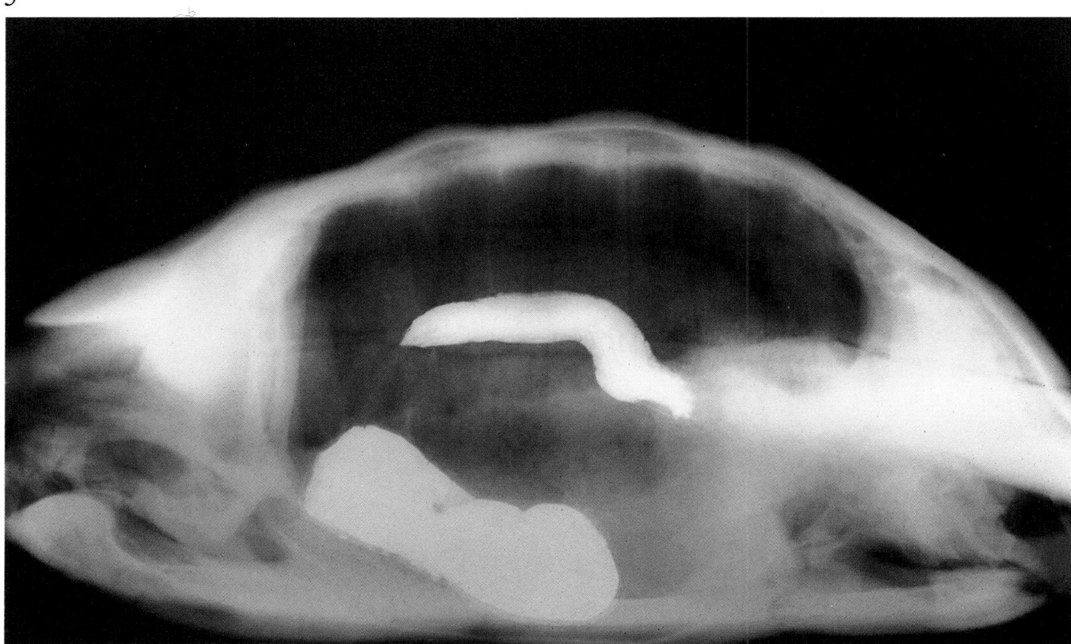

6

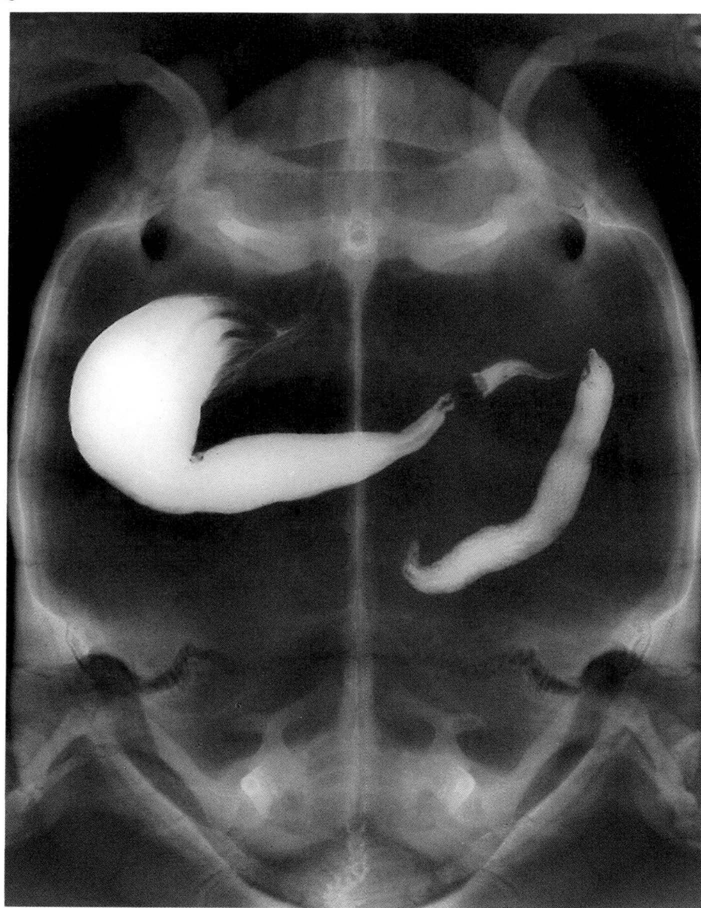

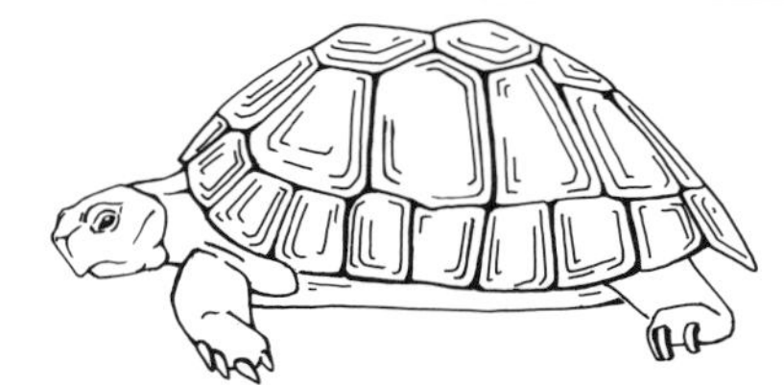

7

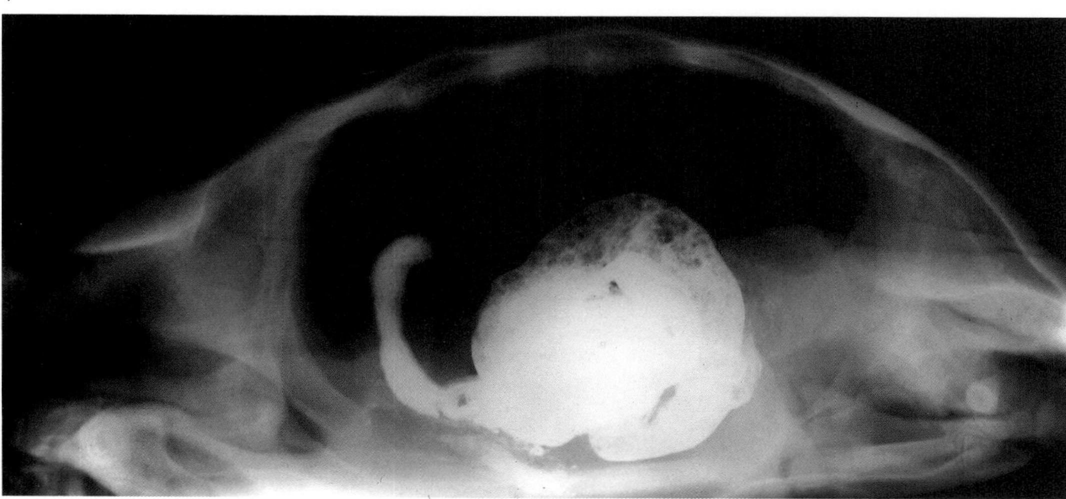

8

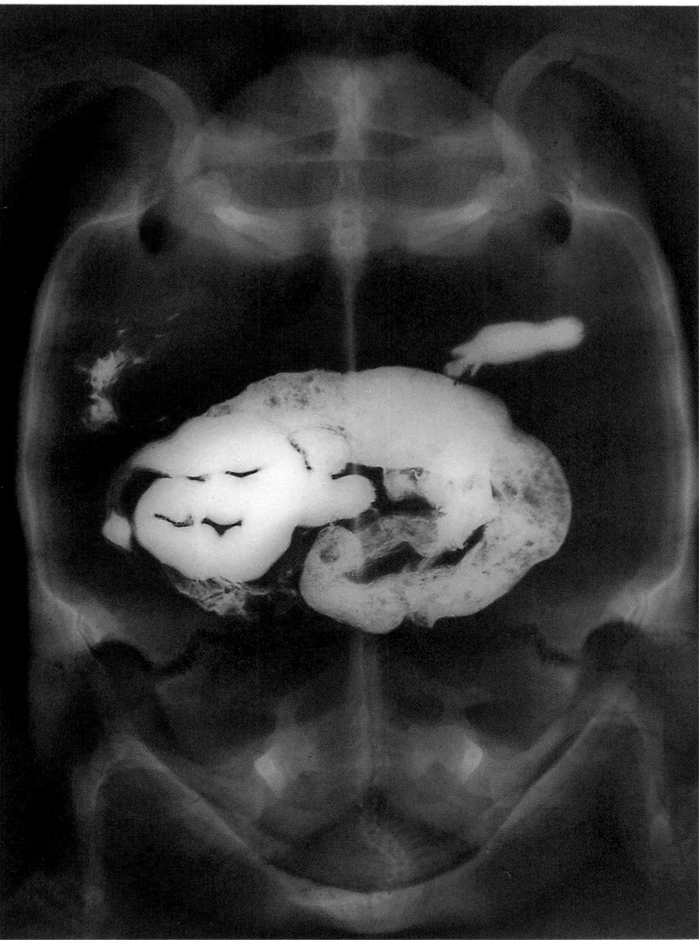

5-8 Normal Radiographic Appearance,
lateral and dorsoventral: contrast study.

Hermann's Tortoise *(Testudo hermanni),* female.

On the lateral radiograph, 10 min. after administration of contrast medium, the stomach is located ventrally and the duodenum more dorsally surrounded by aerated lungs (FIG. **5**).

On the dorsoventral radiograph, the stomach is visible on the left side of the celomic cavity. The duodenum has a right-sided position. A faint trace of the esophagus is visible (FIG. **6**).

On the $7^1/_2$ h lateral radiograph, the duodenum extends dorsally. The rest of the intestines cannot be differentiated due to crowding and superimposition in the celomic cavity (FIG. **7**).

On the $7^1/_2$ h dorsoventral radiograph (FIG. **8**), residues of contrast medium are seen in the stomach on the left side and in the duodenum on the right side. In the midportion of the body, contrast-filled loops of small intestine and the s-shaped large intestinal loop are visible.

For the continuation of the contrast study please turn to the next page (FIG. **9-12**).

9

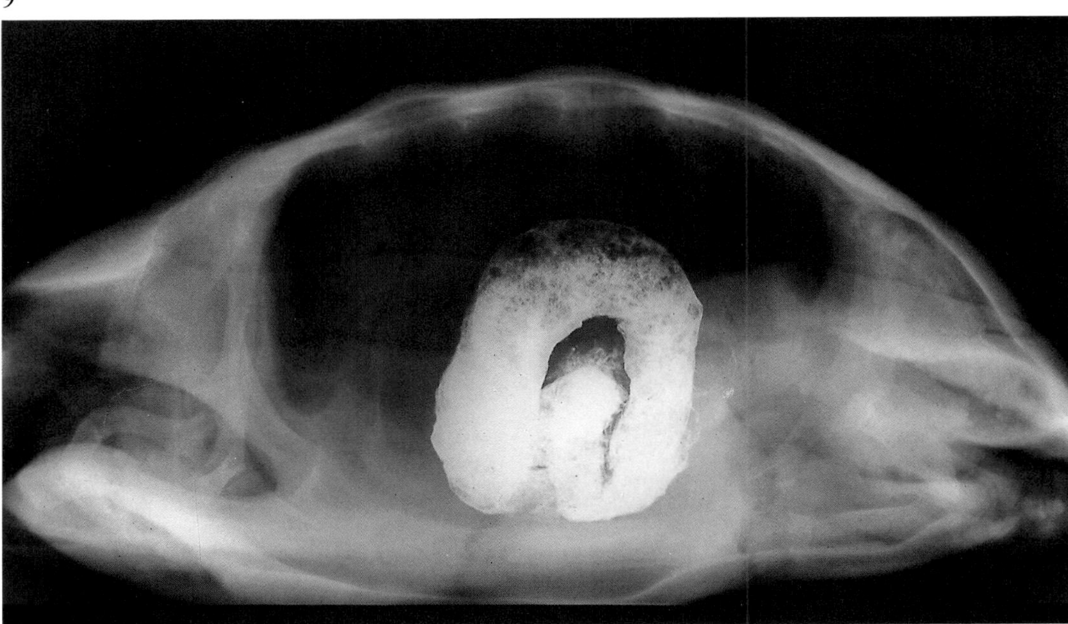

10

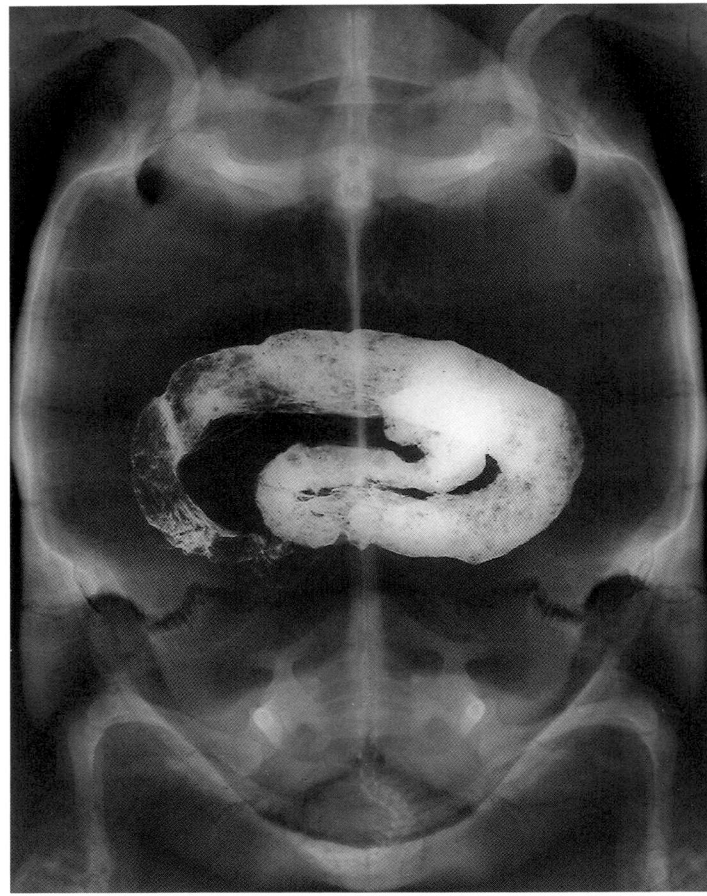

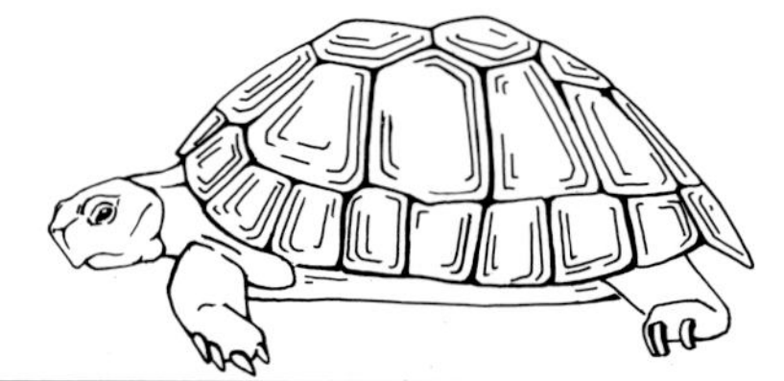

11

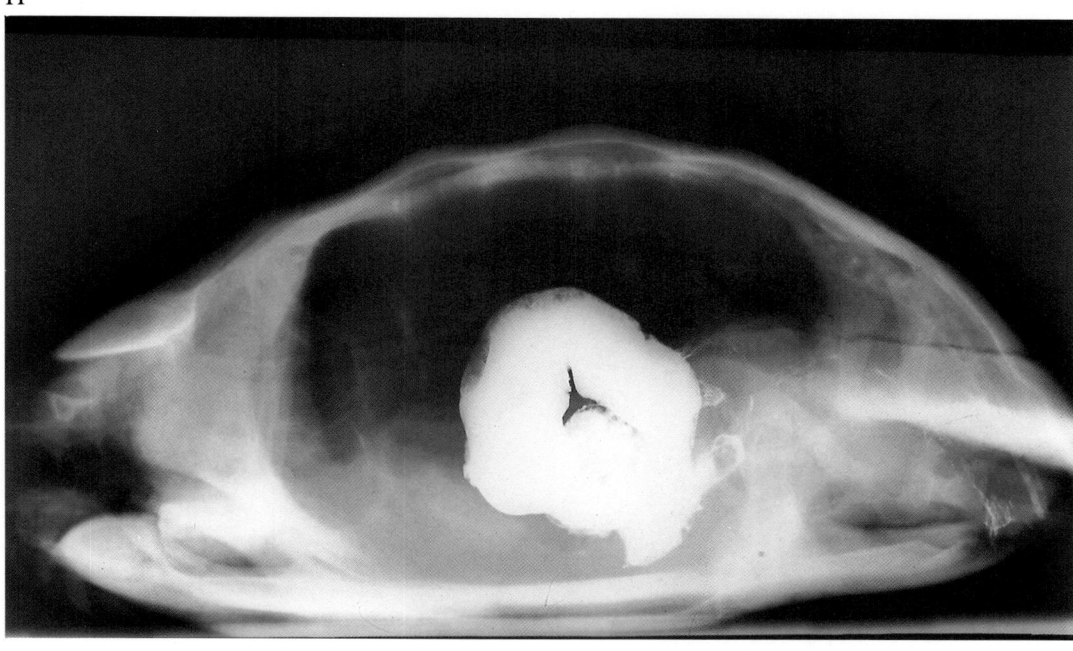

12

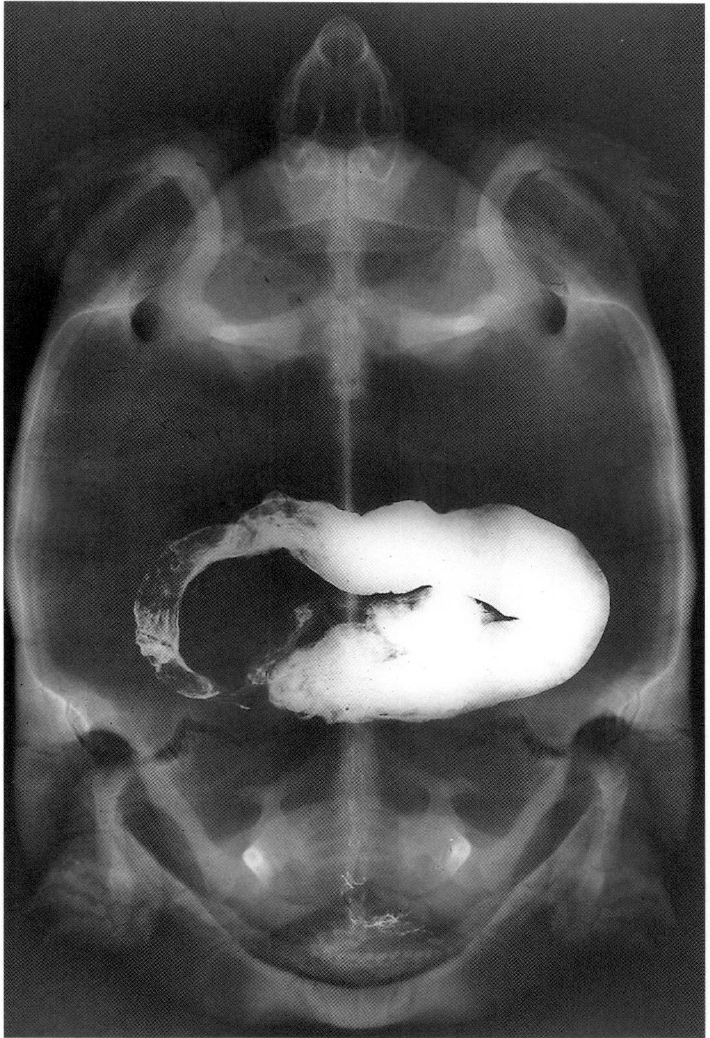

9-12 Normal Radiographic Appearance,
lateral and dorsoventral: contrast study (continuation).

Hermann's Tortoise *(Testudo hermanni),* female.

On the 22 h lateral radiograph, the contrast-filled loop of the large intestine is superimposed on the pulmonary shadow (FIG. **9**).

On the 22 h dorsoventral radiograph, the s-shaped large intestine turns caudally into the rectum (FIG. **10**).

On the lateral radiograph taken after 10 days, a fine line of contrast medium extends from the rectum dorsally into the pelvis and then turns ventrally into the cloaca. This is caused by adherence of barium to the rectal mucosa (FIG. **11**).

On the dorsoventral radiograph of the same time (FIG. **12**), the rectum is filled with contrast medium. A barium residue is present inside the cloaca.

13

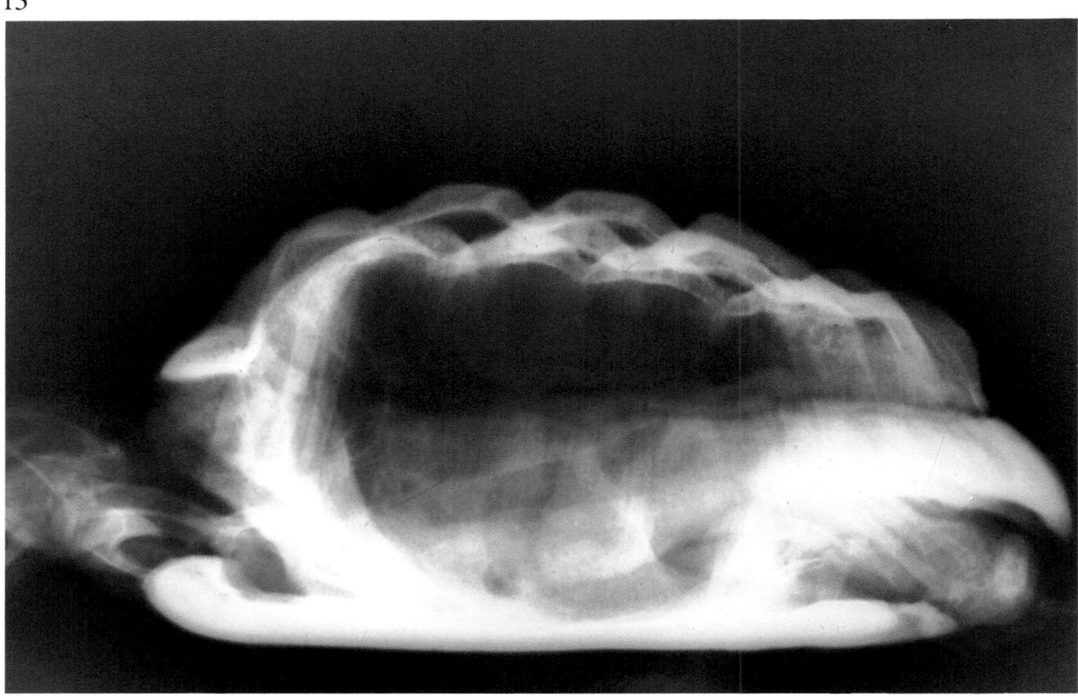

14

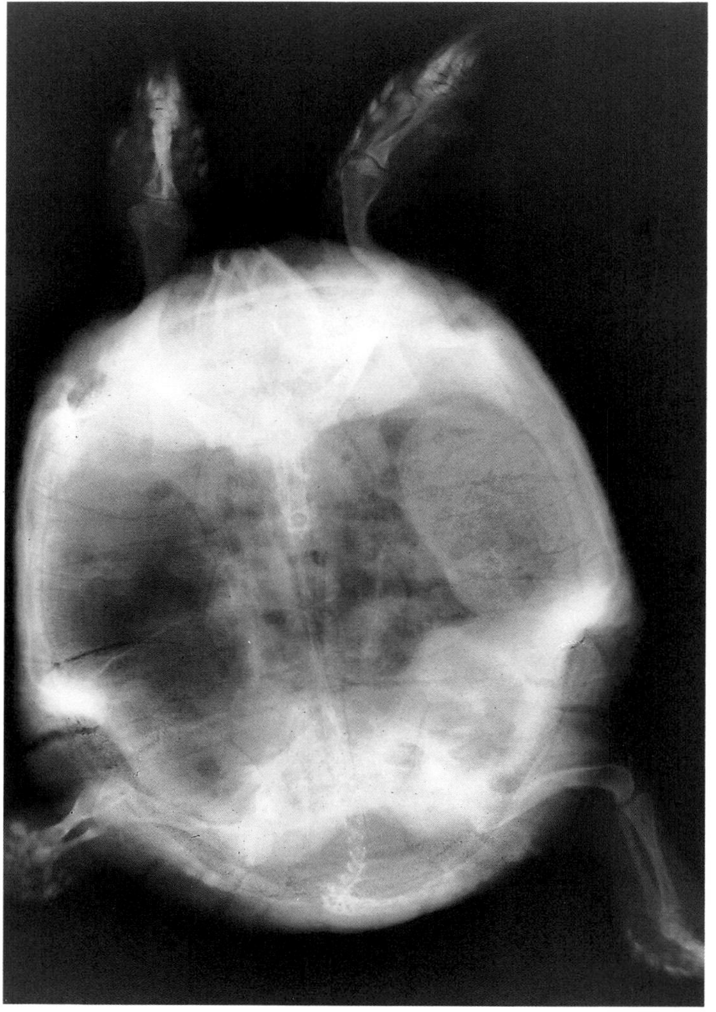

13 Metabolic Bone Disease.

Hermann's tortoise *(Testudo hermanni)*, juvenile.

The bony plates of the carapace are thickened and turned dorsally in a semicircular fashion. This is typical for rickets.

14 Fracture of the shell.

Central Asian Tortoise *(Agrionemys horsfieldii)*.

A transverse fracture line can be seen on the left side of the carapace dorsal to the knee fold. The suture between the lateral plates near the knee is abnormally widened.

This tortoise fell from the third floor of a building onto the stones of the sidewalk.

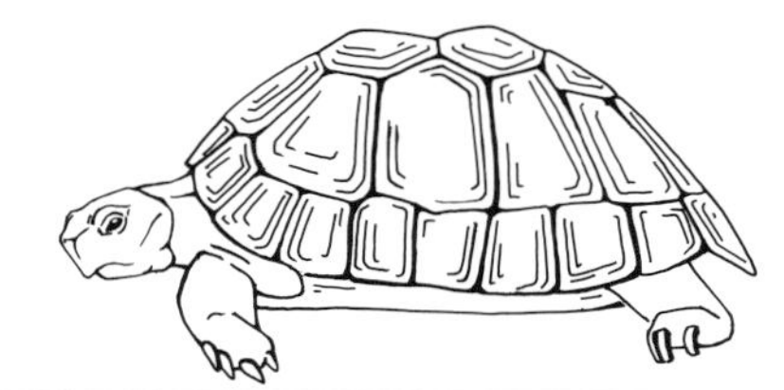

15

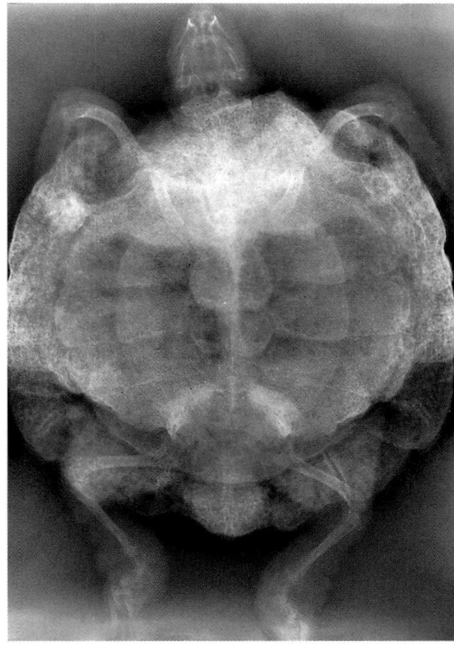

16

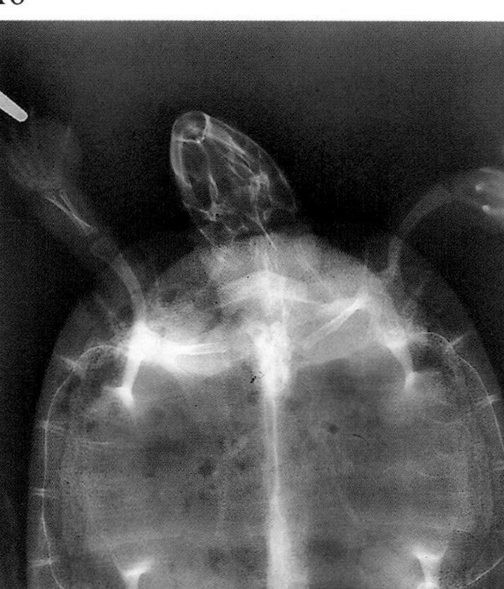

17

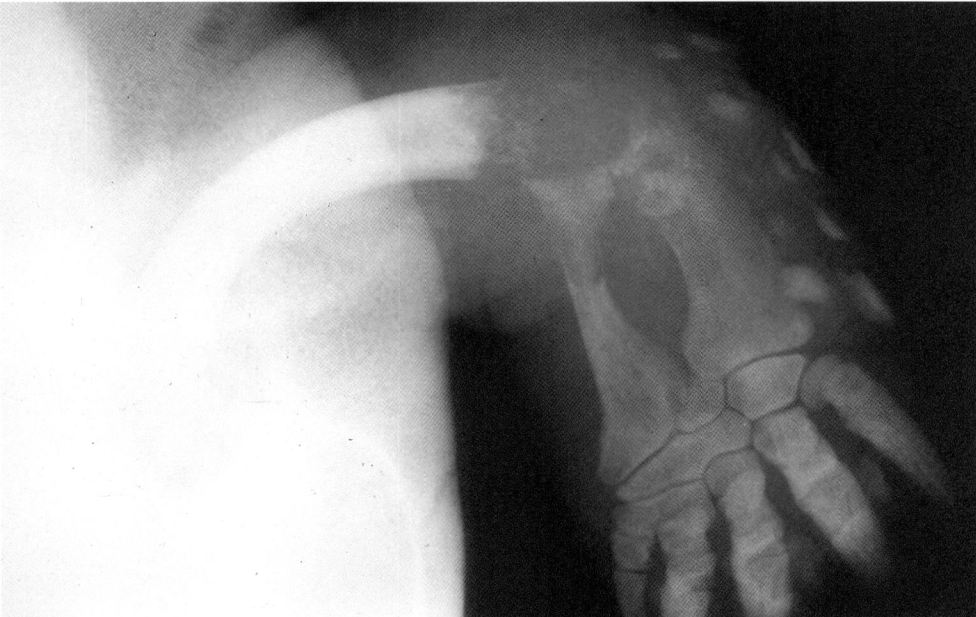

15 Osteodystrophia fibrosa generalisata.

Hermann's Tortoise *(Testudo hermanni).*

The bony shell is demineralized. Only finely-branched bone trabeculae are still visible.

16 Mycotic Osteolysis.

Red Eared Slider *(Pseudemys scripta elegans).*

Mutiple small focal radiolucencies are visible, especially in the front quadrants of the carapace. This is the typical presentation of mycosis with osteolysis.

17 Osteolytic Arthritis.

Hermann's Tortoise *(Testudo hermanni).*

The bones of the elbow joint show severe lytic changes. There is soft tissue swelling around the joint. These are typical signs of an infectious arthritis, in this case caused by Staphylococcus sp.

18

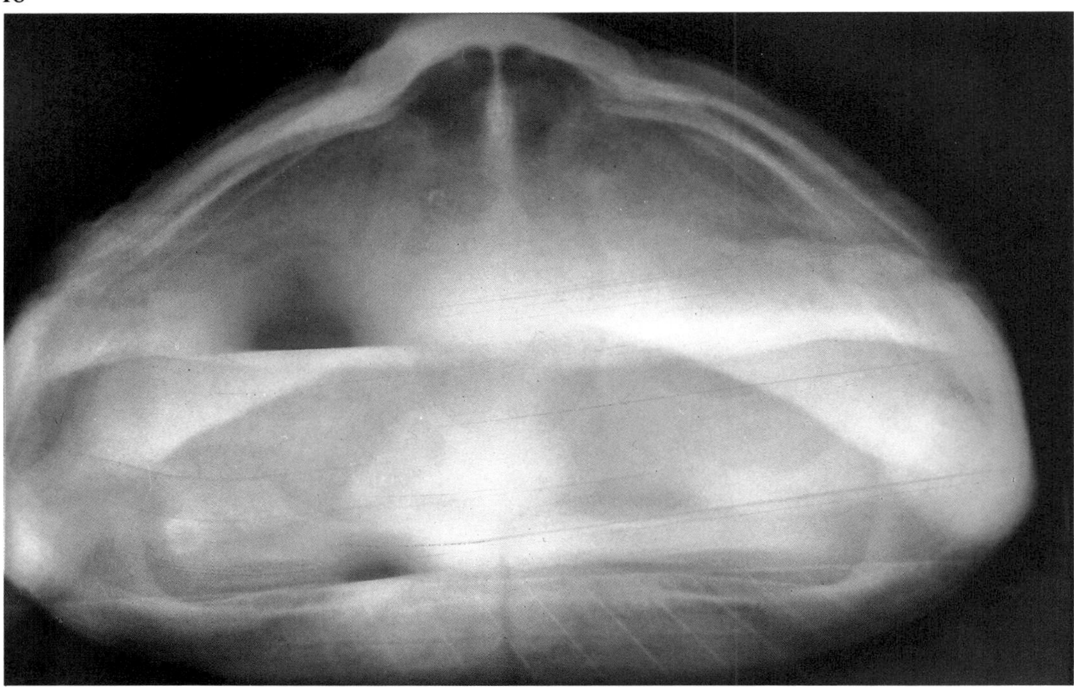

19

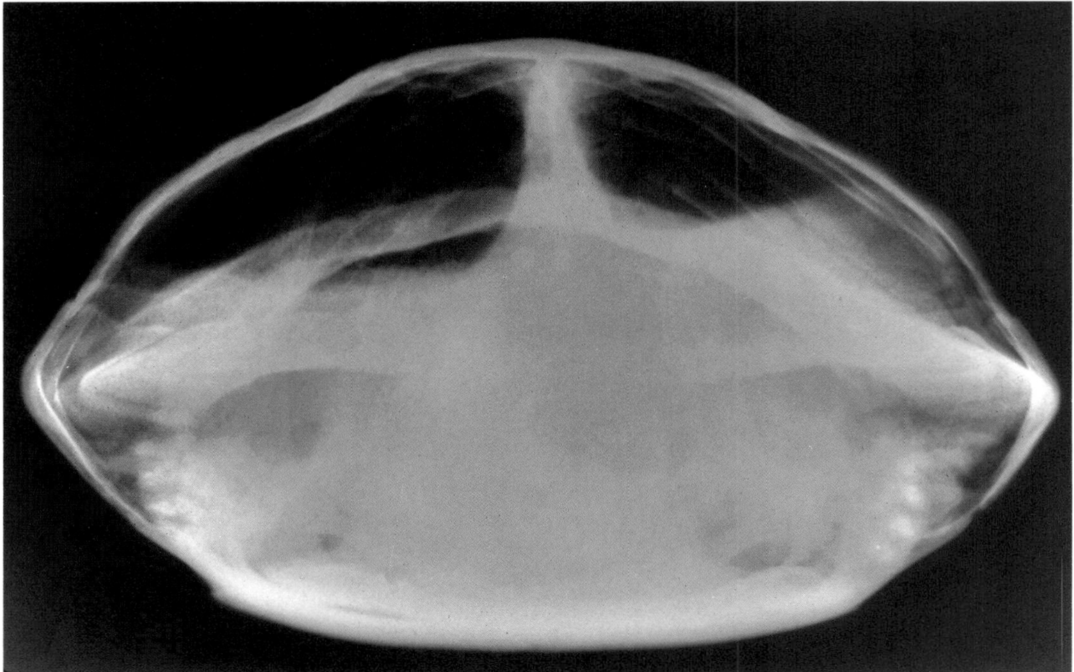

18 Pneumonia.

Hermann's tortoise *(Testudo hermanni).*

On the craniocaudal radiograph, cloudy densities can be seen in both lungs due to a mycotic pneumonia.

Note: The dorsoventral view is of no value for diagnosing pneumonia in chelonians. The lateral view allows no comparison of both lungfields.

19 Unilateral Pneumonia.

Red Eared Slider *(Pseudemys scripta elegans).*

Due to horizontal beam projection, this radiograph shows a horizontal fluid line due to the accumulation of exudates in the left lung. This is the typical radiographic presentation of unilateral pneumonia.

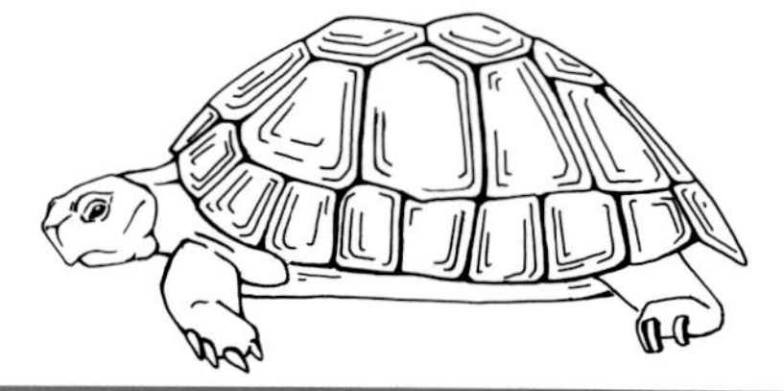

20

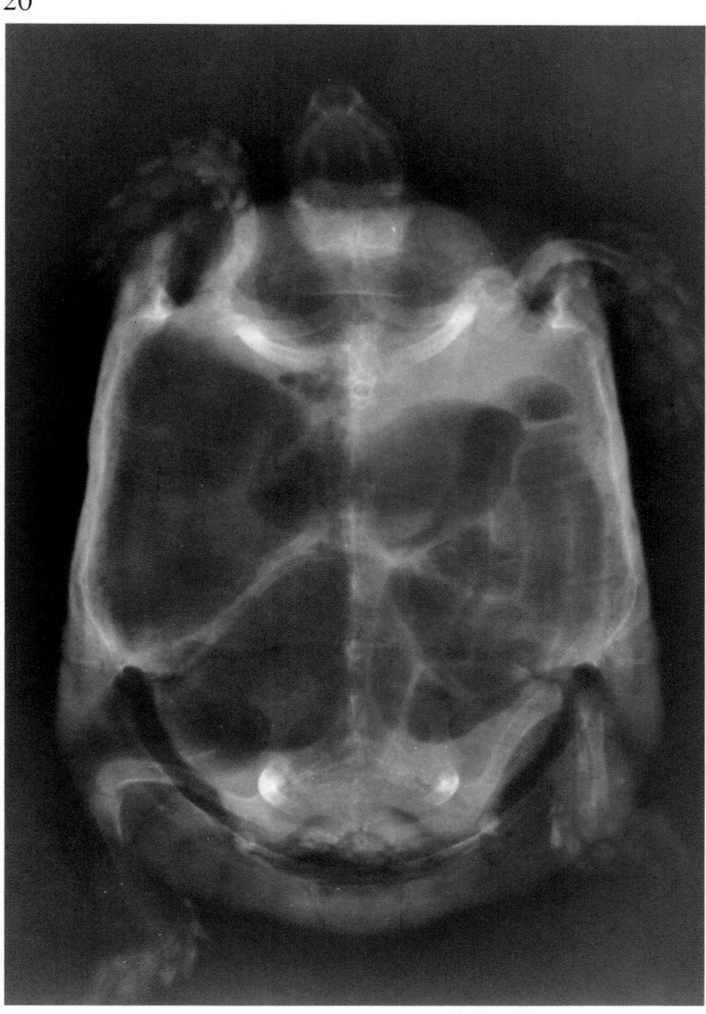

20 Enteritis.

Spur-thighed Tortoise *(Testudo graeca)*.

On the dorsoventral radiograph, gas in the celomic cavity and gaseous distension of the gastrointestinal tract are visible. A similar picture is seen after surgical opening of the celom.

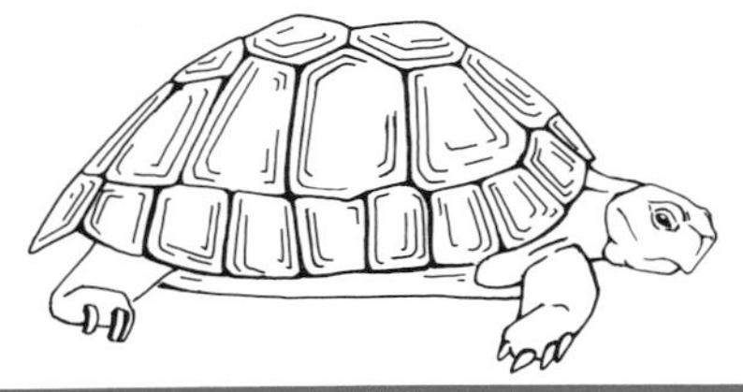

21

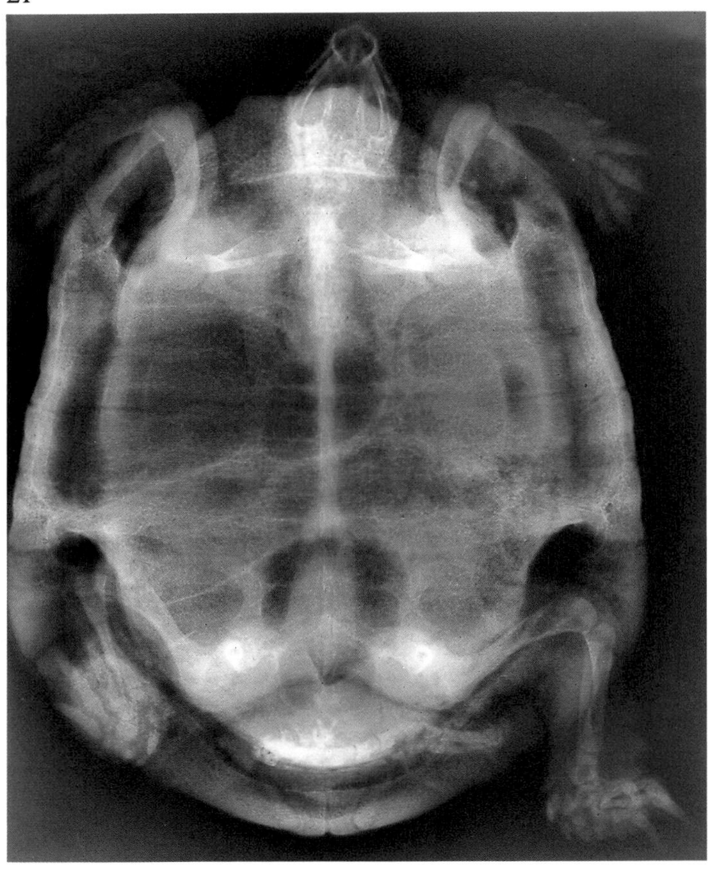

22

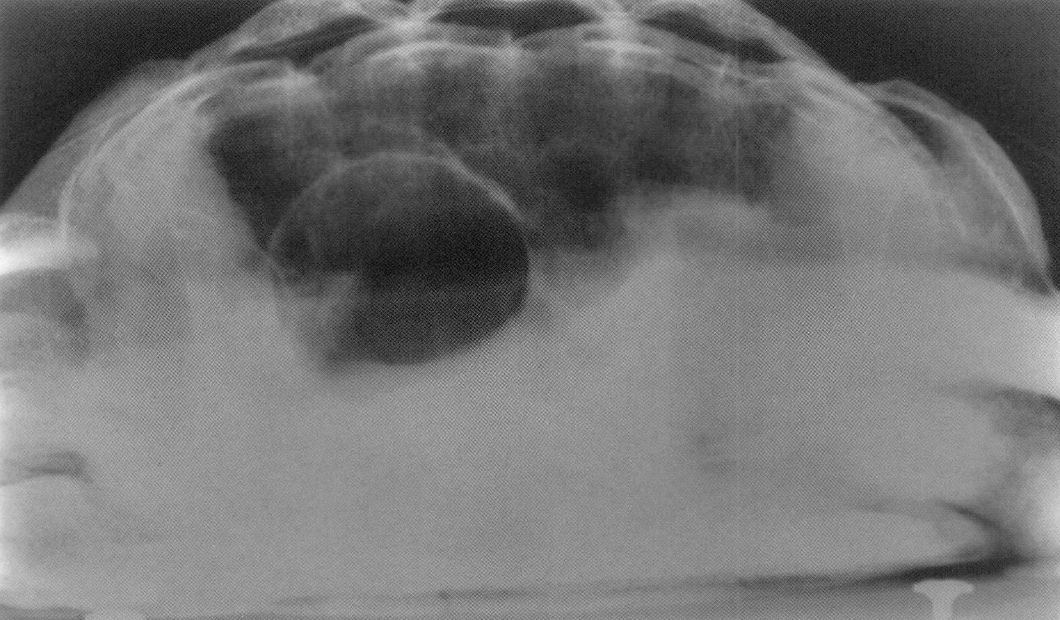

21/22 Gastritis.

Hermann's Tortoise *(Testudo hermanni).*

On the dorsoventral radiograph, an angular-shaped radiolucency is visible in the left half of the plastron. This is the location of the stomach. Accumulation of gas in the stomach is typical for gastritis.

On the lateral radiograph, the globular gas-filled stomach is also visible. The diagnosis was bacterial gastritis.

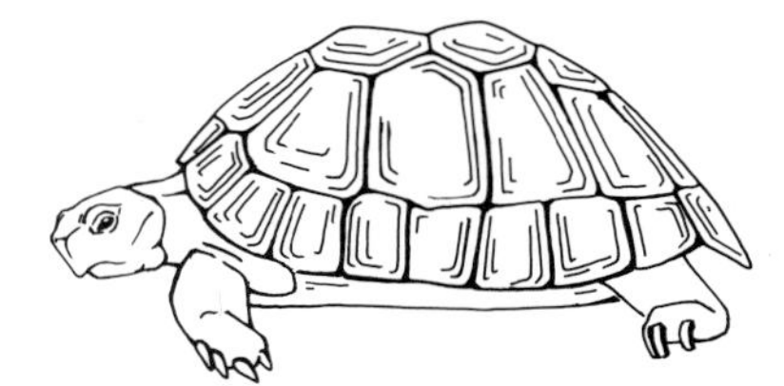

23

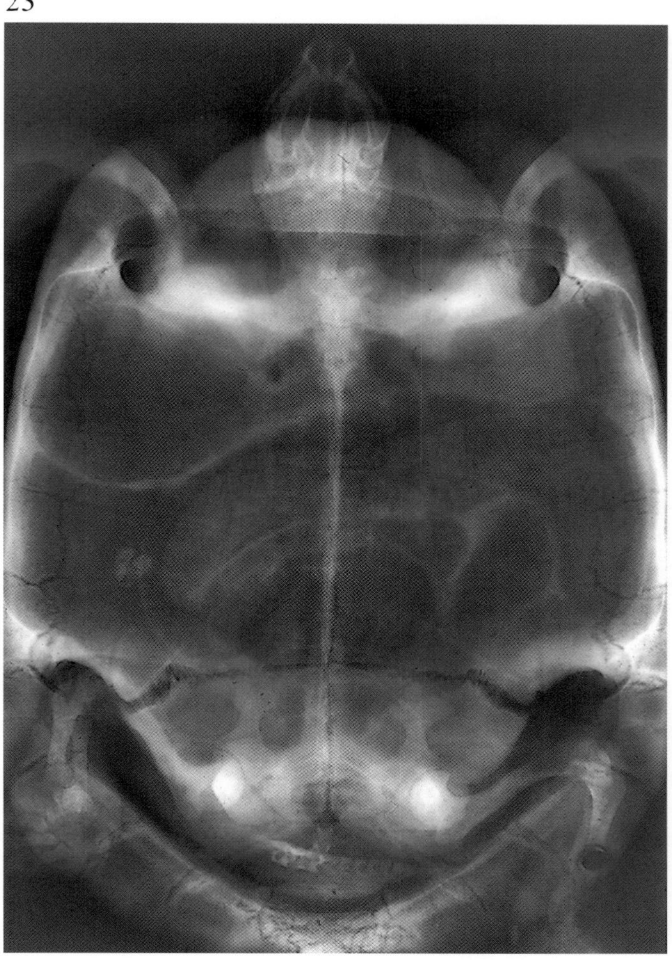

24

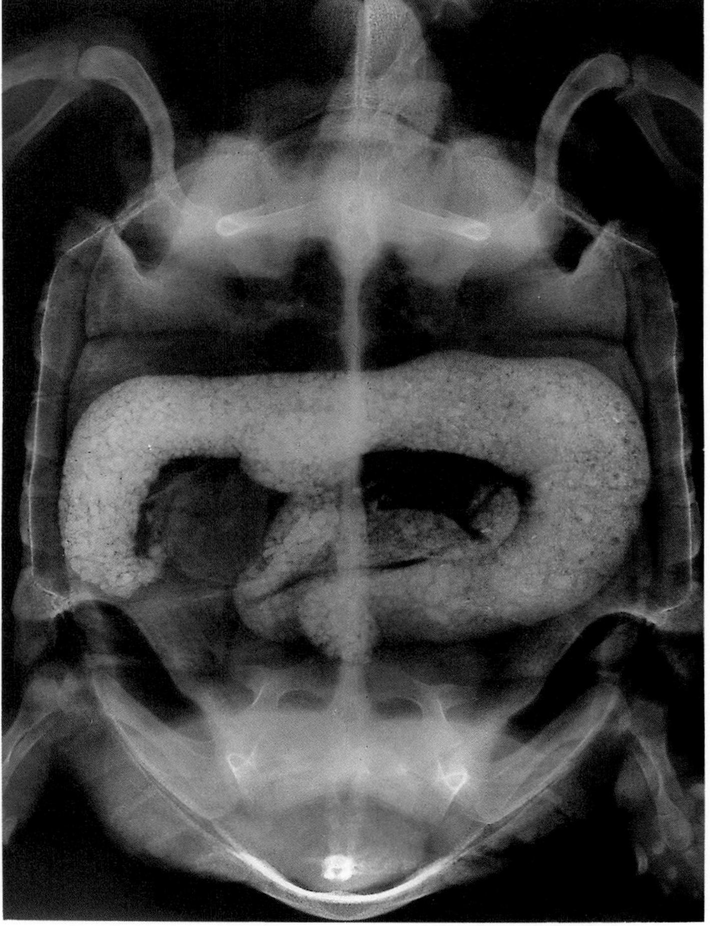

23 Constipation.

Hermann's Tortoise *(Testudo hermanni).*

Inside the transverse loop of the large intestine, impacted ingesta are faintly visible. The collar of gas around the ingesta provides a spontaneous contrast-outlining of the intestinal wall.

24 Constipation caused by foreign bodies.

Gopher Tortoise *(Gopherus polyphemus).*

The entire large intestine is filled with mineral-dense material being cat litter. This resembles barium impaction at the end of a contrast study.

25

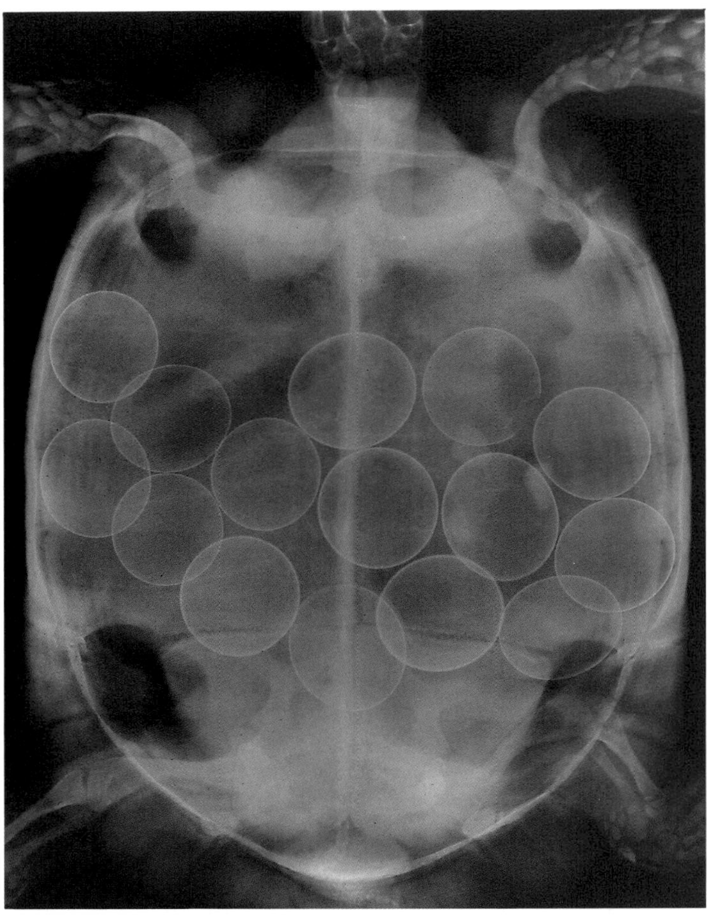

26

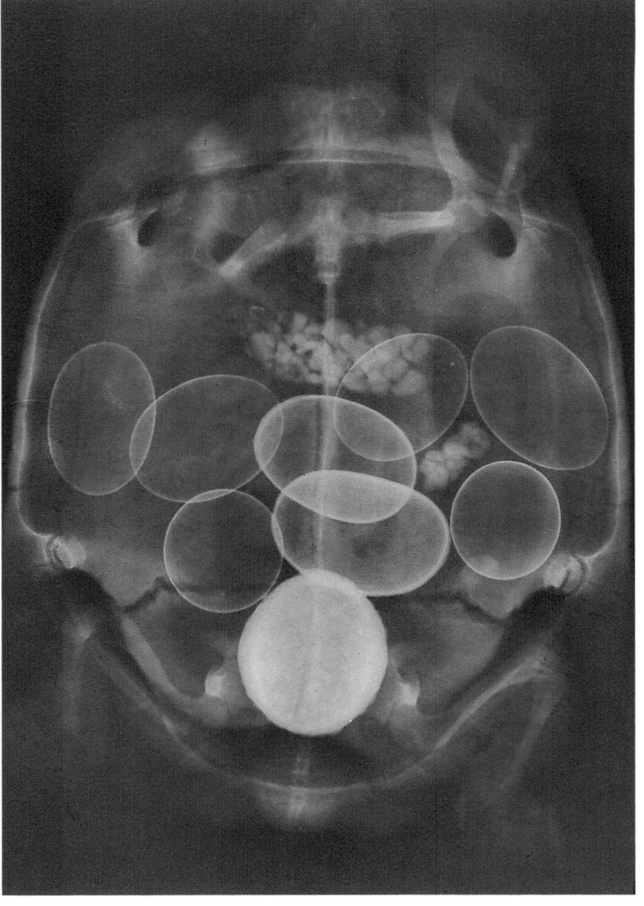

25 Normal Gravidity.

Hermann's Tortoise *(Testudo hermanni).*

Fifteen eggs with calcified shells are seen within the body cavity. The homogeneous form and size of the eggs, that is species-specific, and the homogeneous calcification are indications for a normal gravidity. One egg on the right side has a calcified indentation which can be physiological.

26 Egg Binding.

Spur Thighed Tortoise *(Testudo graeca).*

Six eggs with normal calcification of the shells, and three eggs with abnormal thickening and calcification of the shells are visible. One extremely calcified egg is stuck within the pelvis. This egg is relatively too large and the surface of the shell is rough which impedes normal passage through the oviduct. These findings are an absolute indication for surgical intervention.

Two of the normal eggs present with a round shape as a result of end-on projection by the radiographic beam.

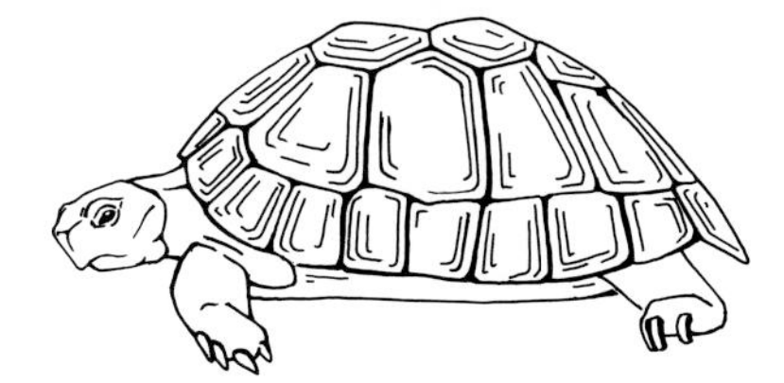

27

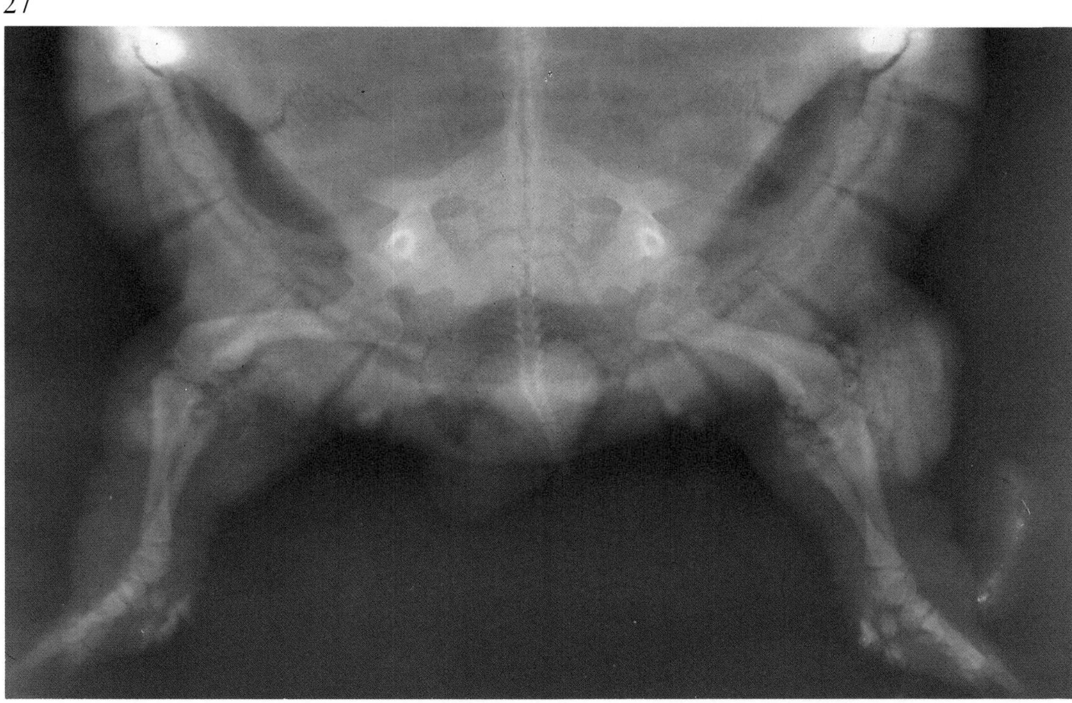

28

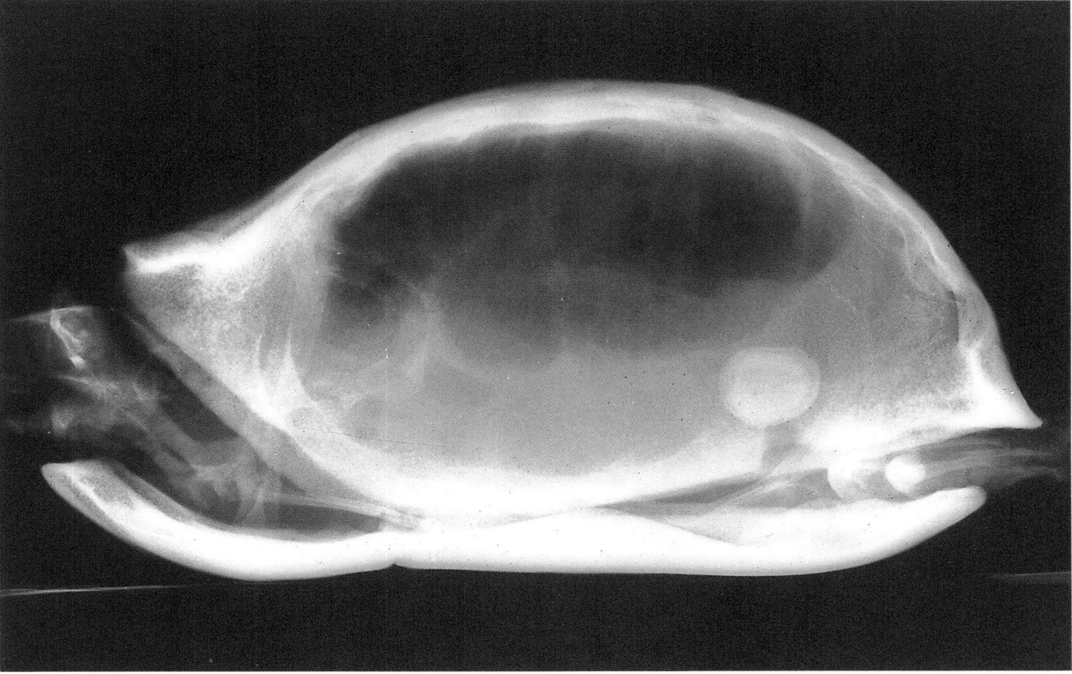

27 Articular Gout.

Spur Thighed Tortoise *(Testudo graeca)*.

Around both stifle joints a large number of small radiopacities are visible in the soft tissues. Similar changes exist around the tarsal joints. The radiopacities proved to be depositions of uric acid.

28 Anal Bladder Calculus.

Box Turtle *(Terrapene carolina)*.

A calculus is seen cranial to the pelvis and ventral to the rectum. It is probably located in the anal bladder.

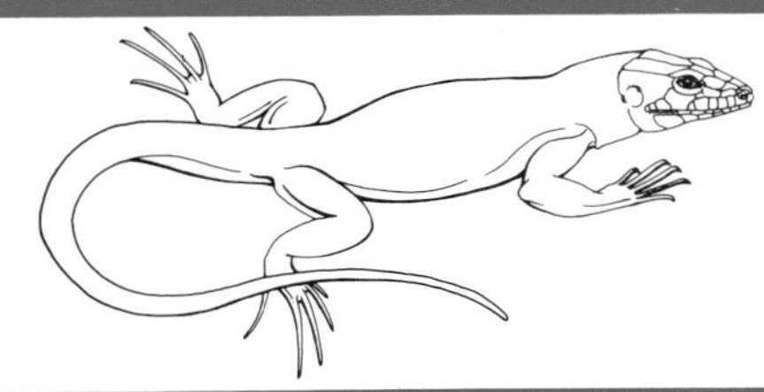

Reptiles: Lizards

Radiographic Anatomy
Internal Organs and Skeleton

29

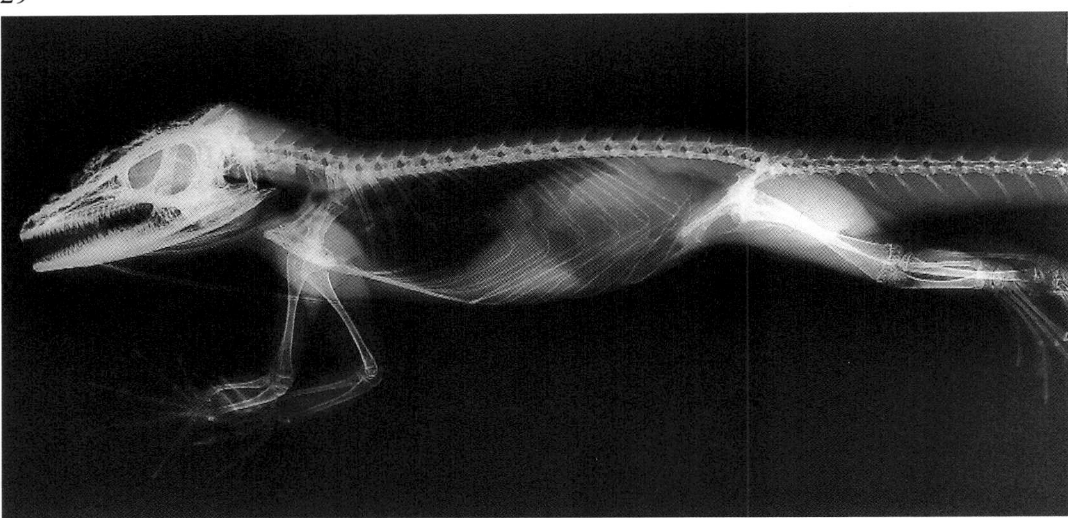

29 A

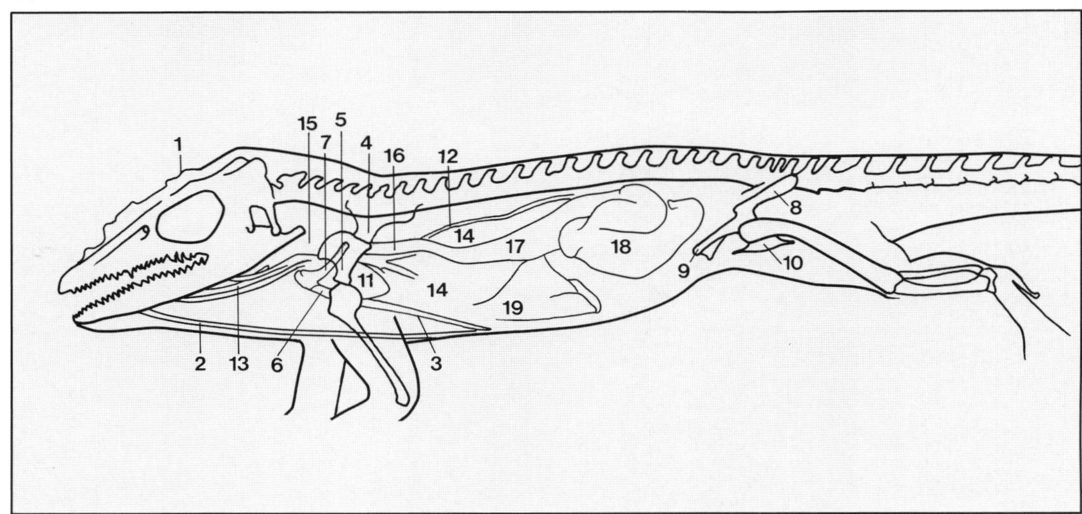

29/29A Normal Radiographic Appearance, lateral.

Cuban Giant Anole *(Anolis luteogularis).*

The bony protuberances on the skull (**1**) are normal in this and other species of lizards such as the chameleon. The cranial area of the hyoid bone (**2**) extends to the middle of the sternum (**3**). It is moveable and supports the large dewlap. The shoulder girdle with suprascapula (**4**), scapula (**5**), coracoid (**6**), clavicle (**7**), and humerus is clearly defined. Ten pairs of ribs connect the vertebral column to the sternum. The ilium (**8**) extends caudodorsally to the spine, the pubis (**9**) cranioventrally, and the ischium (**10**) caudally. The growth plates (physes) of the long bones are well visible.

Only the caudal outline of the cardiac shadow (**11**), that is located far cranially in the celom, is visible dorsal to the sternum. The aorta (**12**) curves caudodorsally from the heart.

Between the middle and the caudal part of the hyoid bone the trachea (**13**) reaches the aperture of the chest. It is easily recognizable dorsal to the heart. The radiolucent lungs (**14**) occupy the cranial portion of the body cavity.

The mouth and the pharynx (**15**) are large and filled with air. Within the centre of the lung shadows the esophagus (**16**) is visible that merges with the stomach (**17**). A few loops of small intestine (**18**) are visible but cannot be differentiated. The liver (**19**) is visible in the mid-central celomic cavity. The kidneys are located within the pelvis and cannot be seen.

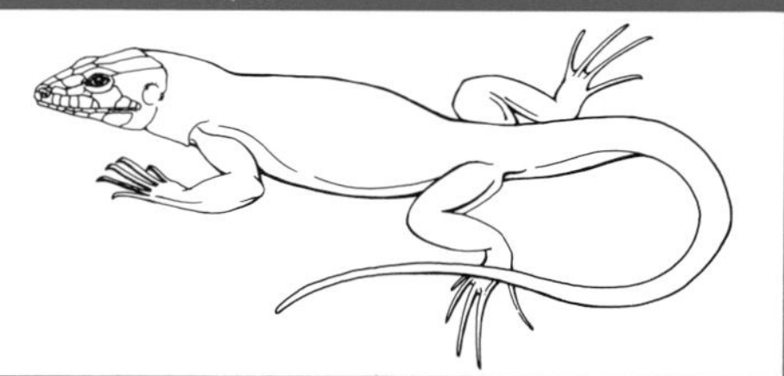

30

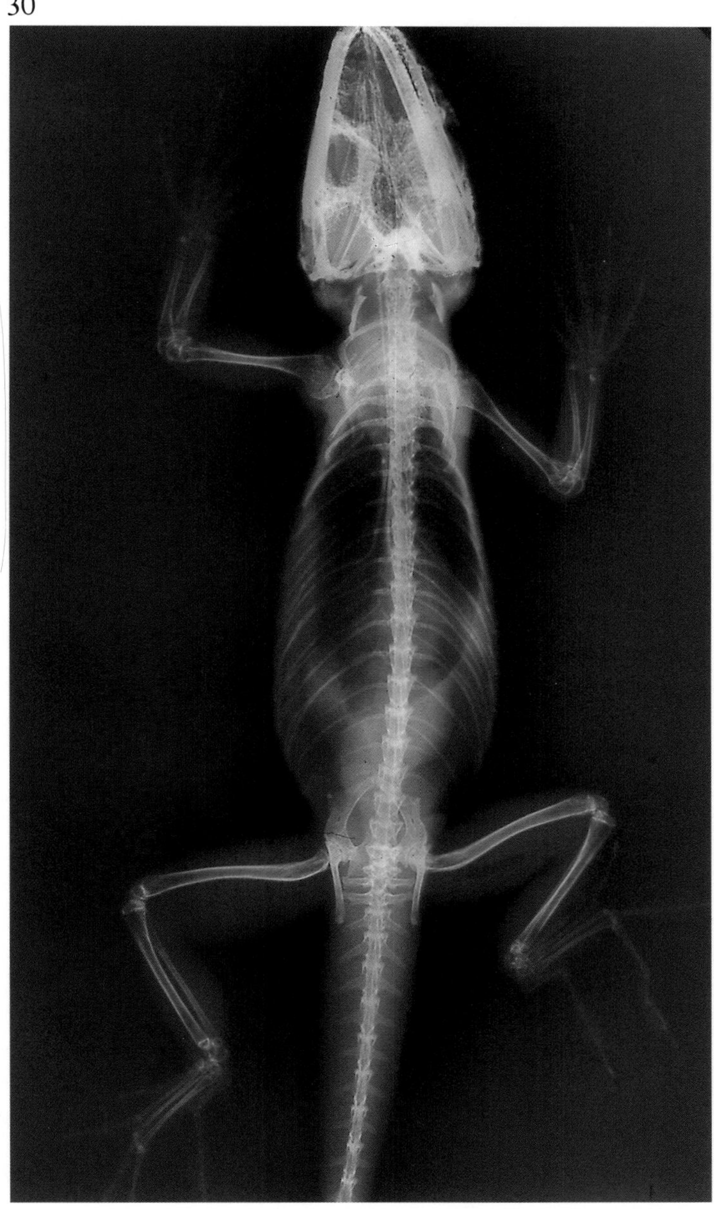

30 A

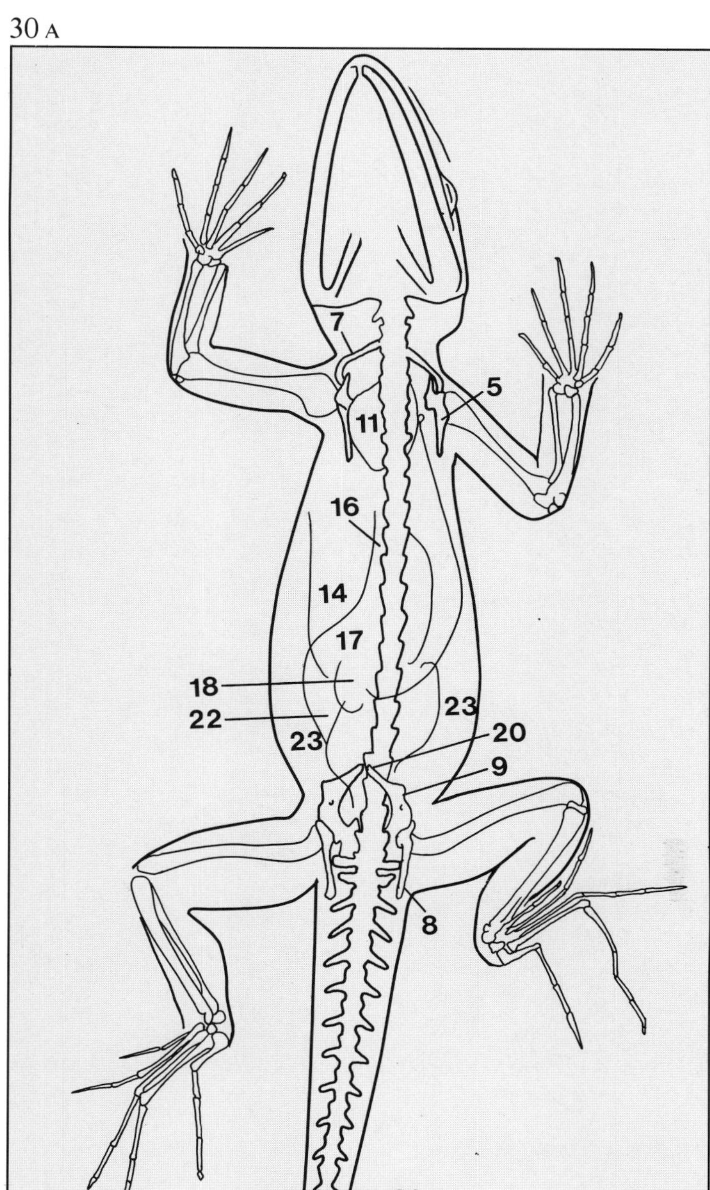

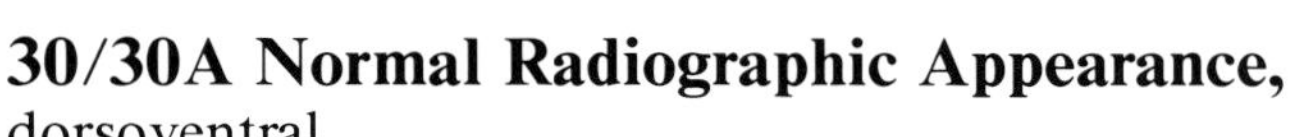

30/30A Normal Radiographic Appearance, dorsoventral.

Cuban Giant Anole *(Anolis luteogularis).*

On the dorsoventral radiograph, the skull, vertebral column, clavicles (**7**) and pelvis can be clearly seen. The ilium (**8**) extends caudodorsally, the pubis (**9**) with its symphysis (**20**) cranioventrally. The last coccygeal vertebra, which is without transverse processes, contains a fine suture (**21**) that serves as a breakline in cases of autotomy. The cardiac shadow (**11**) is clearly visible between the two scapulae (**5**).

The radiolucent lungs (**14**) extend to the caudal third of the body.

In the mid-celomic cavity, the esophagus (**16**) reaches the stomach (**17**). Cranially it is superimposed by the vertebral column. Only the first loop of the small intestine (**22**) can be recognized. The rest of the intestine (**18**) cannot be differentiated.

Laterally, close to the abdominal wall, the paired fat-bodies (**23**) are visible.

31

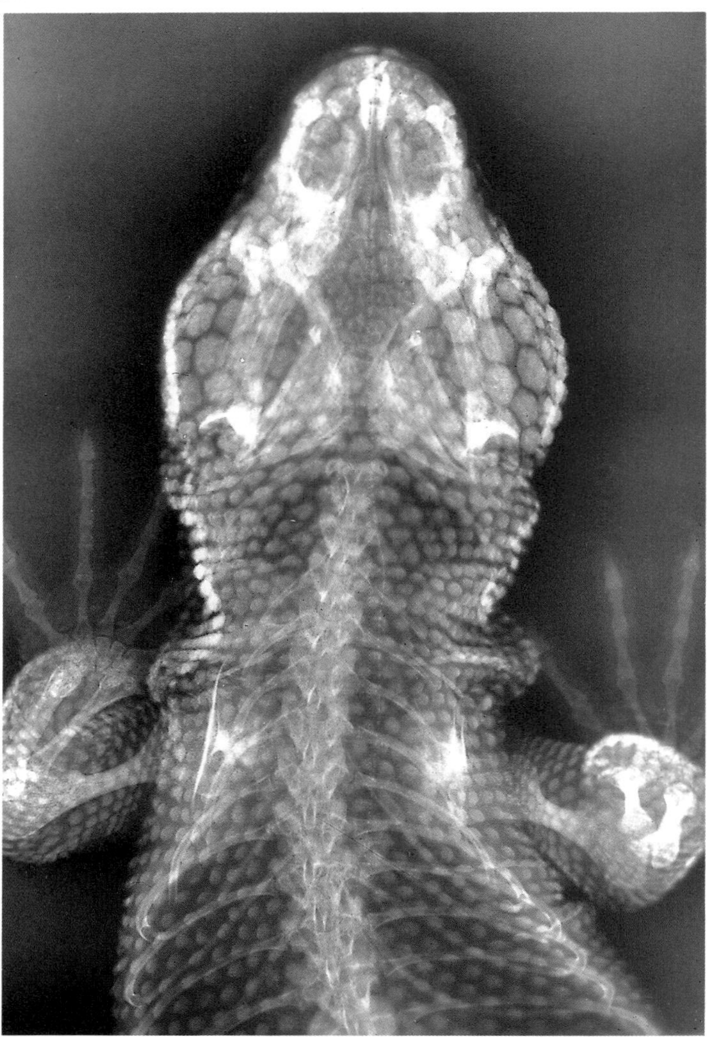

32

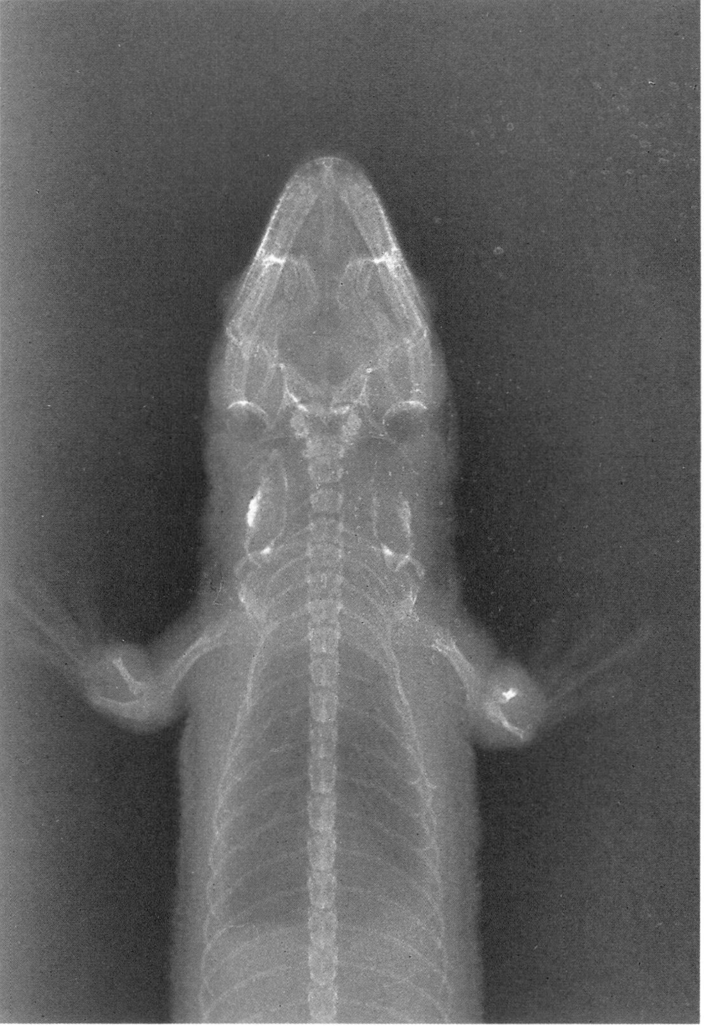

31 Calcified Scales.

Gila Monster *(Heloderma suspectum).*

In many species, calcified scales, especially on the head, complicate radiographic diagnosis. Although the head and neck of a gila monster are recognizable, it is difficult to indentify individual bones of the skull because of the superimposed shadows of the scales and it is impossible to evaluate soft tissues.

32 Calcium Reservoir (Chalk Saccule).

Malagasy Day Gecko *(Phelsuma madagascariensis).*

Some species, especially geckos, are able to store crystalline calcium in reservoirs.

On both sides of the neck an oval structure is displayed. Because the reservoirs are partially filled, only their margins are visible. If they are filled completely, they are much more obvious on radiographs.

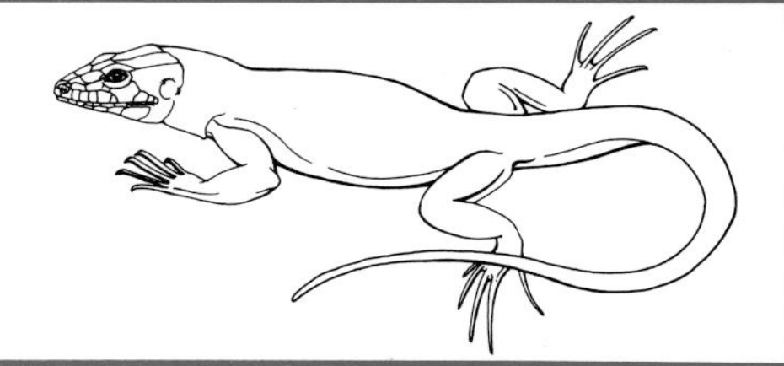

33

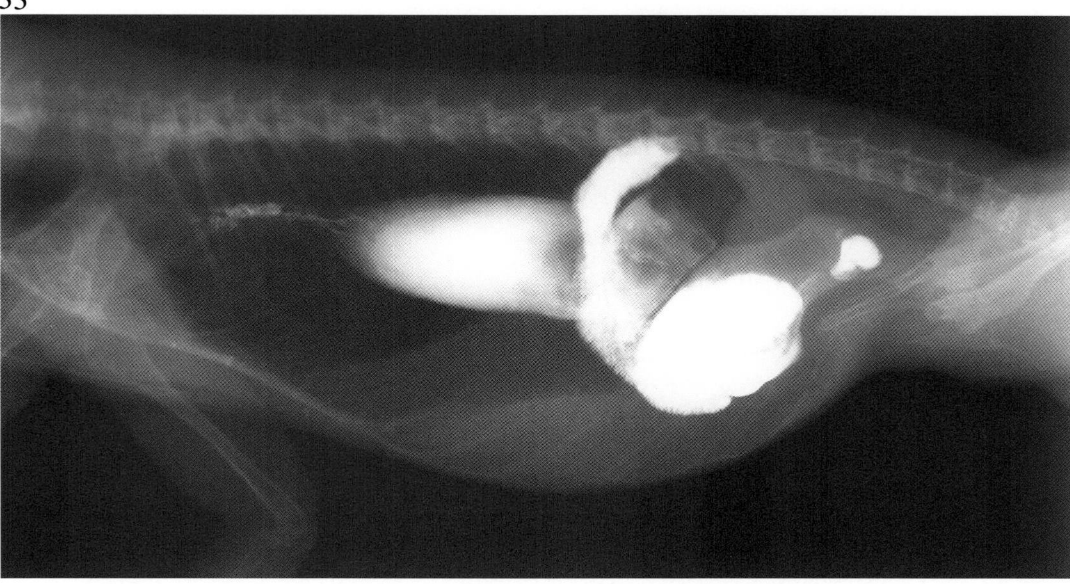

34

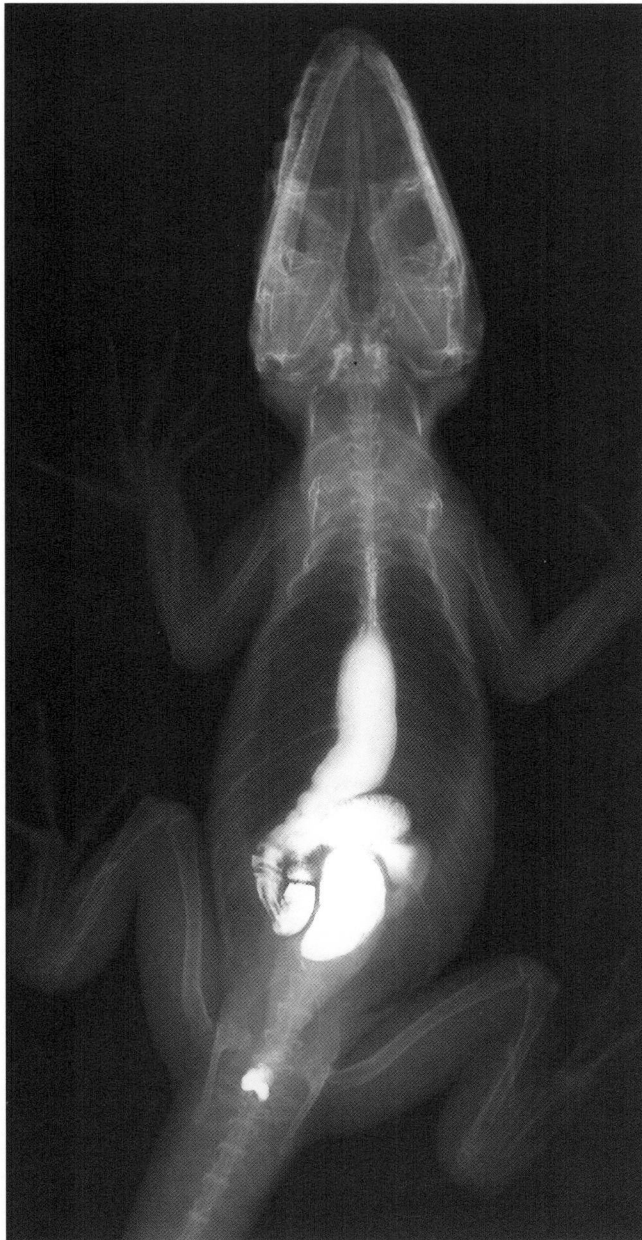

33/34 Normal Radiographic Appearance, lateral and dorsoventral: contrast study.

Cuban Giant Anole *(Anolis luteogularis).*

On radiographs made 4 hours after administration of barium sulfate, the gastrointestinal tract is filled with contrast medium. Stomach, intestines and cloaca are clearly defined. Because of peristaltic activity not all parts of the gastrointestinal tract have the same degree of filling. The rapid filling of the intestinal tract is conditioned by the period of fasting, the environmental temperature and the amount of contrast medium given.

Note: The small intestine is very short (carnivores).

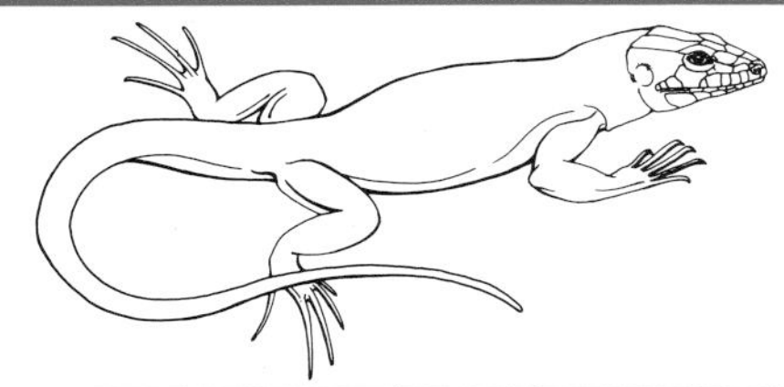

Reptiles: Lizards

Radiographic Abnormalities
Skeleton

35

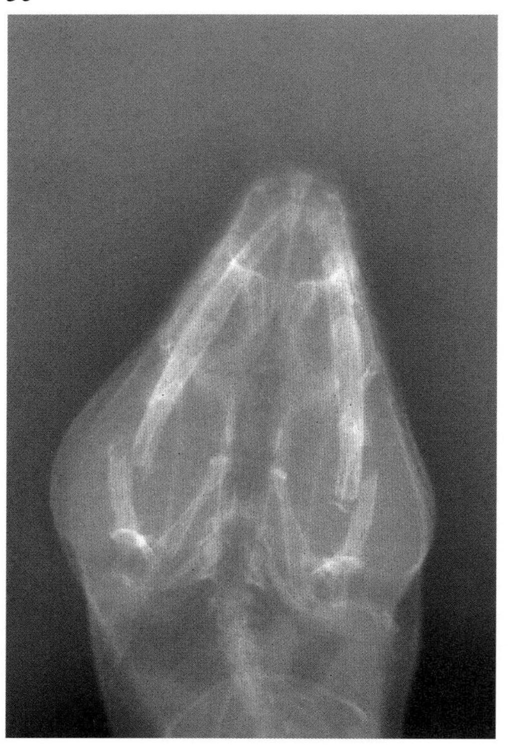

36

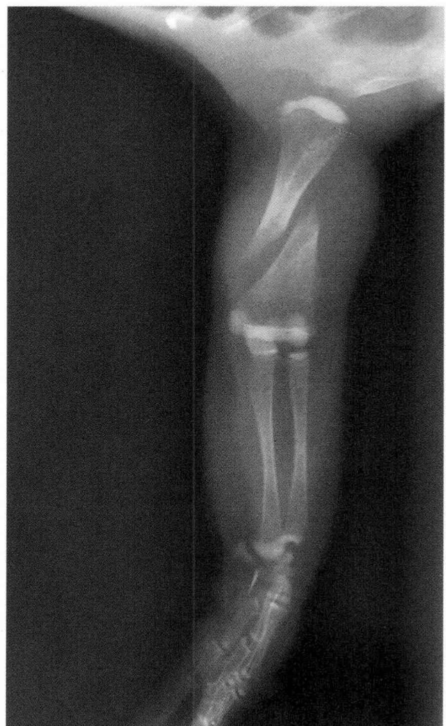

37

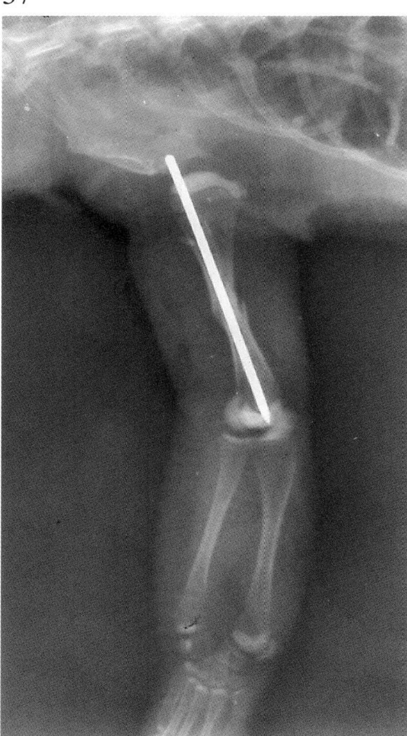

35 Fracture of the Jaw.

Pink-Tongued Lizard
(Tiliqua gerrardii).

The left and right maxillae and the mandibles are fractured symmetrically.

36/37 Fracture of the Humerus.

Two-Banded Monitor *(Varanus salvator).*

A diagonal mid-shaft fracture of the humerus is visible.

FIG. **37** has been taken after an intramedullary pin has been inserted into the marrow cavity of the bone from proximal to distal.

Note: Intramedullary pinning is a practical method for fracture repair in reptiles in spite of chondral ossification that is specific to reptiles.

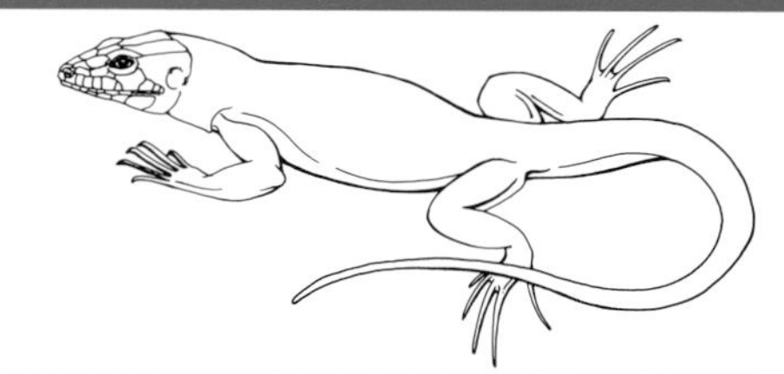

38

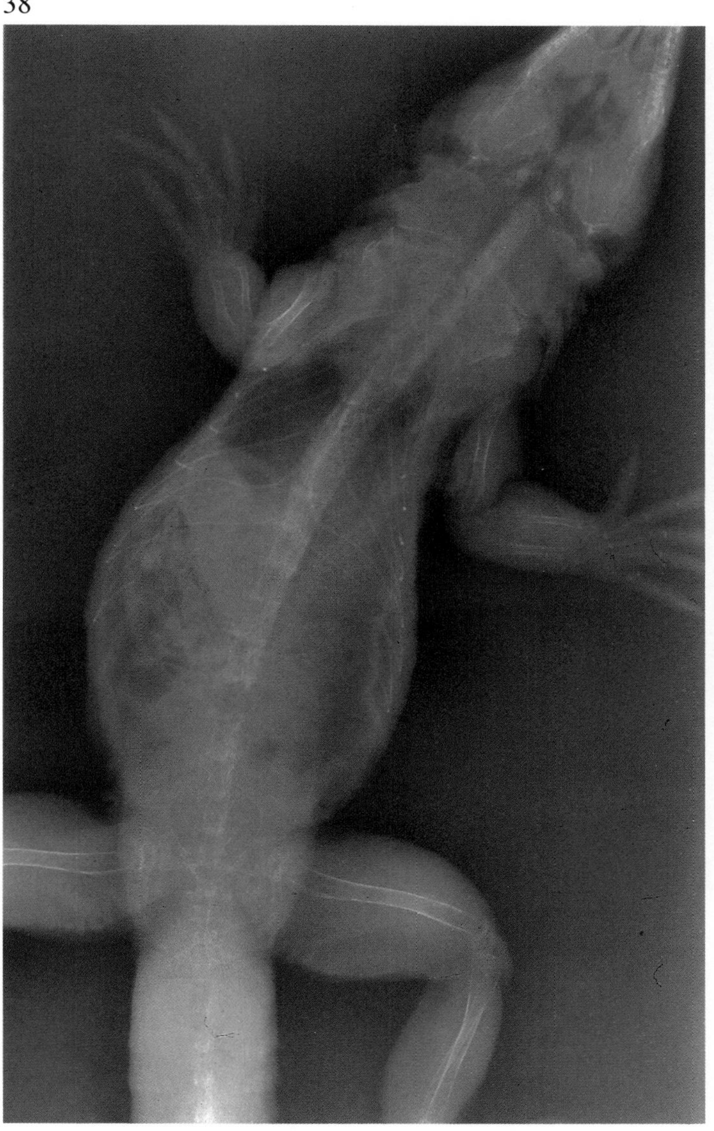

39

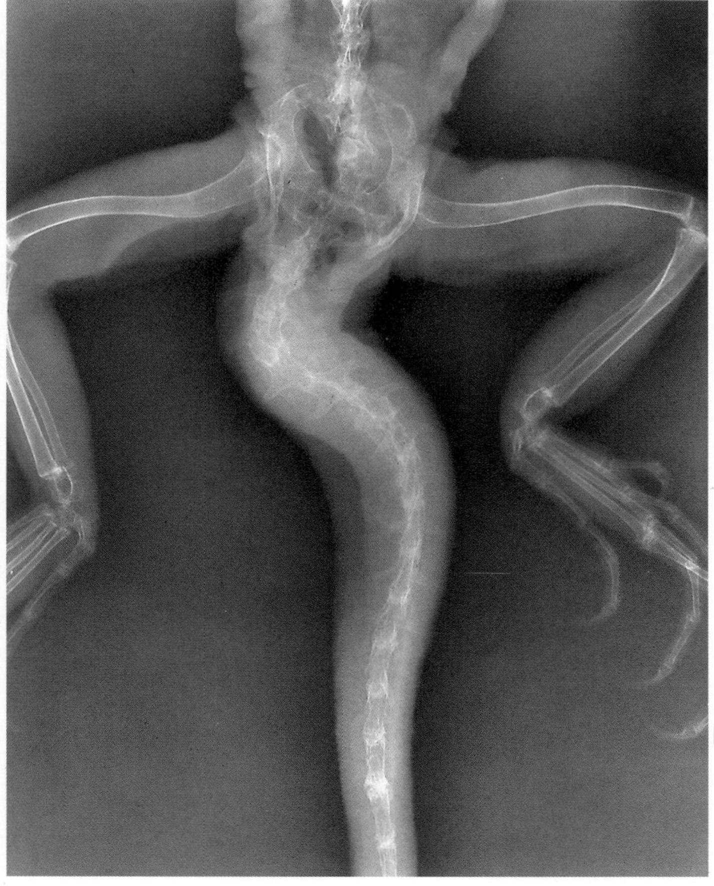

39 Metabolic bone disease.

Green Iguana *(Iguana iguana).*

Deformation of coccygeal and sacral vertebrae are a characteristic late consequence of rickets.

38 Generalized Fibrous Osteodystrophy.

Black Iguana *(Ctenosaura sp.).*

Most of the skeletal structures, especially the skull, the spine and the epiphyses, are difficult to see. The poor bone density is the result of severe demineralization of the skeleton due to chronic vitamin D_3 and calcium deficient diet. The soft tissues of the limbs are swollen and relatively radiodense due to the thick fibrous tissue cuffs around the long bones.

This picture is characteristic for generalized fibrous osteodystrophy, found especially in iguanid lizards.

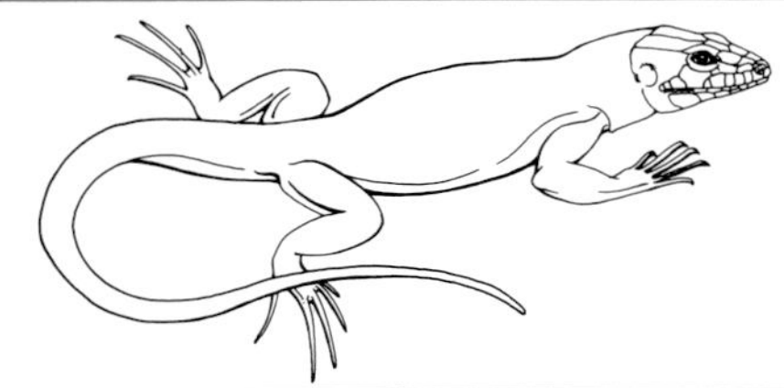

40

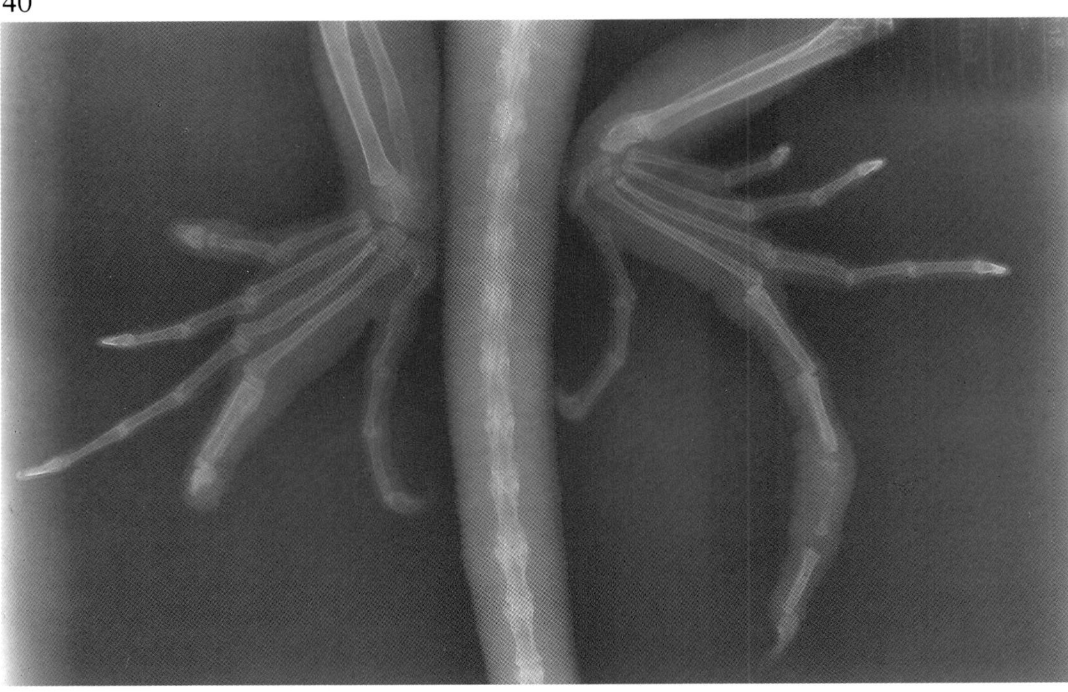

41

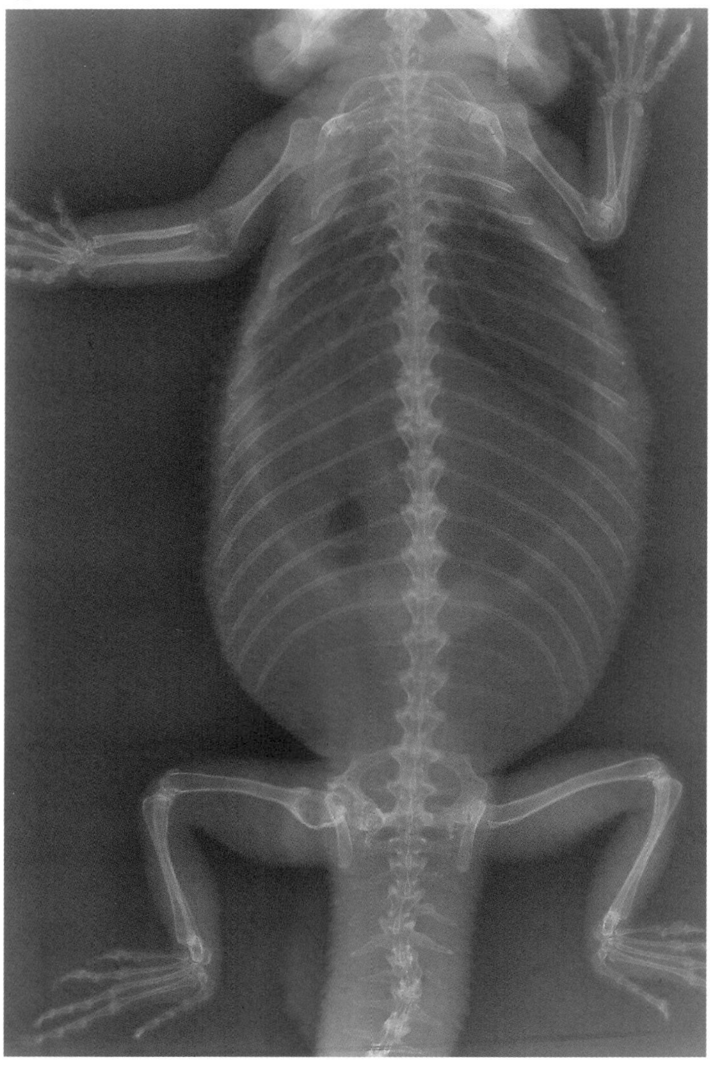

40 Osteomyelitis.

Green Iguana *(Iguana iguana).*

Of the right hind limb, one phalanx is osteolytic. The soft tissues are swollen and radiodense. These changes are characteristic for osteomyelitis caused by a bite-wound.

41 Septic Arthritis.

Midland Bearded Dragon *(Amphibolurus vitticeps).*

The bony parts of the elbow show severe bone destruction. In addition, the head of the left femur is expanded due to metastatic infection. These findings are typical for an infectious arthritis that developed after a bite-wound.

In the tail, multiple fractures of transverse processes are present. Some vertebrae are fused by callus formation.

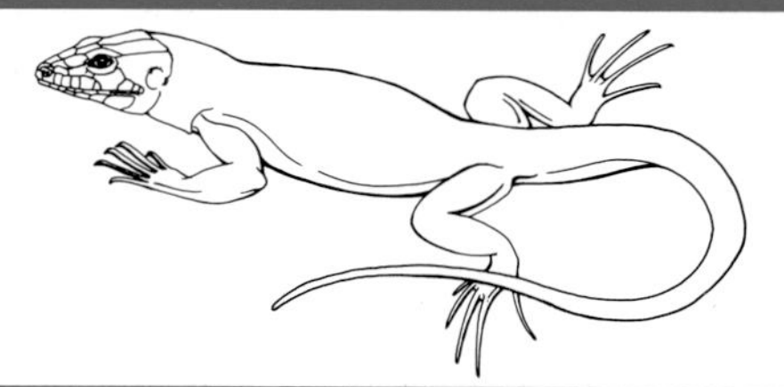

42

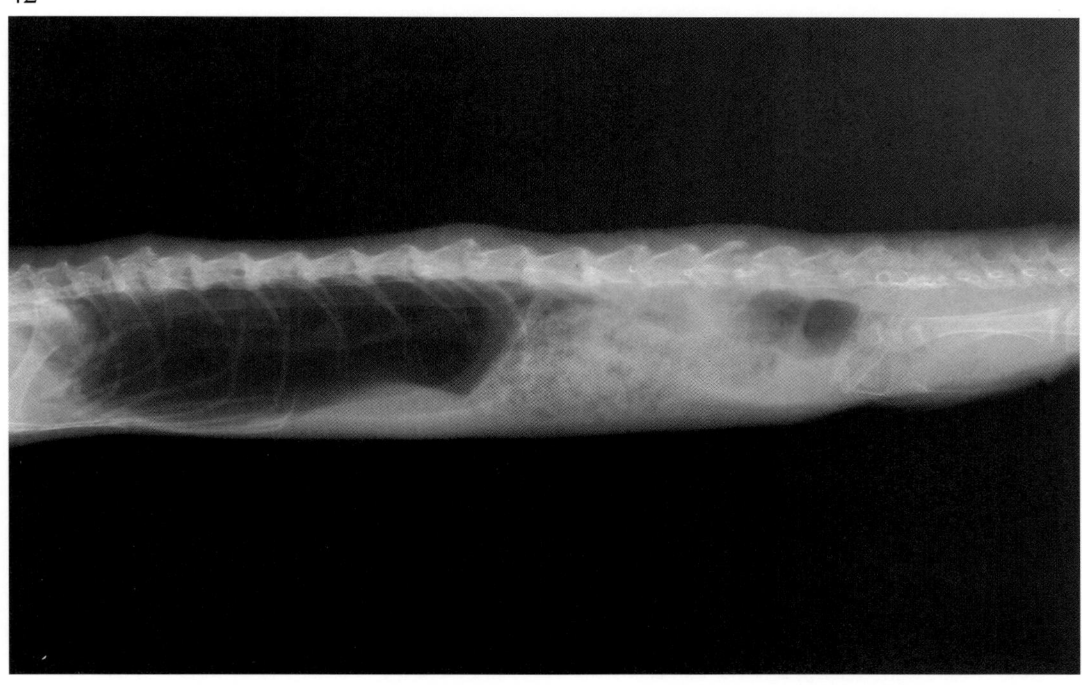

42 Calcinosis.

Indian Spiny-Tailed Lizard *(Uromastix hardwicki).*

In the region of the thoracic vertebral column, two soft tissue humps are noticed. The vertebrae in that region are fused and have a swollen appearance. The aorta is clearly visible.

These signs are characteristic of calcinosis with alterations of the bones and vessels caused by chronic intake of high dosages of vitamin D_3 and calcium.

43

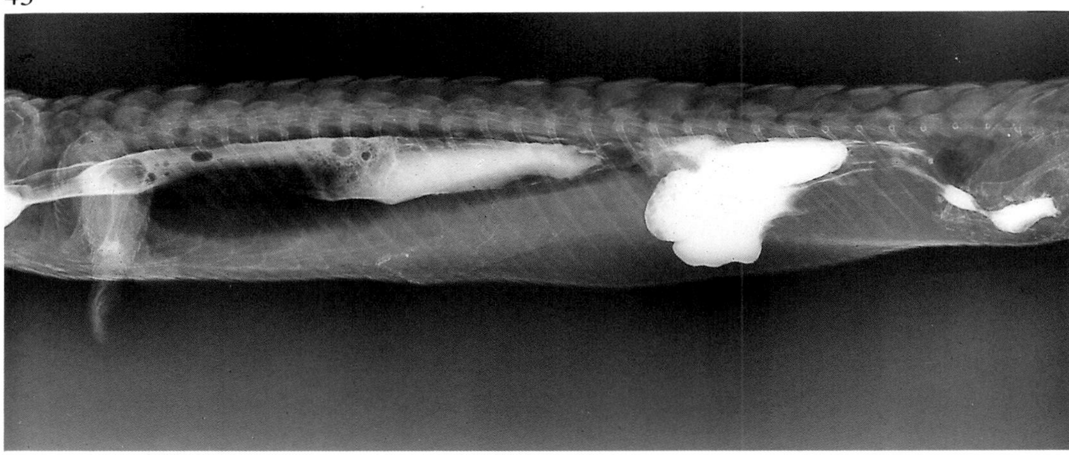

44

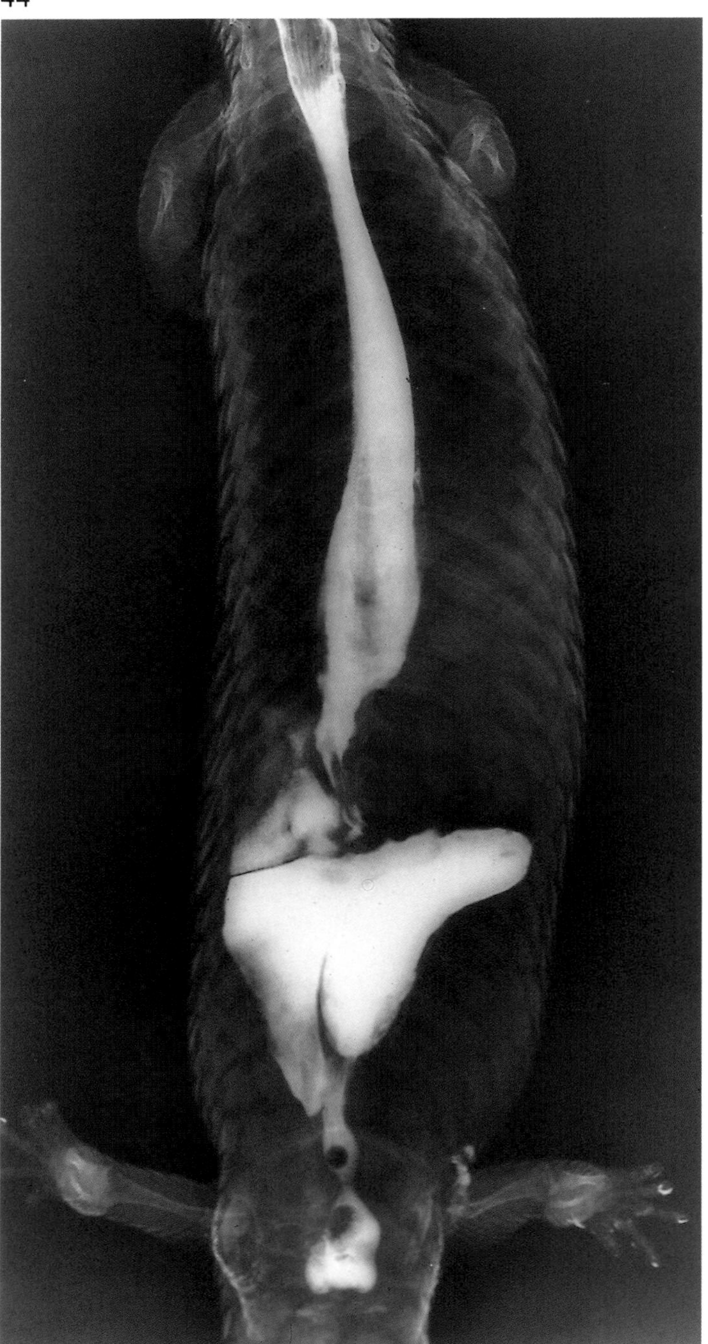

43/44 Enteritis: contrast study.

Shingle-Back *(Trachydosaurus rugosus)*.

On the lateral radiograph, 6 h after the administration of barium sulfate, a dilated esophagus is visible. It is difficult to distinguish the esophagus from the stomach that begins approximately in the middle of the pulmonary region.

The barium sulfate suspension has passed through the entire digestive tract within 6 h. This is much too fast and indicates intestinal inflammation. The normal passage time in this species is 3 to 6 weeks, depending on feeding, environmental temperature and activity.

The enteritis was caused by a candida infection.

In this species, also calcified bony scales are visible.

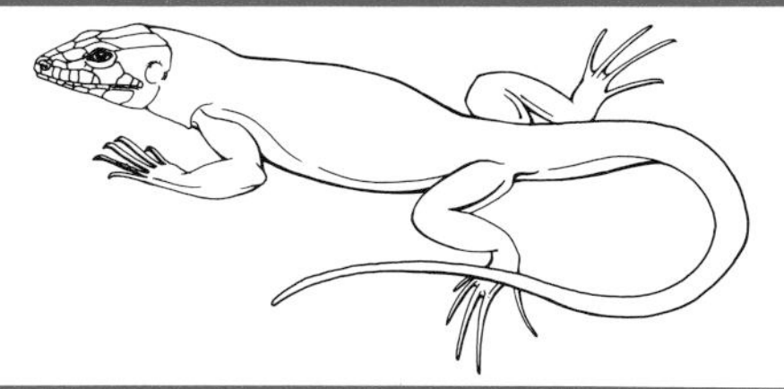

45

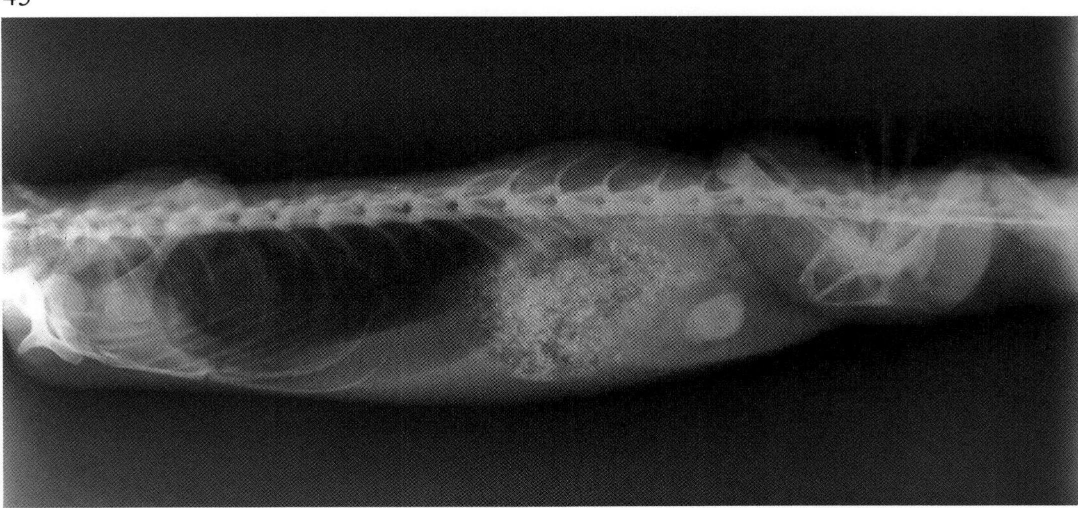

46

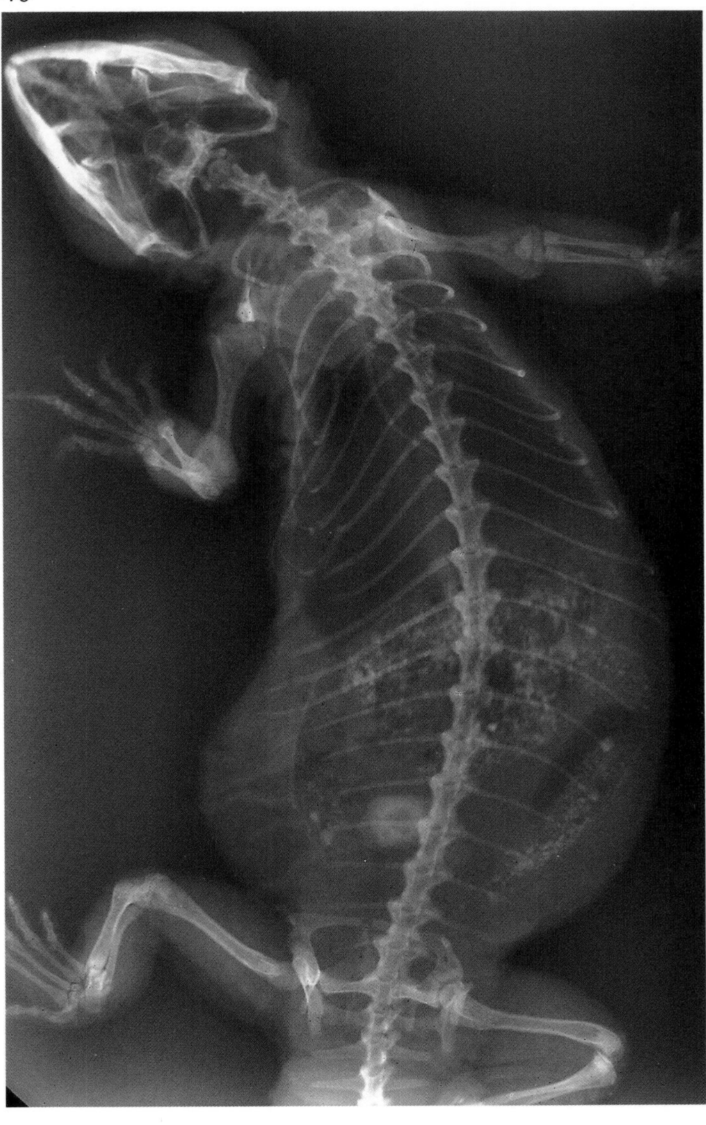

45/46 Constipation.

African Spiny Tailed Lizard *(Uromastix acanthinurus)*.

The large intestine is filled with impacted sand and little stones. On both radiographs, an anal bladder calculus is visible just cranial to the pelvis.

Note: In addition, the lizard has multiple old fractures of the ribs.

47

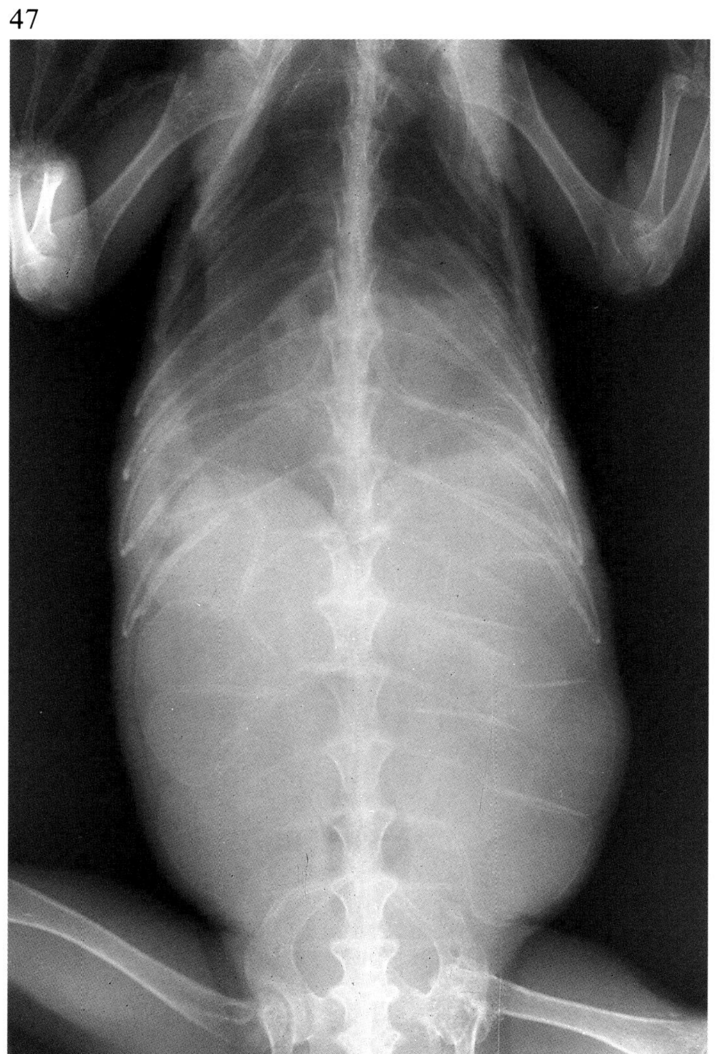

47A

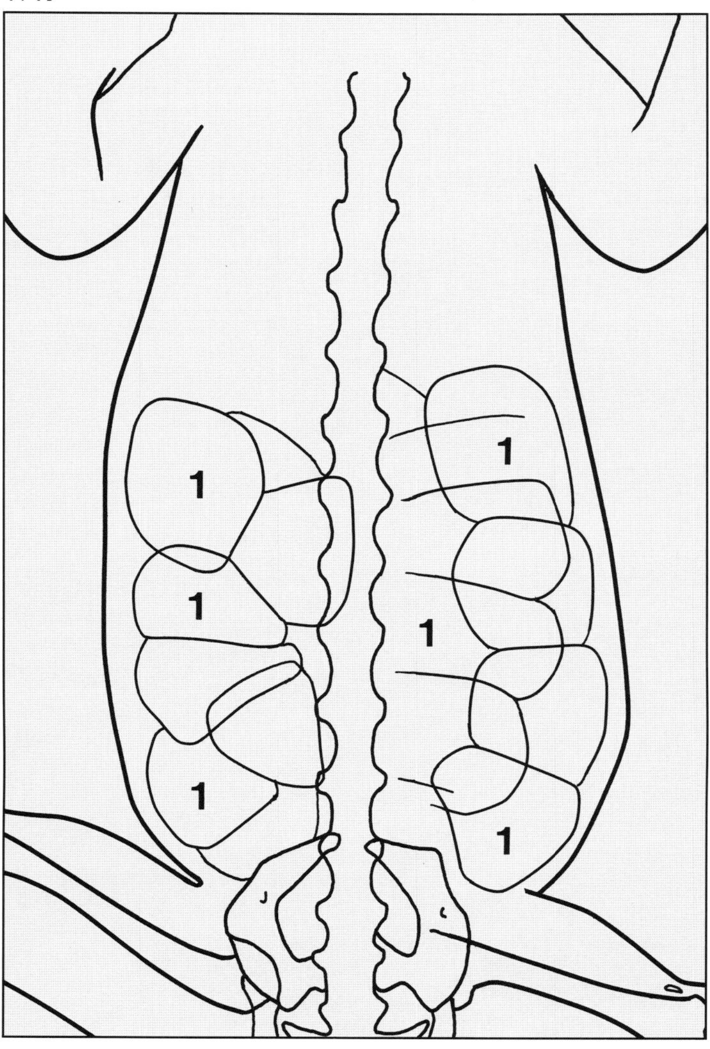

47/47A Normal Gravidity.

Green Iguana *(Iguana iguana).*

Several incompletely calcified eggs (**1**) that seem to be quadrangular and present in a "roll of money"-like alignment are visible. This indicates an early stage of gravidity.

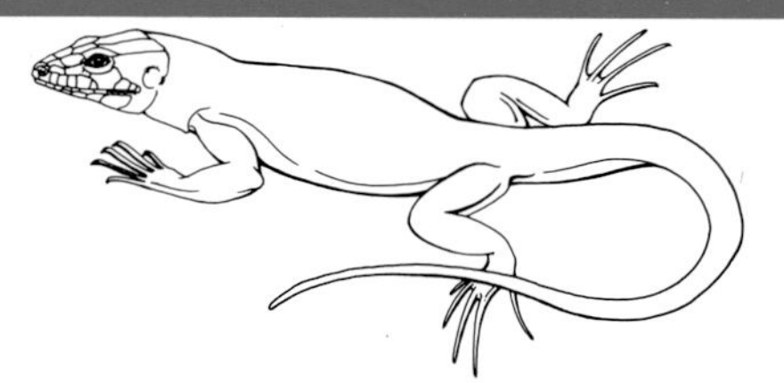

48

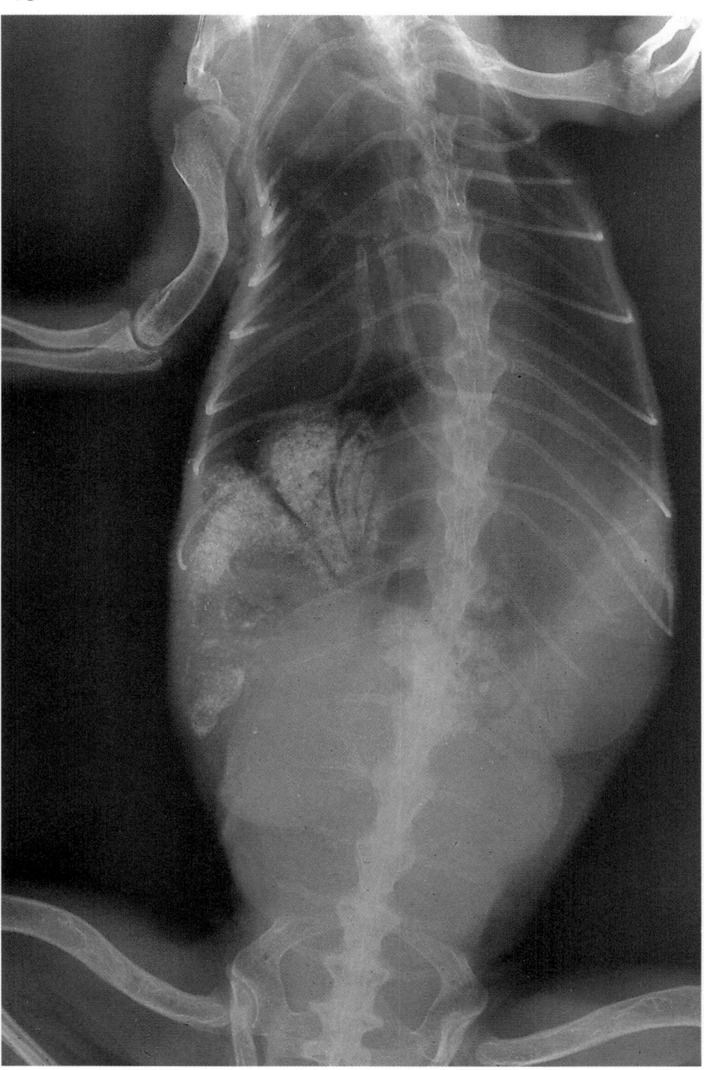

49

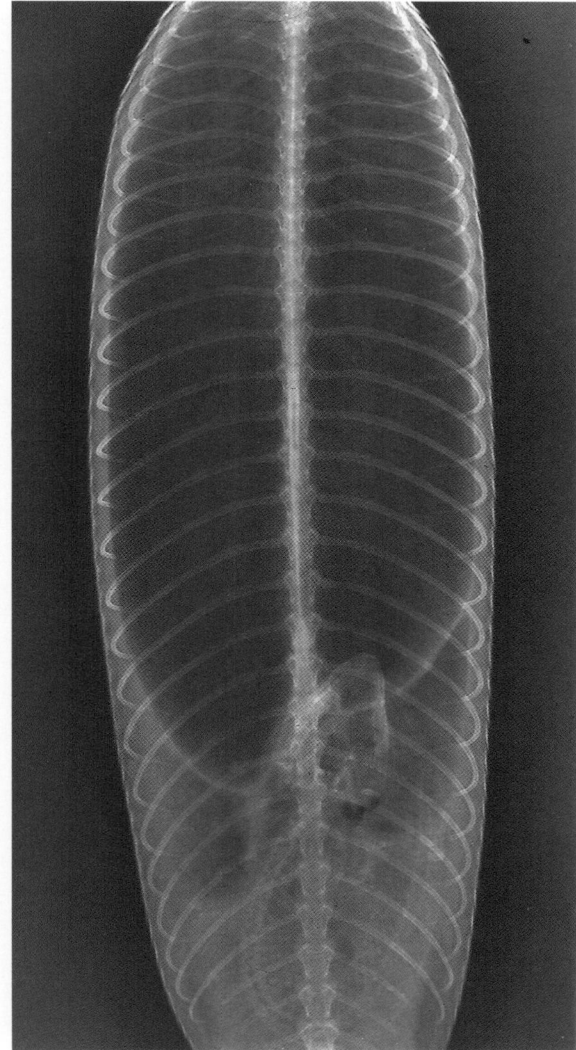

48 Egg Binding.

Green Iguana *(Iguana iguana).*

In the caudal part of the body, ovoid and round calcified eggs are visible. The large intestine is filled with impacted ingesta (constipation). Along with the clinical symptoms, this finding confirms the diagnosis of egg binding.

Note: In this herbivorous species, the large intestine is segmented into compartments similar to the omasum of cattle.

49 Ovoviviparous Gravidity.

Blotched Blue-Tongued Lizard *(Tiliqua nigrolutea).*

The skeleton of a mature fetus is visible.

Note: In this species, the embryos develop within the body cavity. The egg membranes rupture during birth. In this case, the embryo died as a result of mal-positioning. Because it was known that the lizard gave birth to two young animals two weeks previously, this single fetus had to be dead. This was the indication for immediate surgery.

50

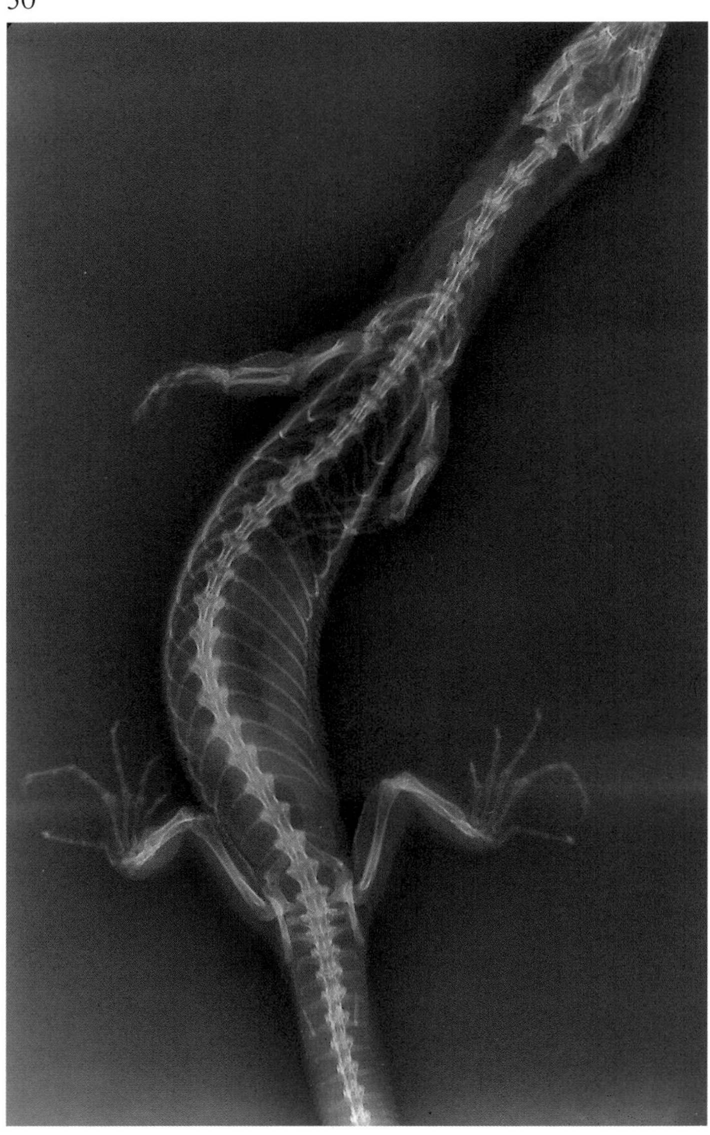

51

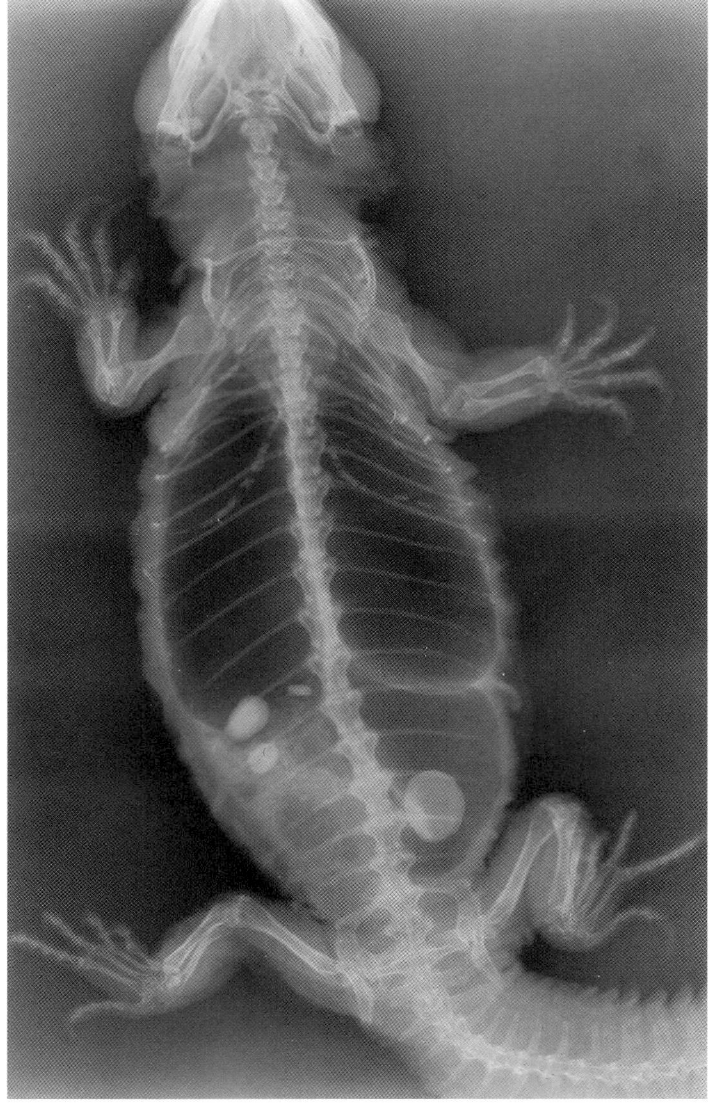

50 Calcified Hemipenes.

Timor Monitor *(Varanus timorensis).*

The calcified cylindrical hemipenes are visible posterior to the pelvis, on both sides of the vertebral column.

In some species, this is a method to determine the sex of a lizard.

51 Anal Bladder Calculus.

African Spiny Tailed Lizard *(Uromastix acanthinurus).*

Caudal to the pulmonary radiolucencies, a congested large intestine is visible on the left side and a round radiodense structure surrounded by gas is visible on the right side. An anal bladder calculus was found at surgery.

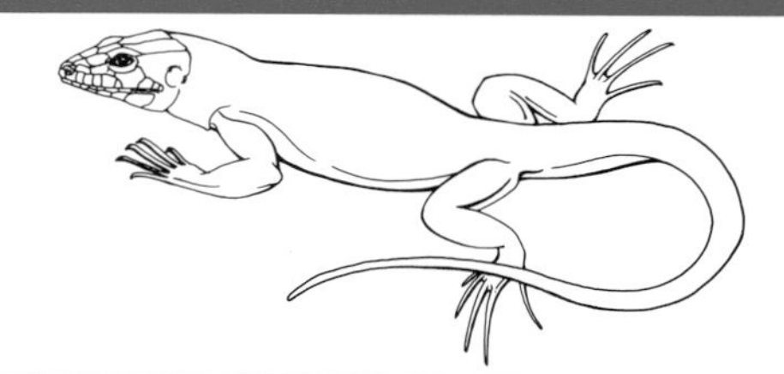

52

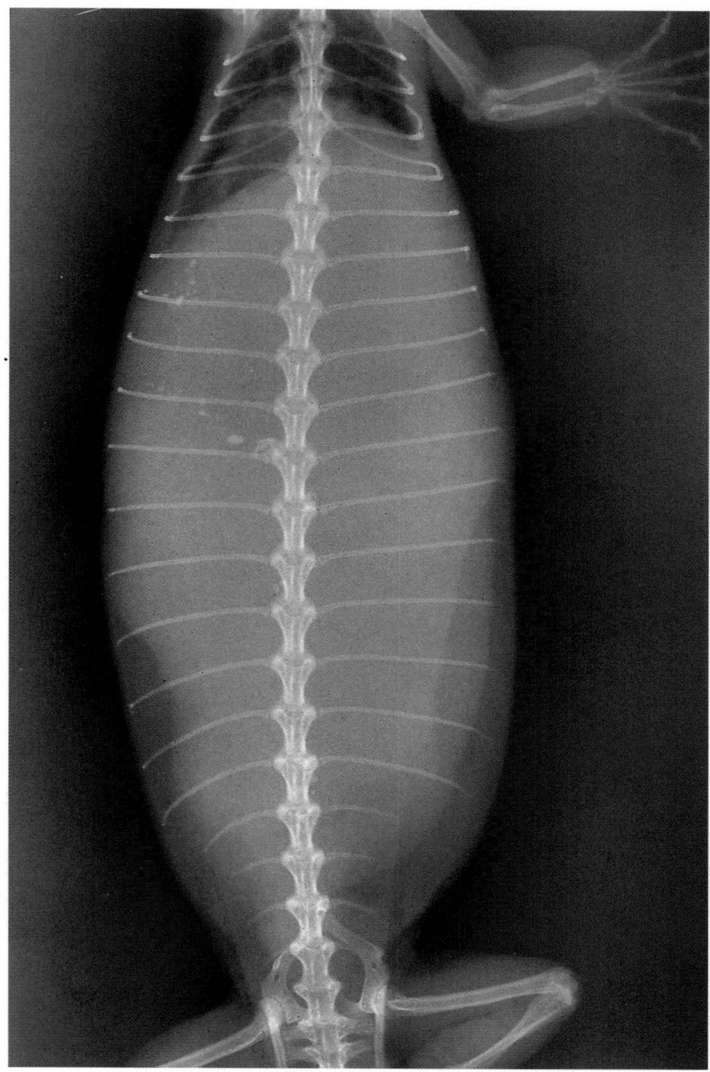

53

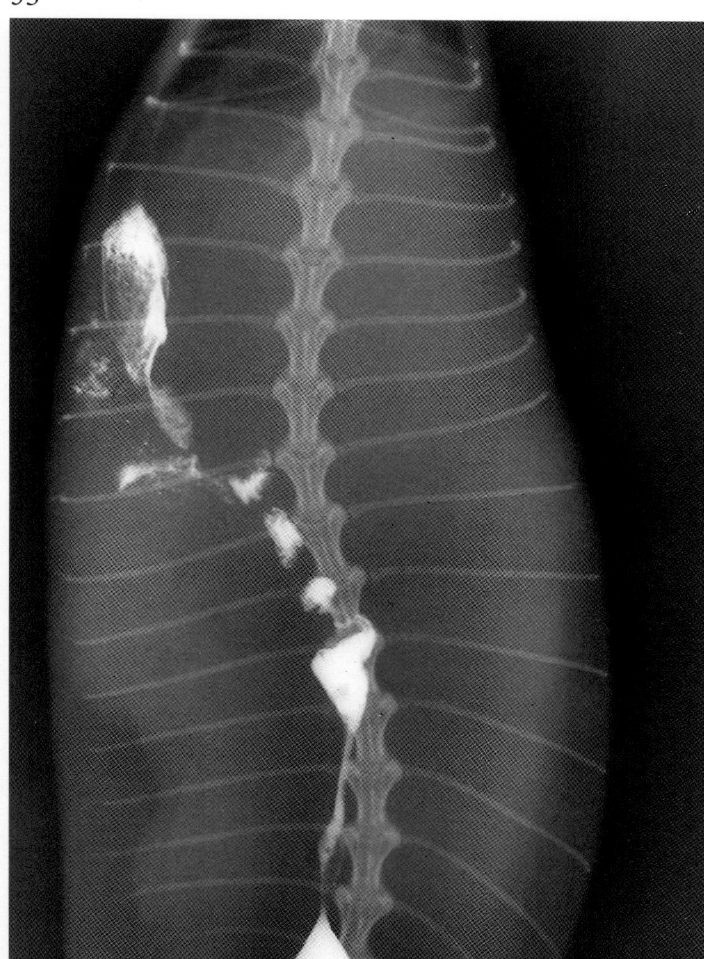

52/53 Ascites.

Timor Monitor *(Varanus timorensis).*

The entire celomic cavity presents with a ground-glass appearance. Caudolaterally and close to the wall of the body the radiolucent shadows of the fat bodies are visible.

FIG. **53** shows that a barium sulfate suspension has passed unimpeded through the digestive tract, 24 h after administration. There seems to be no cause-and-effect connection between the gastrointestinal tract and the generalized density of the celomic cavity.

The opacity proved to be the result of ascites due to hepatic degeneration.

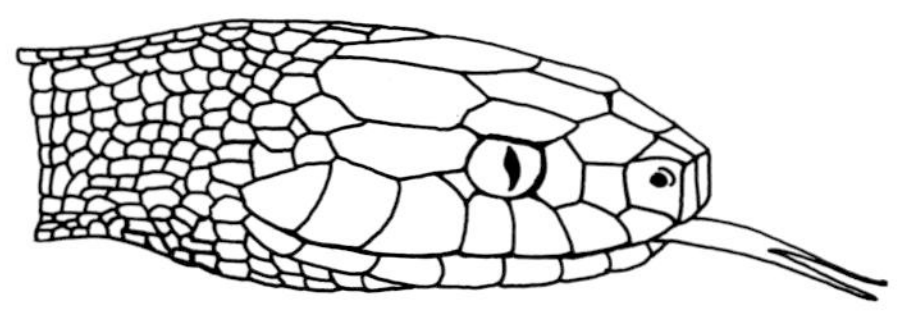

Reptiles: Snakes

Radiographic Anatomy
Internal Organs and Skeleton

54-1

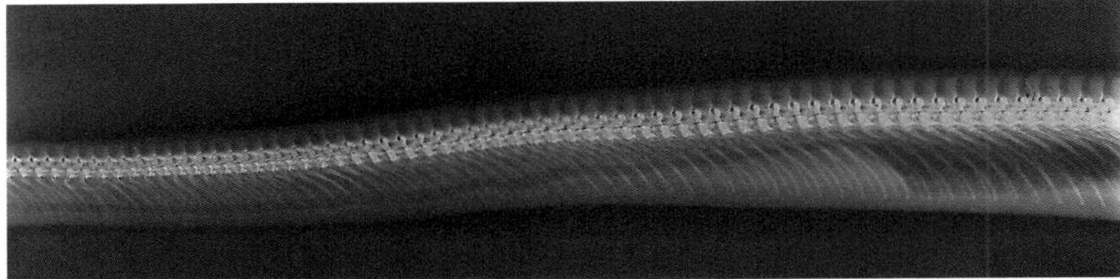

54-1 A

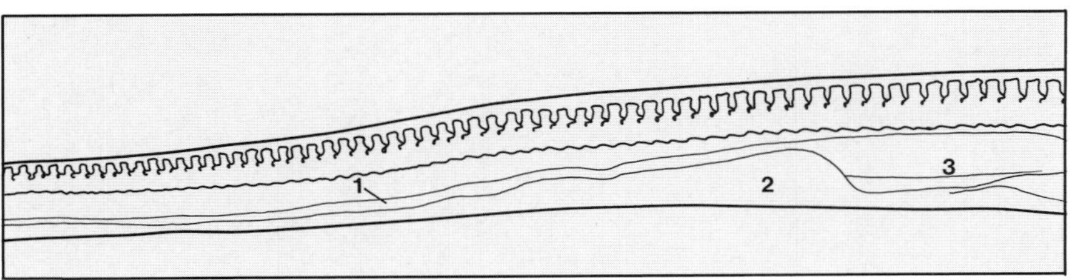

54-2

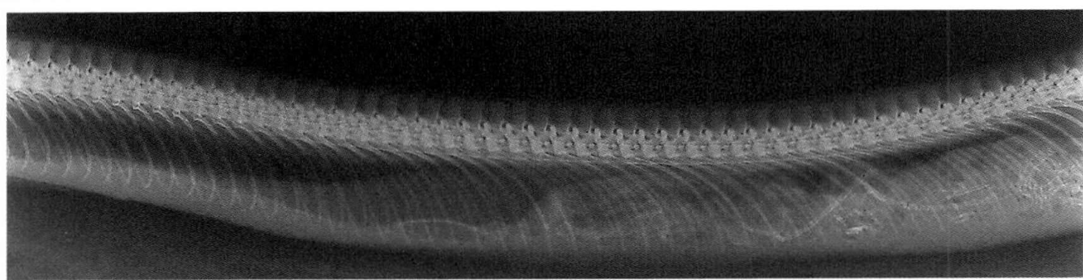

54-2 A

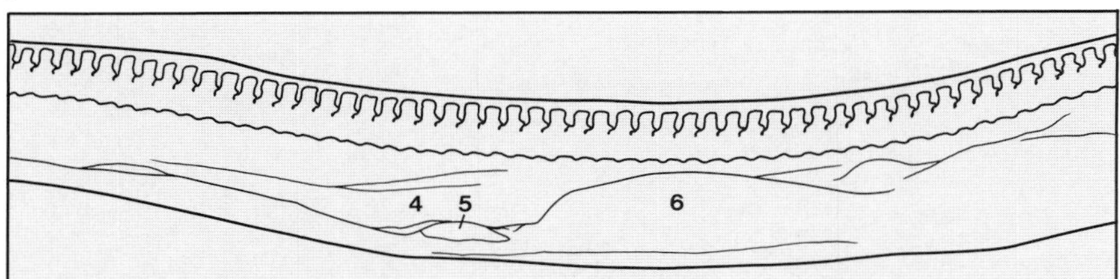

54-3

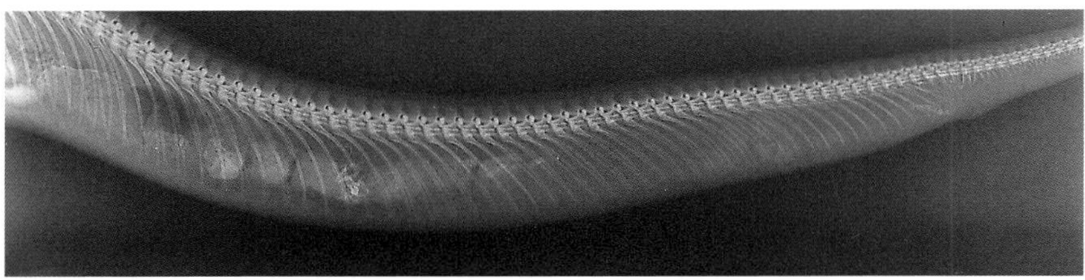

54-3 A

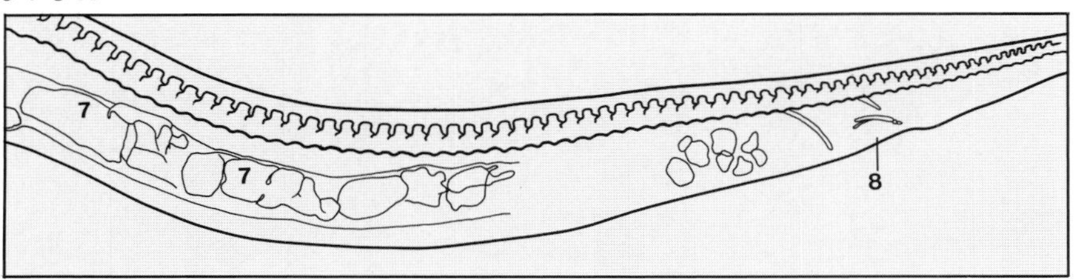

54-1/54-1A/54-2/54-2A/54-3/54-3A Normal Radiographic Appearance, lateral.

Royal Python *(Python regius).*

The cranial third of the snake's body is placed on top, the middle third in between, and the caudal third below.

On these radiographs, the trachea (**1**) is visible beginning slightly caudal to the head. Curving around the shadow of the heart (**2**) it extends to the lungs (**3**).

The liver (**4**) is located ventral to the lungs. Caudal to the liver the gallbladder (**5**) is visible as a separate shadow. Caudal to the lungs, the stomach (**6**) is filled with two mice. It fades into the intestines (**7**), that are filled with impacted ingesta. Ventral to the intestine, the paired fat bodies are visible. They contain the gonads and the kidneys that cannot be seen as seperate structures.

Boid snakes possess a rudimental pelvis (**8**) that is visible ventral to the last three pairs of ribs.

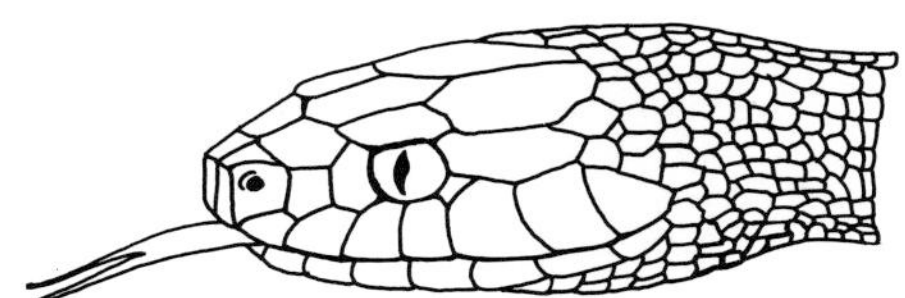

55

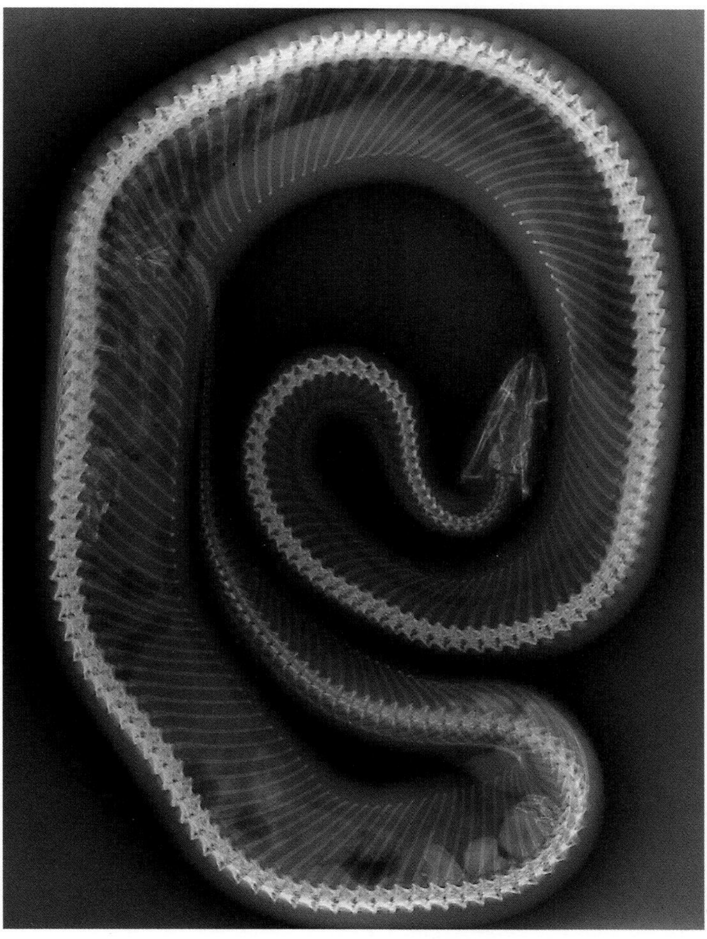

55 A

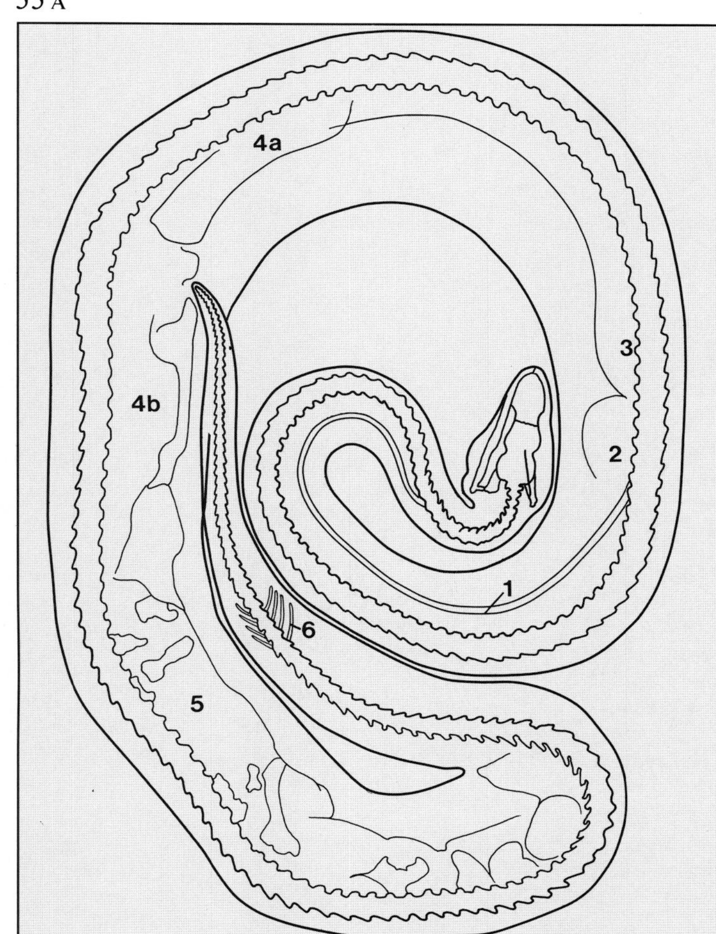

55/55A Normal Radiographic Appearance, dorsoventral.

Royal Python *(Python regius).*

In the cranial third part of the body, the trachea (**1**) extends from the head to the cardiac shadow (**2**) and the lungs (**3**). In some species, the lungs extend into the caudal third part of the body. Caudally, the lungs extend into an air sac without respiratory epithelium, similar to the air sacs of birds.

The stomach is located in the middle third part of the body. In this snake it contains two mice (**4a, 4b**) which can be identified by their skeletons. The intestines (**5**) are filled with impacted ingesta and gas. The last pair of ribs (**6**) indicates the position of the cloaca.

In snakes, total immobilization is necessary for exact dorsoventral positioning; during routine radiography partial rotation of the body is unavoidable most of the time.

56

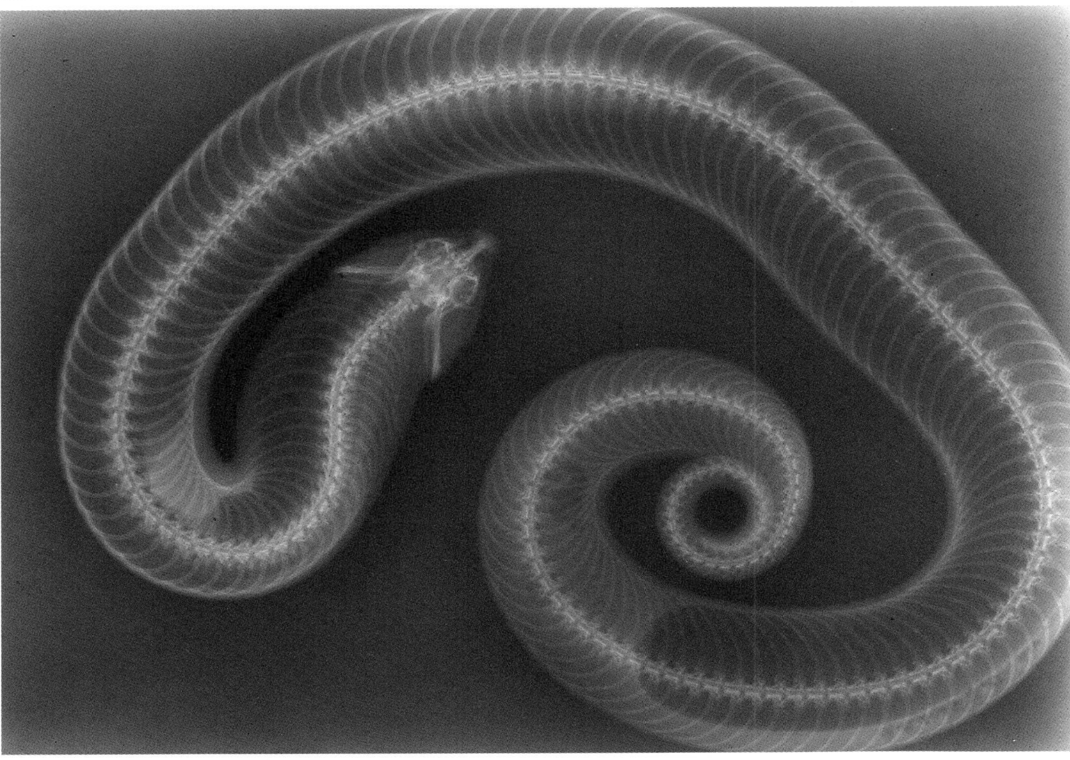

57

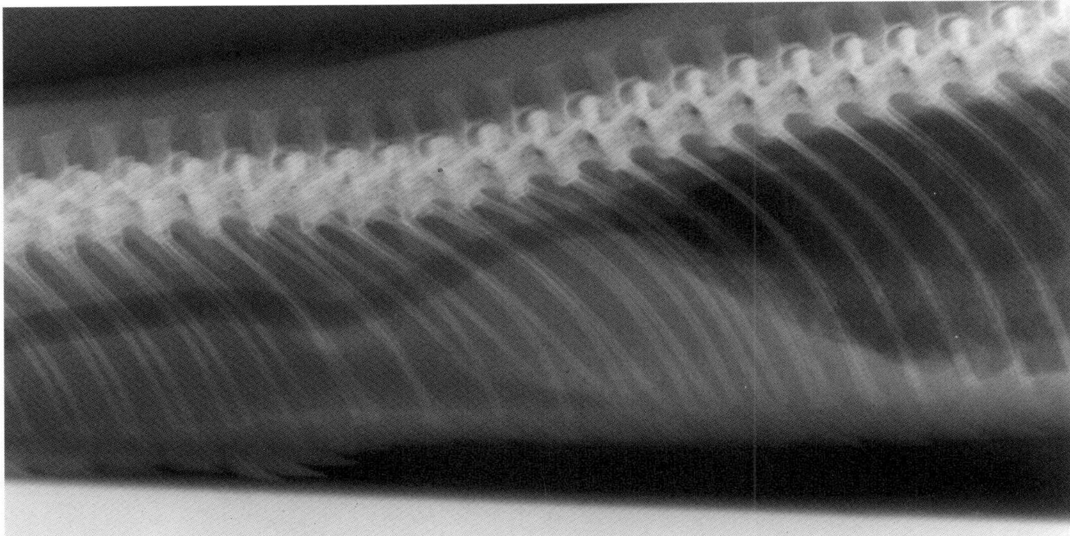

56 Lungs: Normal Radiographic Appearance, dorsoventral.

Western Shovel Nosed Snake *(Heterodon nasicus gloydii).*

In this species, the right lung and air sac extend to the caudal third of the body. In many species, a similar situation is physiologic. It is not due to hyperinflation.

57 Heart: Normal Radiographic Appearance, lateral.

Boa constrictor *(Boa constrictor).*

The trachea curves dorsally to pass over the heart. Cranial to the cardiac shadow the thyroid gland is visible. Within the contours of the right lung, the radiolucent cylindrical shadow of the rudimentary left lung is displayed.

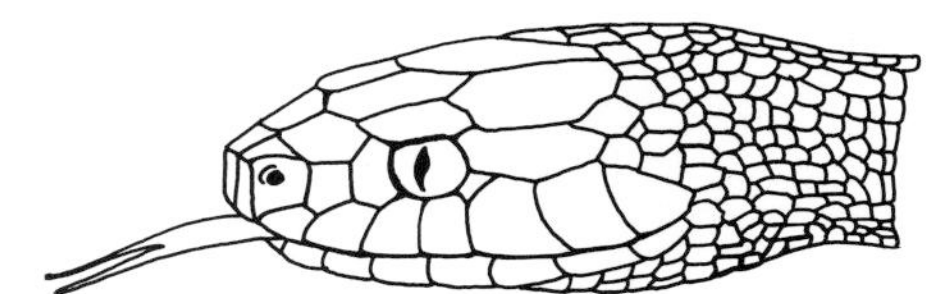

58

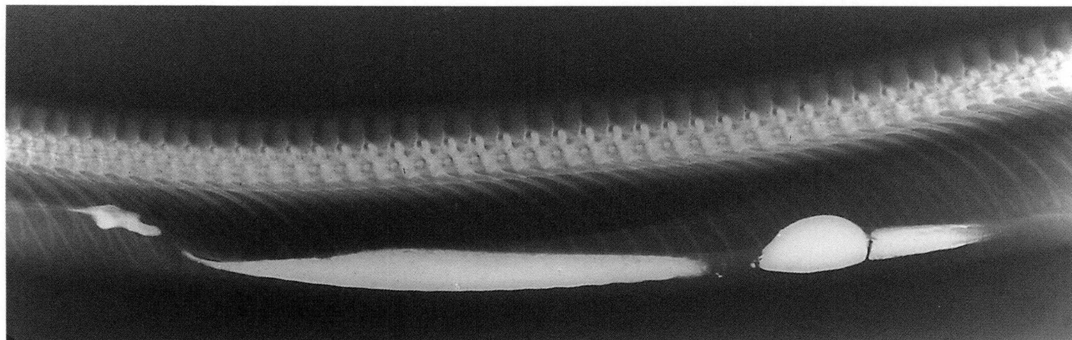

59

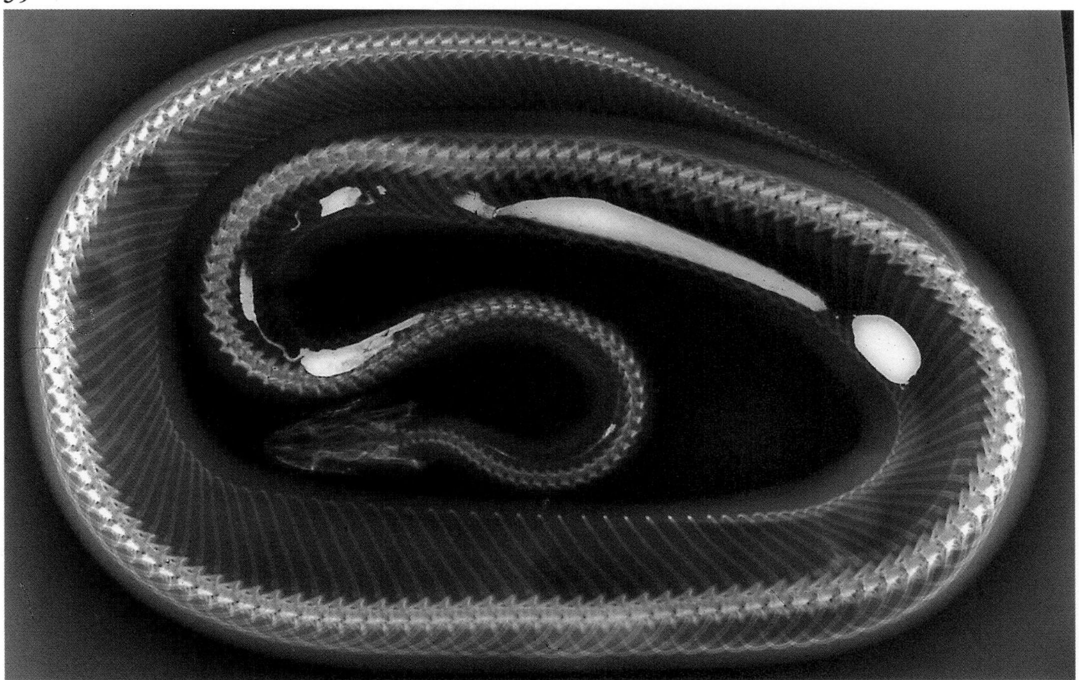

58/59 Normal Radiographic Appearance,
lateral and dorsoventral: contrast study.

Royal Python *(Python regius)*.

On the lateral 30 min. contrast radiograph, the esophagus can be seen directly dorsal to the cardiac shadow, then turning ventrally and blending into the stomach. The first small intestinal loop lies horizontally. Peristaltic segmentation can be noted.

On the dorsoventral radiograph, the esophagus can be seen as a small stripe, with some dilated segments. The elongated stomach is clearly outlined by the contrast medium and the surrounding lungs. One loop of the small intestine contains contrast medium.

60

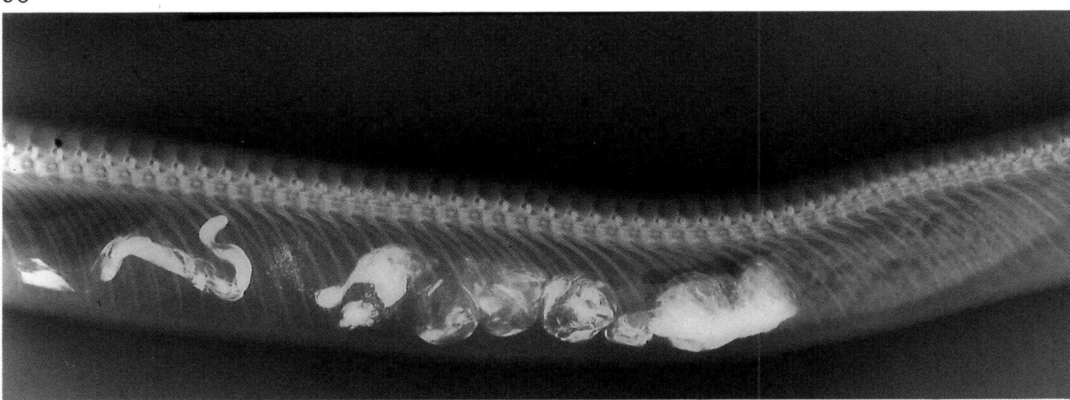

61

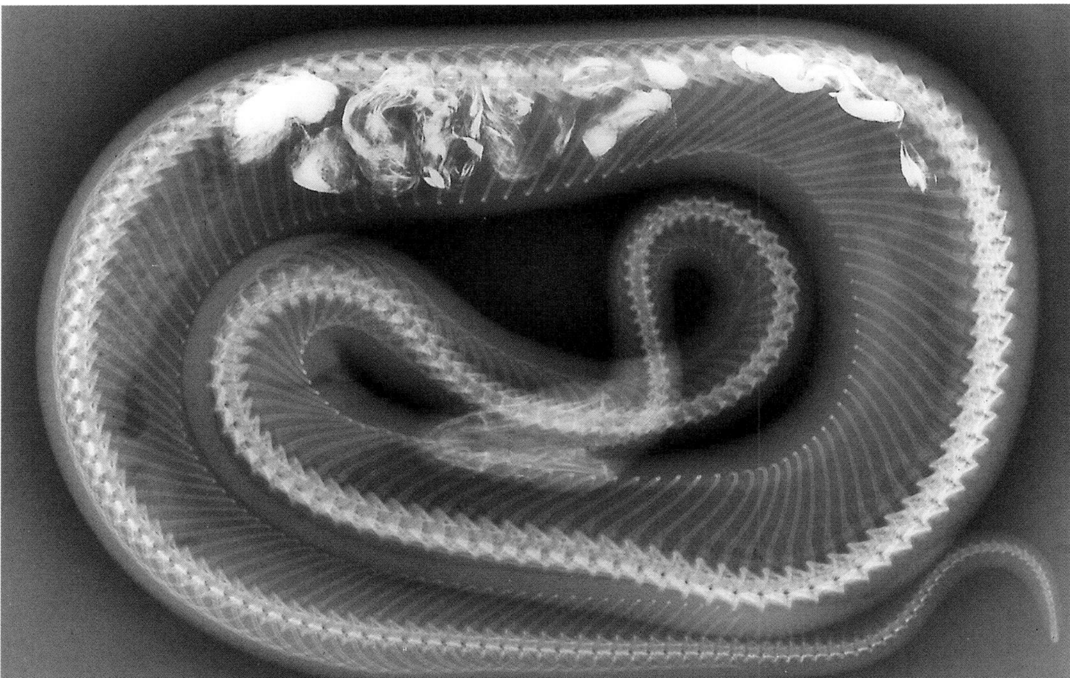

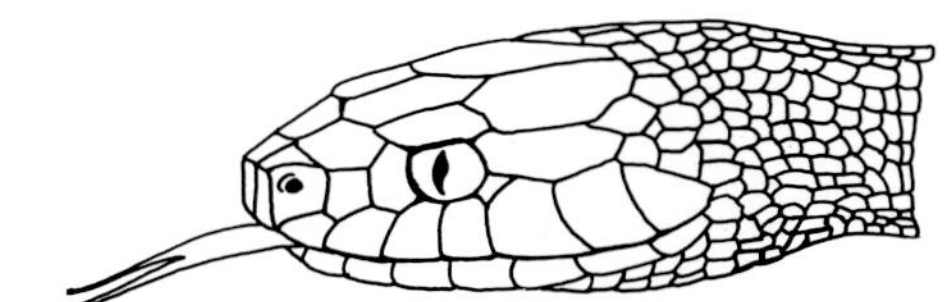

62

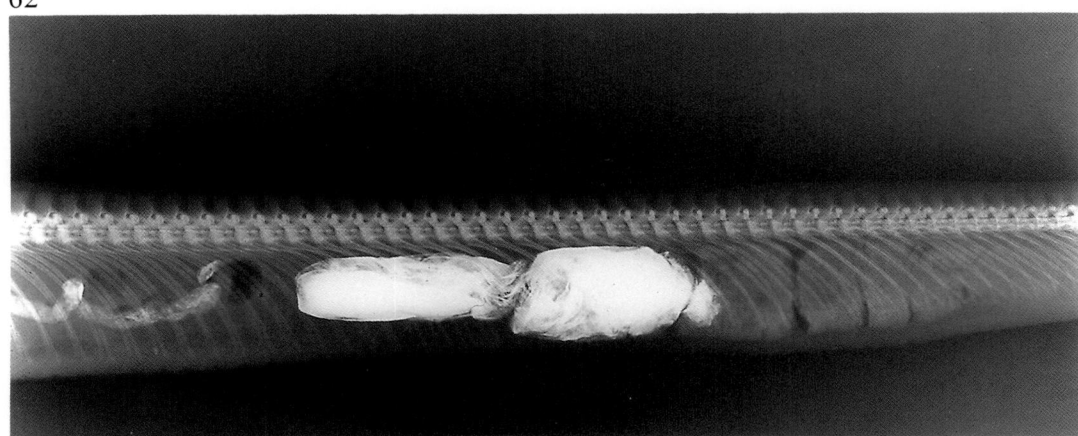

63

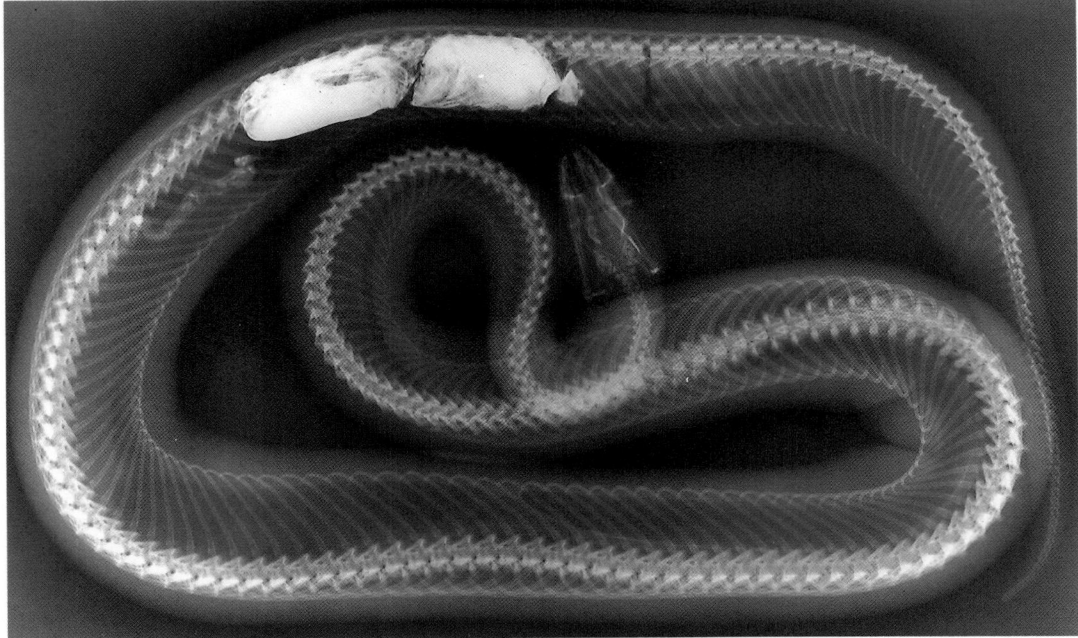

60-63 Normal Radiographic Appearance,
lateral and dorsoventral: contrast study.

Royal Python *(Python regius)*.

24 h after barium sulfate administration, several small intestinal loops are opacified, both in lateral (FIG. **60**) and in dorsoventral (FIG. **61**) projection.

On the lateral radiograph, taken 14 days later (FIG. **62**), the septation of the ingesta is obvious.

On the dorsoventral radiograph (FIG. **63**), the caudal portions of the small intestine and the large intestine are outlined. The disintegration of the ingesta is physiologic in most of the species.

64

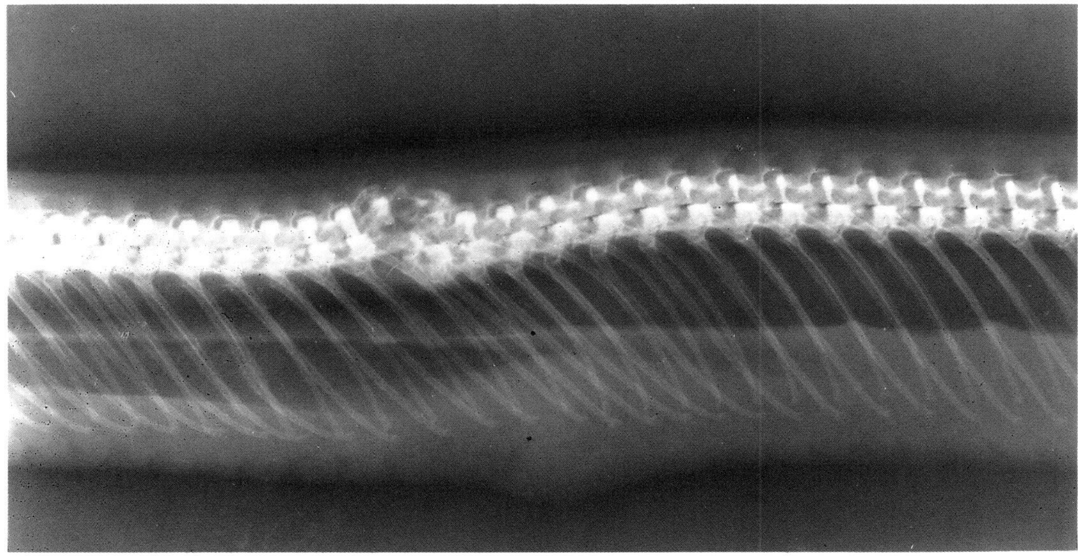

65

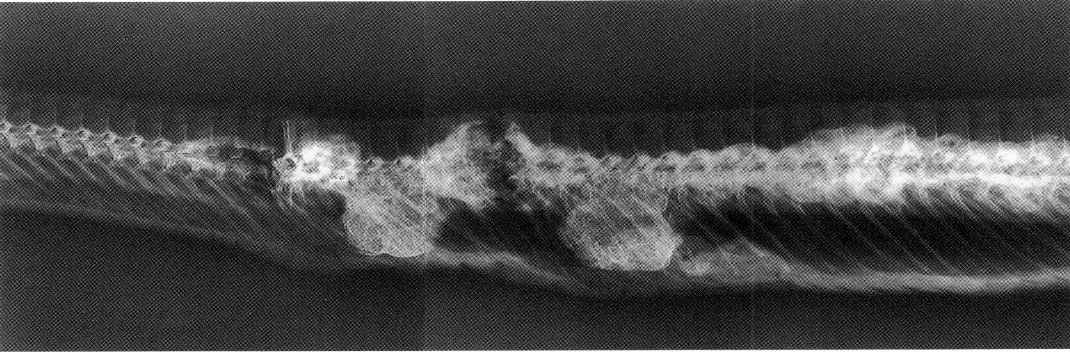

64 Fracture of the Vertebral Column.

Boa constrictor *(Boa constrictor)*.

A vertebral fracture with dislocation is present. Some callus formation is visible dorsally.

65 Osteitis deformans (Paget's Disease).

South American Rattlesnake *(Crotalus durissus)*.

Groups of vertebrae are fused and amorphous bone formations protrude into the body cavity. The etiology of this disease is unknown.

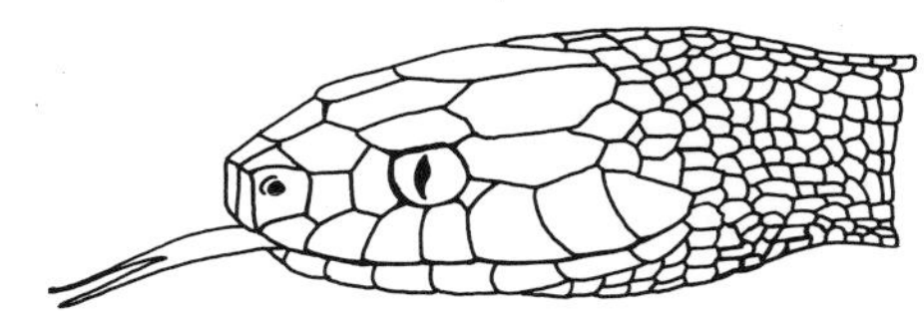

66

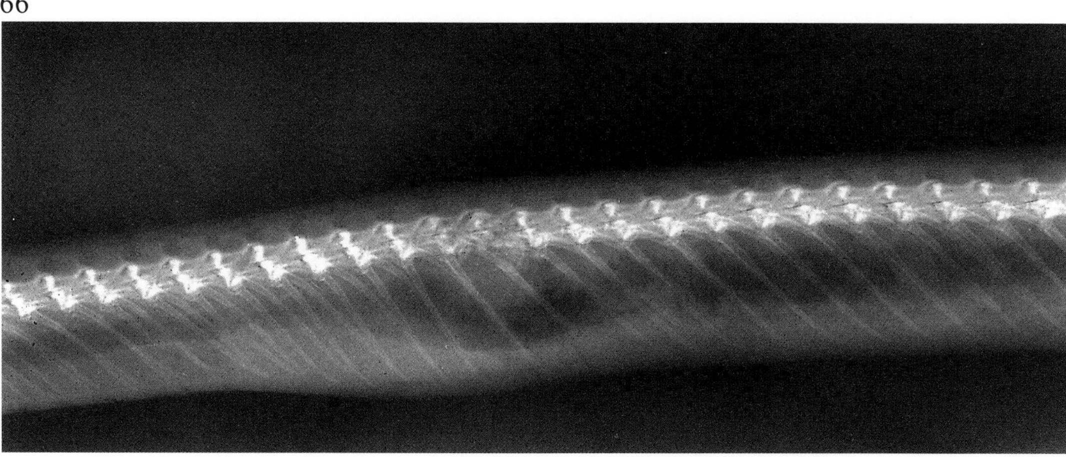

67

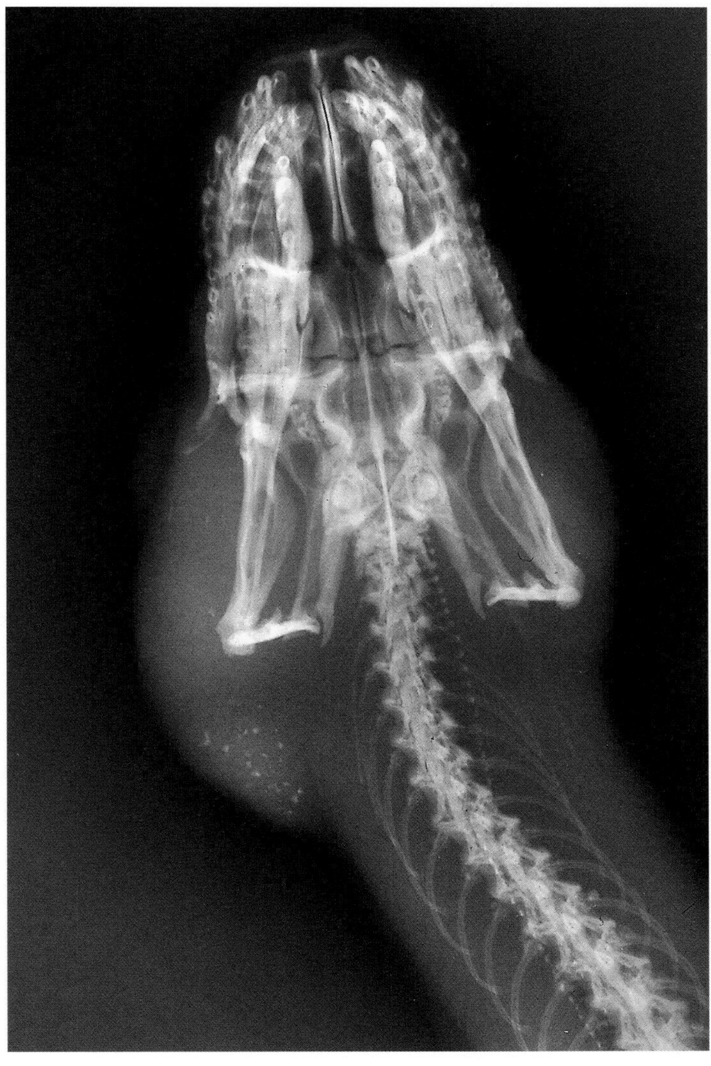

66 Vertebral Osteomyelitis.

Chilean Racer *(Dromicus chamissonis).*

Caudal to the cardiac shadow several vertebrae present with signs of severe bone destruction. Ventral to the area of vertebral destruction a spherical soft tissue density is visible.

The cranial areas of the lung contain multiple solitary densities.

The vertebral lesions and the pulmonary densities were caused by mycobacterial infection.

67 Mandibular Abscess.

Boa constrictor *(Boa constrictor).*

A soft tissue swelling is visible close to the left mandibular articulation. Flaky radiopacities are recognizable in the caudal part of the density. These are radiographic signs of an abscess with calcifications.

68

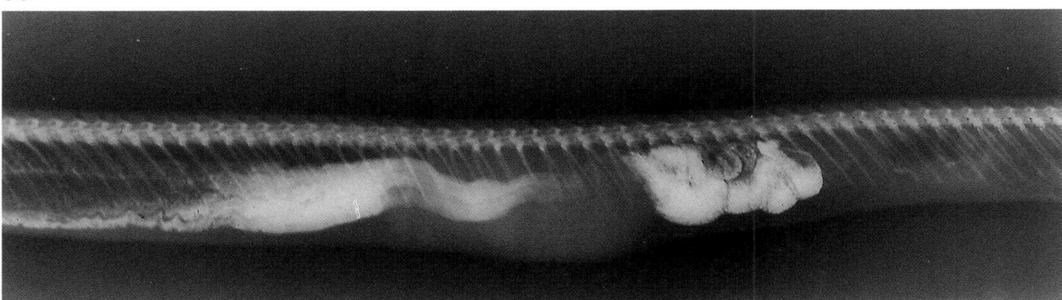

69

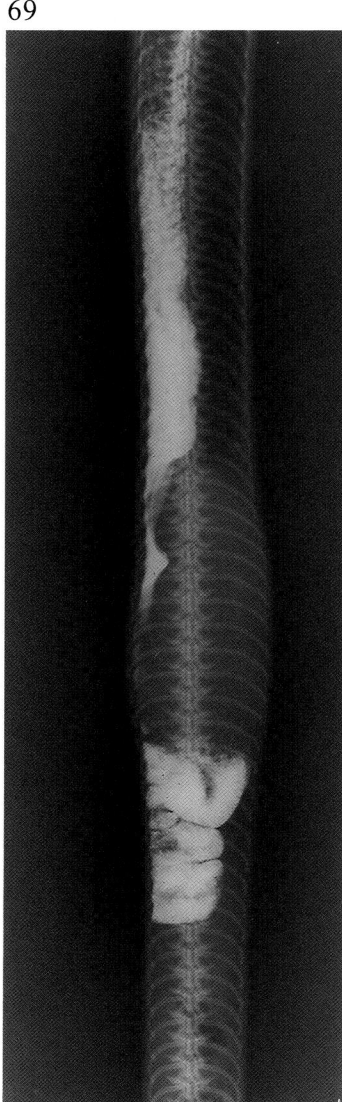

68/69 Abscess of the Intestinal Wall, contrast study.

Corn Snake *(Elaphe guttata).*

On the lateral radiograph, the contrast examination reveals a space-occupying soft tissue lesion, just caudal to the stomach, that compresses and displaces the first intestinal loop. The passage of contrast medium is maintained. At the oral side of the mass, the stomach is visible. At the aboral side, the contrasted small intestinal loops are present.

On the dorsoventral radiograph, the lumen of the intestine is compressed against the body wall.

At surgery, the mass turned out to be an abscess caused by Salmonella sp.

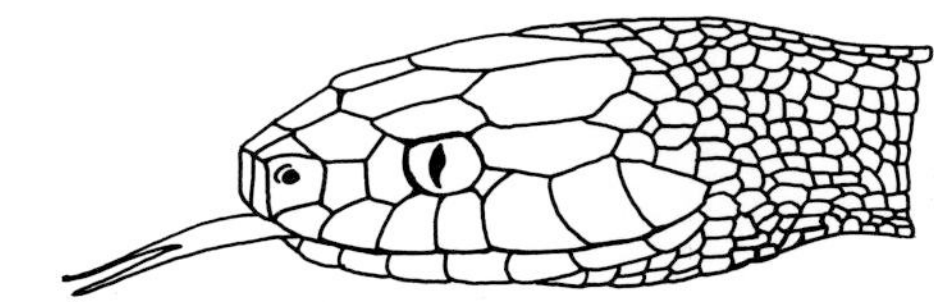

70

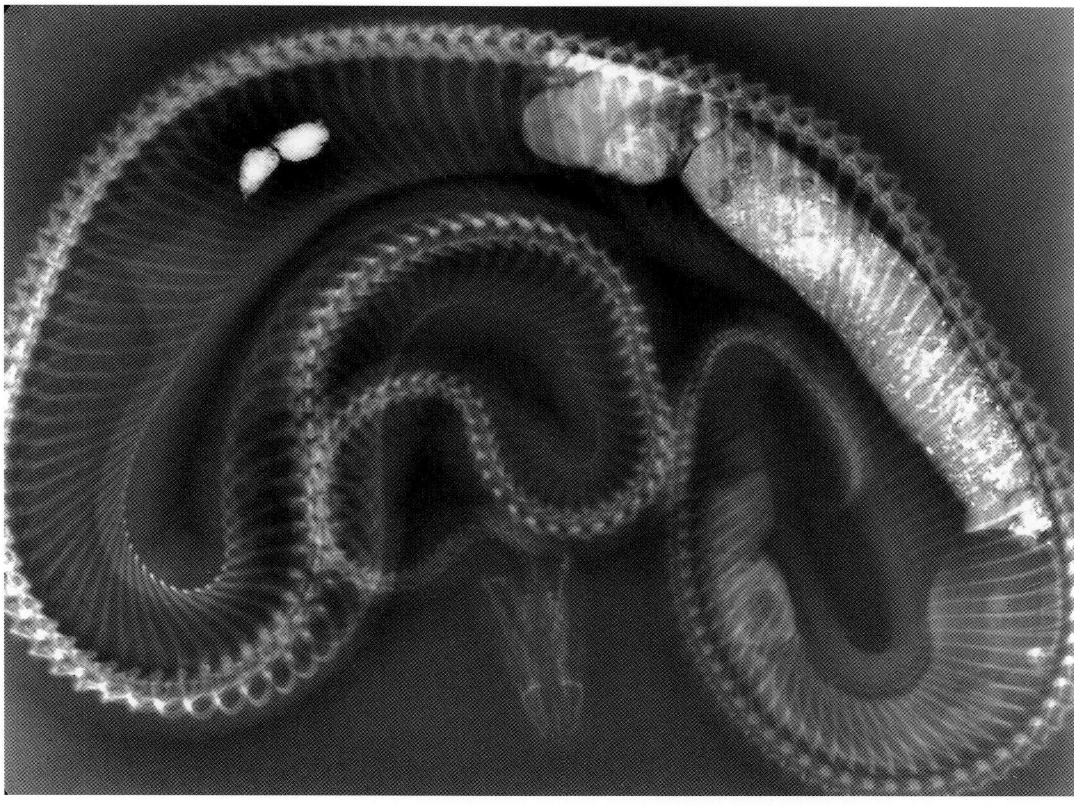

71

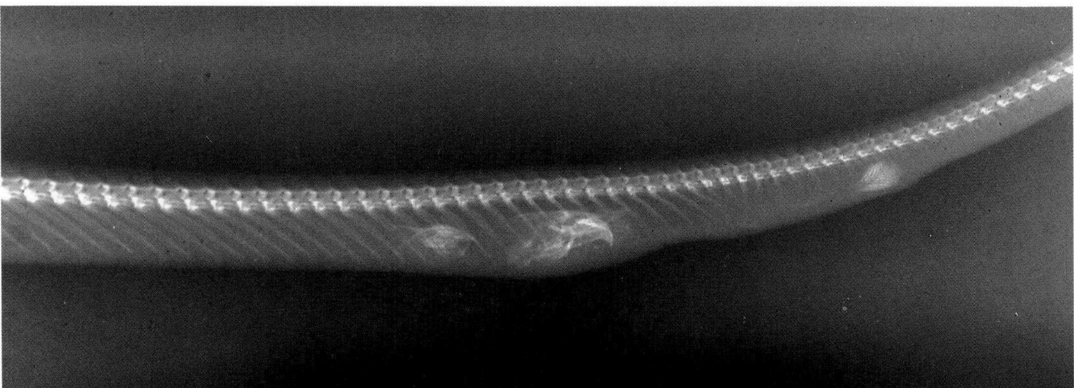

70 Constipation, contrast study.

Royal Python *(Python regius).*

Four days after administration, the contrast medium accumulates in the constipated large intestine. There are no small intestinal loops opacified.

71 Foreign Body.

Eastern King Snake *(Lampropeltis getulus).*

In the last third part of the body, fragments of a lower and upper jaw of a mouse are visible. The body of the snake is obviously swollen. Both bony fragments penetrated into the intestinal wall and had to be removed surgically.

Note: This is a male. The calcified hemipenes are clearly visible.

72

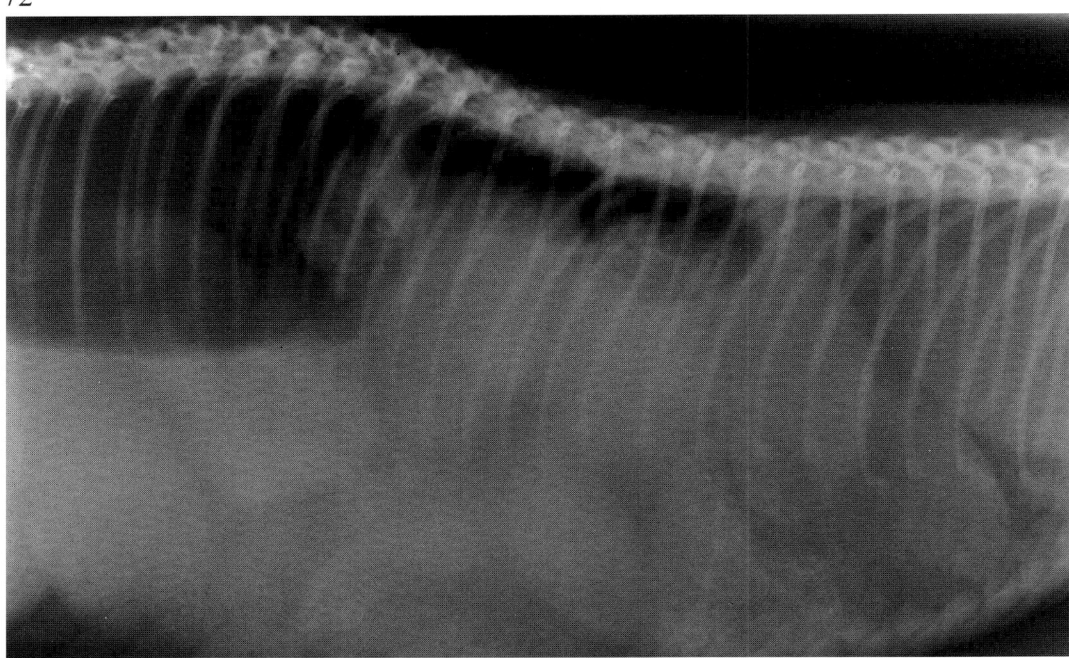

73

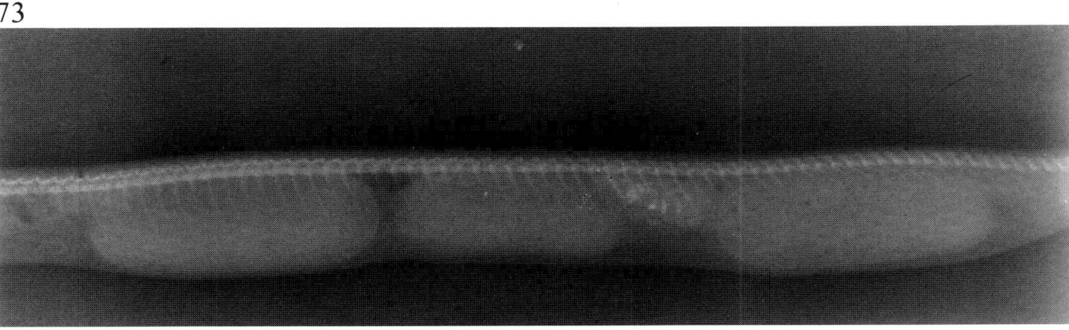

72 Normal Gravidity.

Boa constrictor *(Boa constrictor).*

Ovoid eggs are visible ventral to the lung. Within the eggs, parts of fetal jaws and skulls are recognizable. Because this species is ovoviviparous, no calcified egg shells are present.

73 Egg Binding.

Corn Snake *(Elapha guttata).*

In snakes, egg shells are usually less calcified than in other reptiles. In this animal, the variety in size and calcification of the eggs, in combination with the clinical signs of depression and dehydration, indicates egg binding.

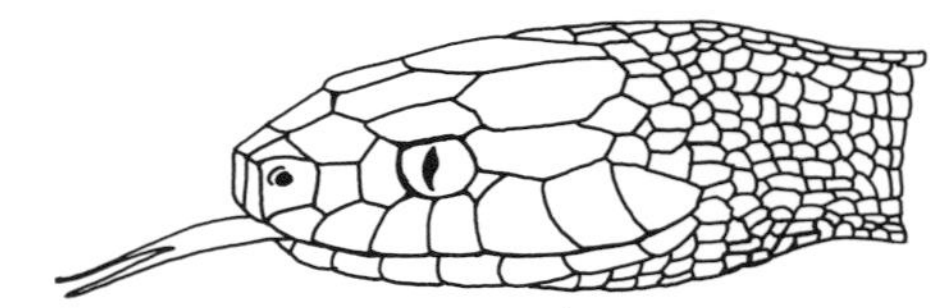

74

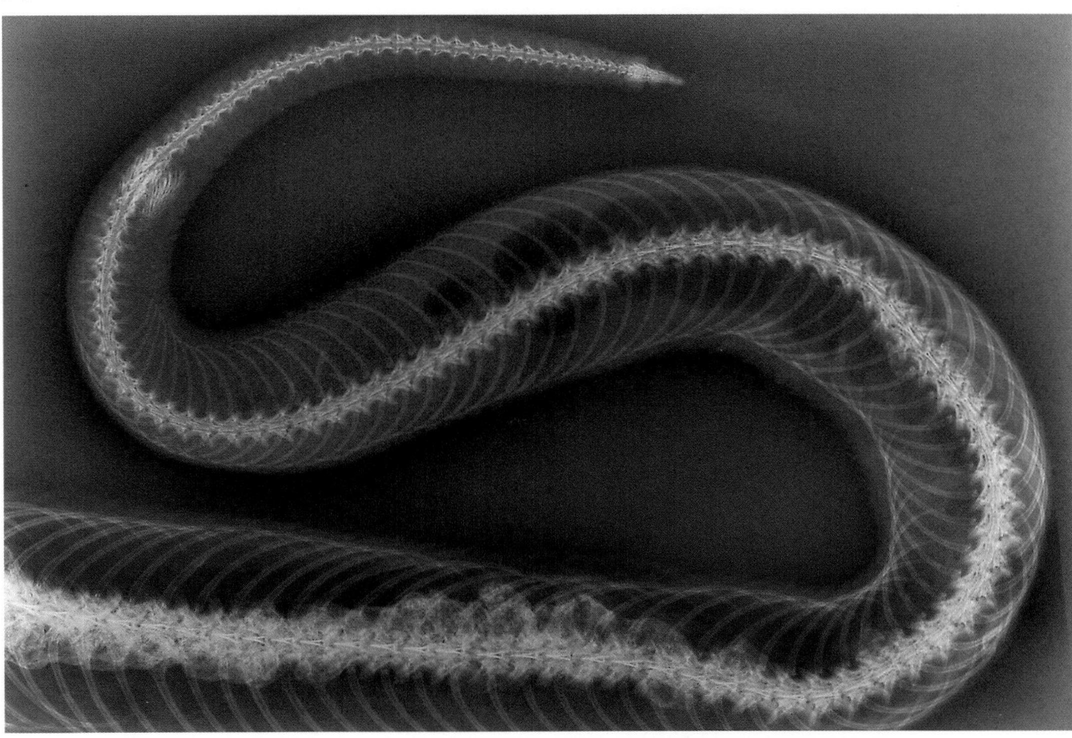

75

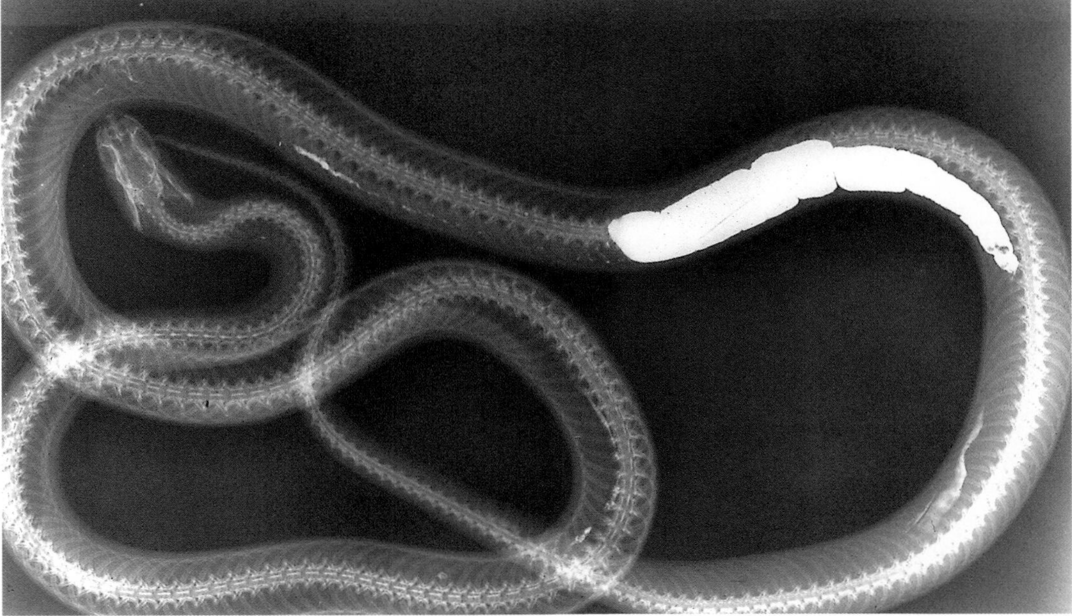

74 Calcified Hemipenes.

South American Rattlesnake *(Crotalus durissus).*

On both sides, caudal to the cloaca the calcified structures of the hemipenes are visible. This is a normal finding in some species and can be used for sex determination.

Vertebral ostitis is present.

75 Kidney Tumor, contrast study.

Milk Snake *(Lampropeltis triangulum).*

Passage of the barium column is obstructed by a mass that permits only small amounts of contrast medium to pass into the caudal intestinal loops.

The mass was a renal tumor.

76

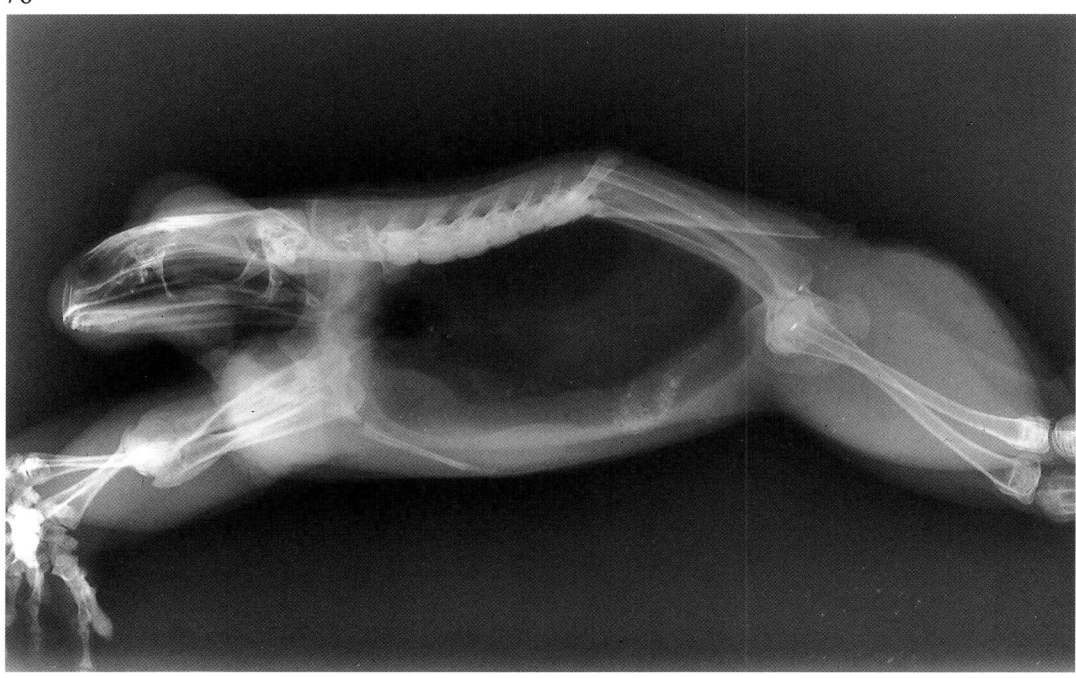

76 A

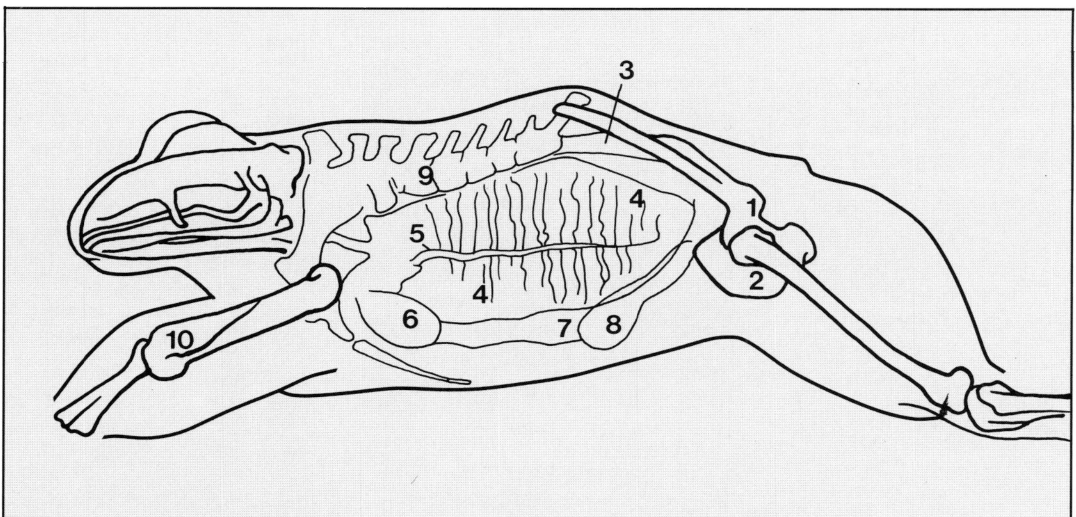

76/76A Normal Radiographic Appearance, lateral.

South American Bullfrog *(Leptodactylus pentadactylus)*, male.

The short spine is supported by the two ilia (**1**). The two halves of the pelvis are fused to a disc-like structure (**2**). The sacrum (**3**) passes caudally between the two ilia. Dorsal to the shoulder joint the trachea passes and extends into the lungs (**4**). The pulmonary vasculature is distinctly outlined (**5**). Ventral to the lungs and dorsal to the sternum the cardic shadow (**6**) is visible. Caudal to the heart the liver shadow can be seen (**7**). In the caudoventral part of the celom grainy intestinal contents are recognized (**8**). The spinal bone formations (**9**) and spherical elbow joints (**10**) are better visible on the dorsoventral radiograph.

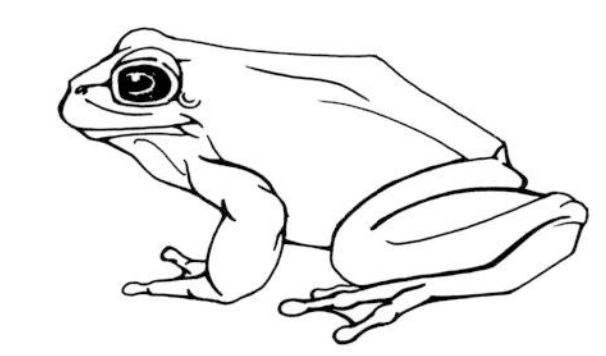

77

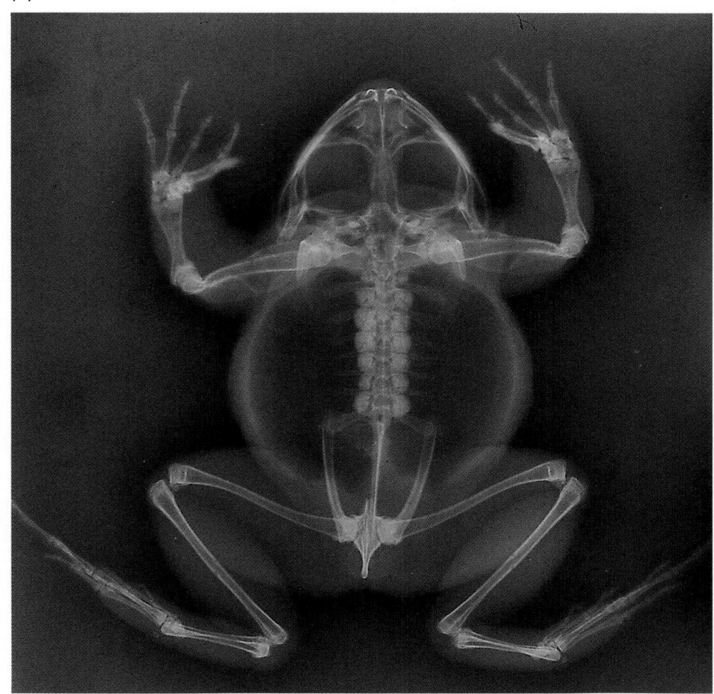

77 A

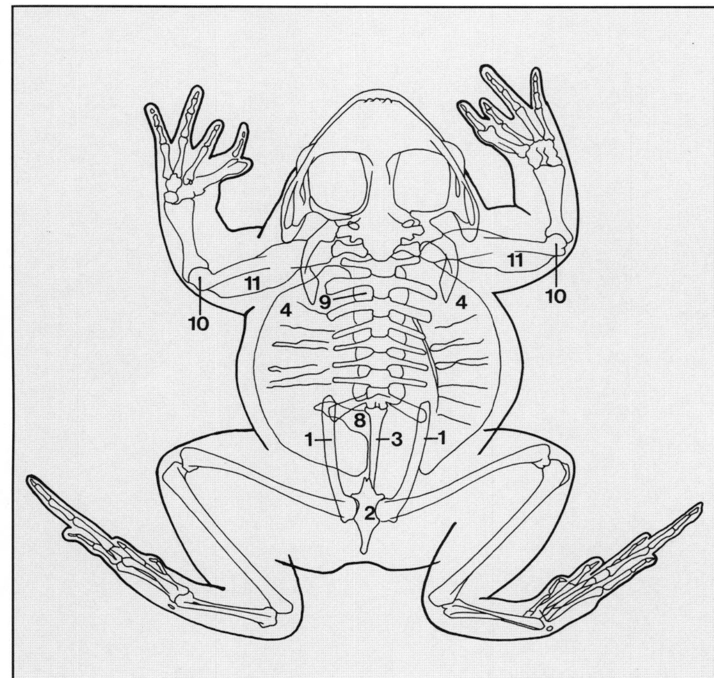

78

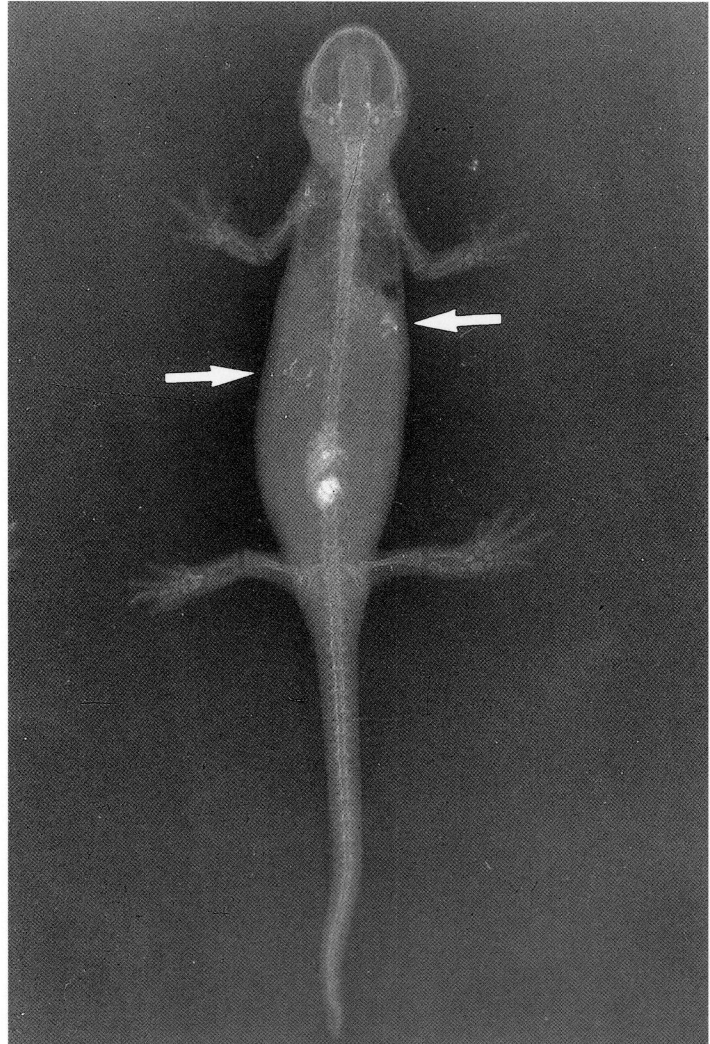

77/77A Normal Radiographic Appearance, dorsoventral.

South American Bullfrog *(Leptodactylus pentadactylus)*, male.

Lateral to the spine spheric bone formations are visible (**9**). They function probably as stabilizing elements for the spine when frogs jump. The ilia (**1**) extend far cranially and the two halves of the pelvis are fused (**2**). The thumb of the fore limb is distinct and supplied with a horny plug. The elbow (**10**) is formed as a spheric joint. In the area of the biceps distinct tendon plates are visible (**11**). These anatomical structures are used for the prolonged clinging to the female during mating. During inspiration, the lungs (**4**) occupy the entire celomic cavity. Within the lungs, fine pulmonary vessels are recognizable. In the caudal area, the instestines that contain grainy densities (**8**) are visible.

78 Gravidity.

Alpine Salamander *(Salamandra atra)*, female, adult.

This radiograph shows a salamander with two larvae in its body cavity. The larval skull bones and parts of the spine can be distinguished.

79

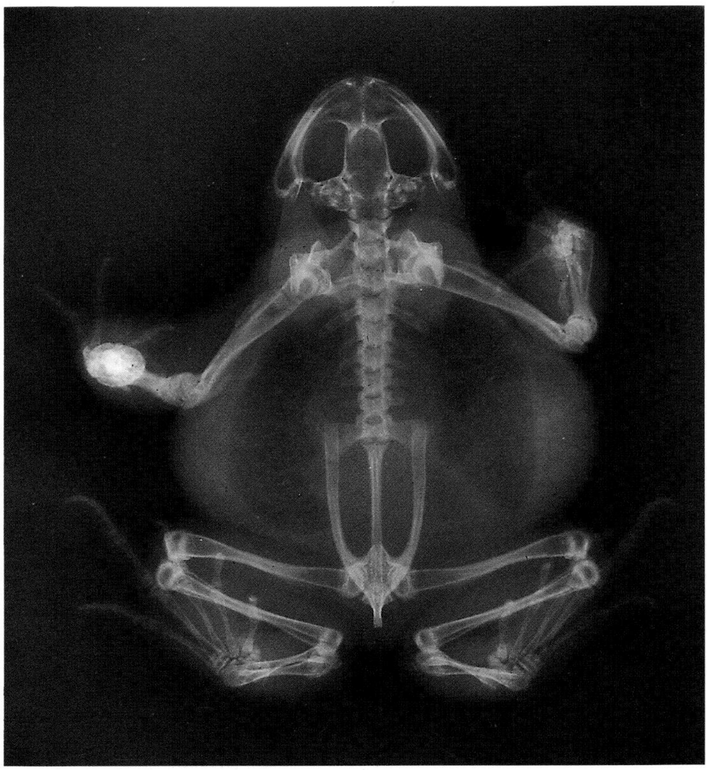

80

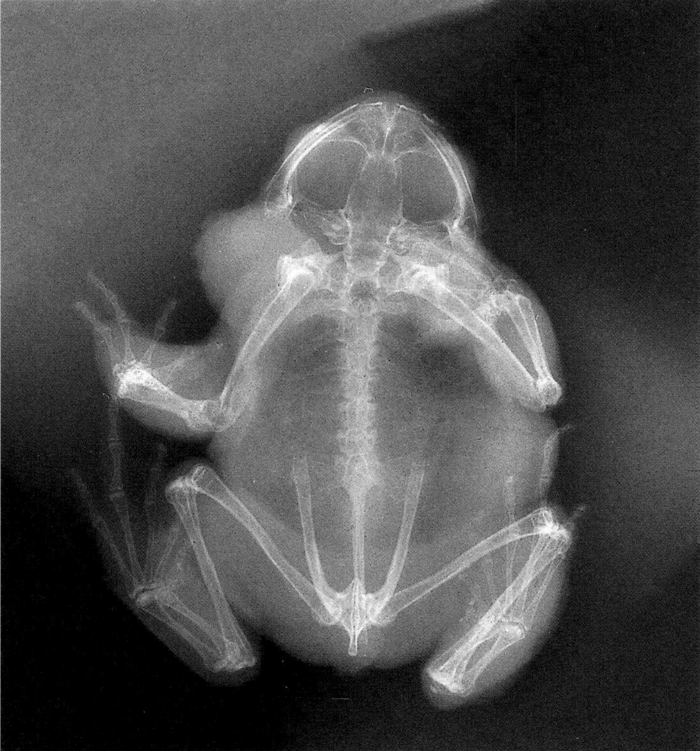

81

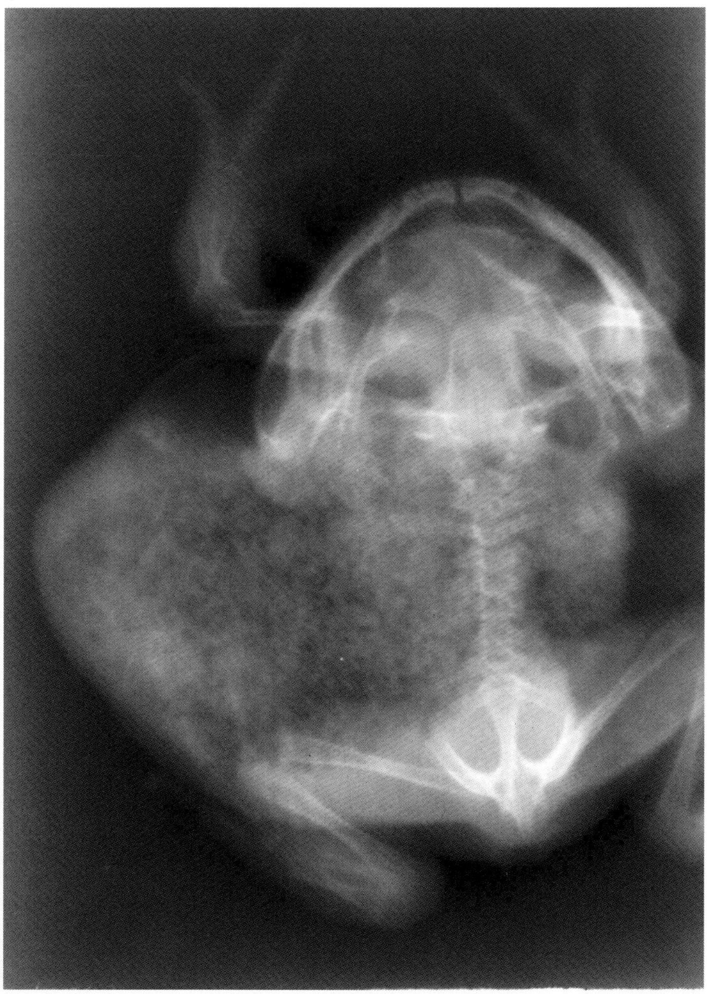

79 Osteosarcoma.

Eurasian Toad *(Bufo bufo)*, adult.

A proliferative bone lesion of the radius and ulna is clearly visible. Histological examination following biopsy revealed an osteosarcoma.

80 Adenoma.

Green Toad *(Bufo viridis)*, adult.

There is a large soft tissue mass on the left side of the neck. The underlying bones are uninvolved. After surgical removement histological examination revealed a cystadenoma.

81 Foreign Body.

Ornate Horned Frog *(Ceratophrys ornata)*, juvenile.

On the left side of the body and in the region of the stomach, a large granular appearing mass extends beyond the normal borders of the celomic cavity. The mass proved to be a piece of foam rubber in the stomach that could be removed through the mouth.